NITROUS-OXIDE INJECTION

BY DAVID VIZARD

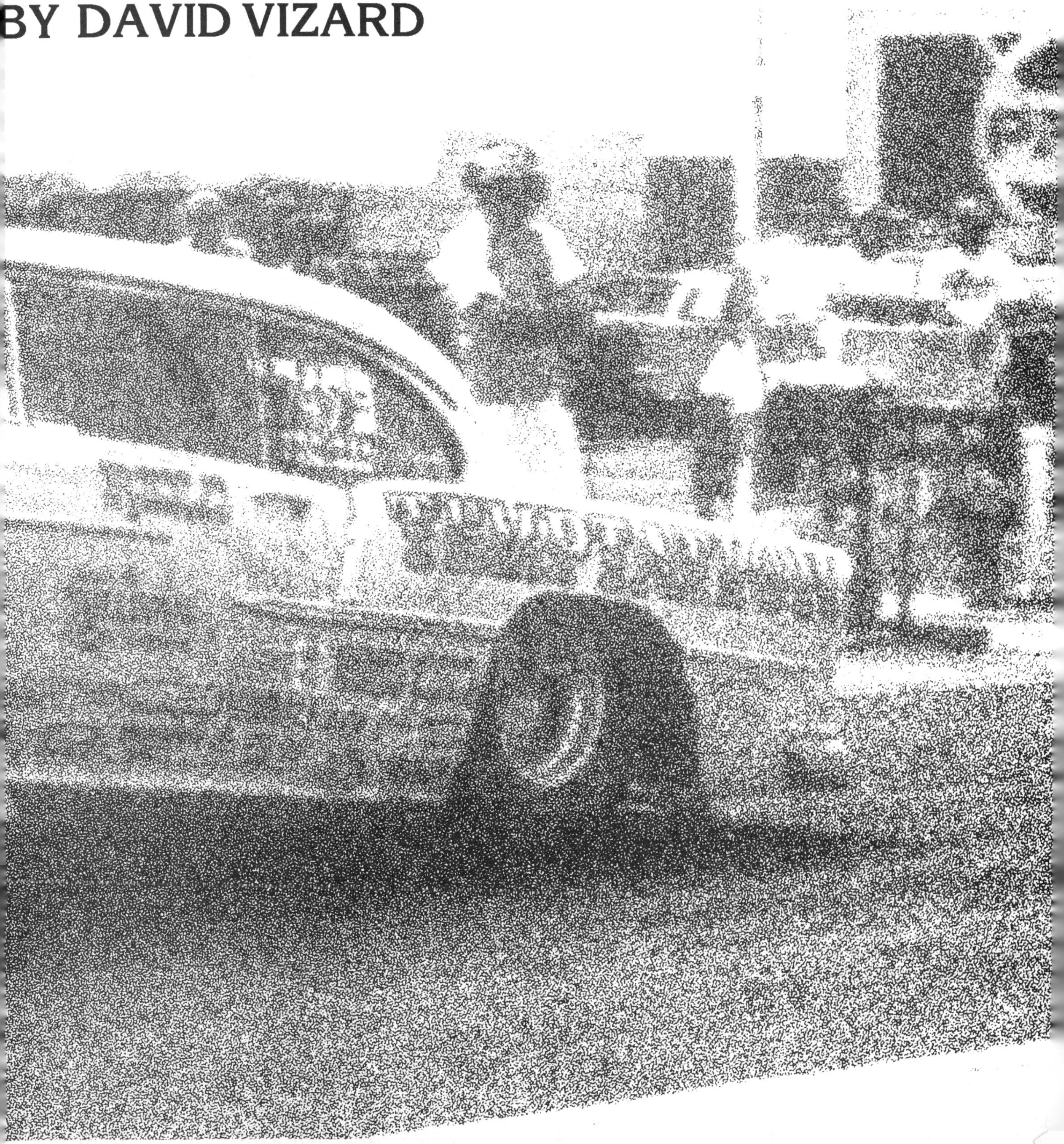

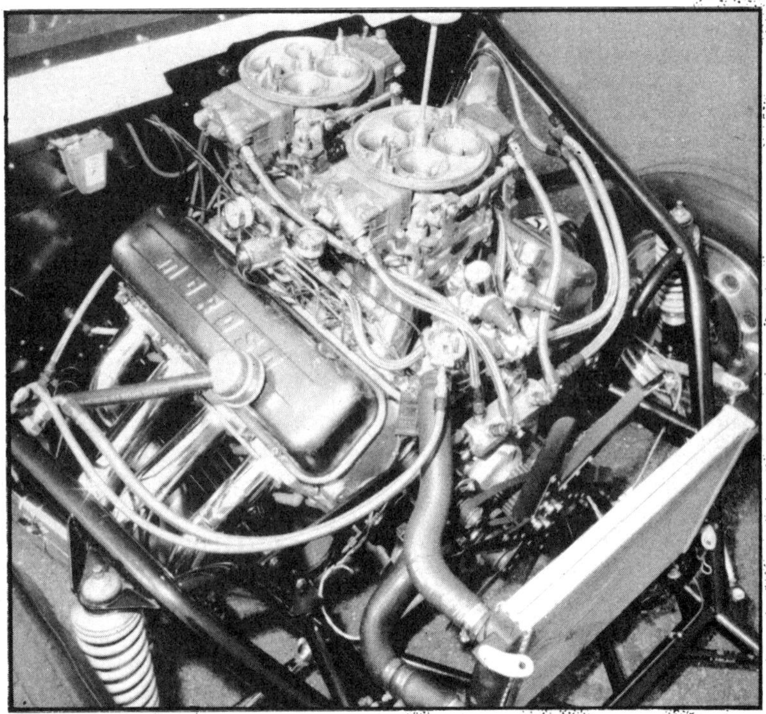

Charles Carpenter's 5/8 scale '55 Chevy ultra match racer. This tube-chassis killer is powered by a 540 cid aluminum head Chevrolet, built by Gene Fulton. Assisted by nitrous-oxide injection, it has run 7.27 ETs at over 190 mph.

NITROUS-OXIDE INJECTION

EDITED BY
LARRY SCHREIB

PRODUCTION BY
LARRY ATHERTON

ISBN 0-931472-16-4
Part No. 16-4

ADDITIONAL TECHNICAL EDITING BY
LARRY ATHERTON
MIKE PARRY

DRAWINGS BY
JIM DENNEWILL

S-A DESIGN BOOKS, 515 WEST LAMBERT, BLDG E, BREA, CA 92621-3991

CONTENTS

INTRODUCTION

Nitrous-oxide was first isolated and identified in 1772 by Joseph Priestly, an English scientist. Though he recorded its existence, nitrous-oxide did not greatly interest Priestly. His main concern was to systematically search for chemical elements and compounds, probably in the hope of finding some with obvious medical or scientific uses. The properties of gaseous nitrous-oxide were not immediately evident (the equipment for liquefying nitrous-oxide--a form in which it is commonly used today--did not exist), so for many years the lack of apparent practical usefulness prevented serious study of nitrous-oxide.

The next historical record of nitrous-oxide is associated with Sir Humphrey Davy. This English scientist is better known for the invention of the Davy miner's lamp. In the days before electricity, coal miners had to carry oil-flame lanterns into the mines to light their work. Unfortunately, this flame would occasionally ignite trapped gases and the result was usually a disastrous explosion. The Davy's lamp was a useful means of eliminating this danger.

Davy's other work with nitrous-oxide was far removed from the ingenious lamp. Davy found that if nitrous was inhaled in certain quantities it acted as a mild anesthetic. This discovery was ignored for quite some time, but it was a minor landmark in medical history. Today nitrous-oxide is used extensively as an anesthetic, especially in dentistry.

WARTIME DEVELOPMENT

Although positive evidence is hard to find, it would appear that the use of nitrous-oxide in combustion engines was first investigated after World War I. However, it wasn't until World War II that major research was undertaken to determine whether nitrous could successfully augment engine power.

By 1942 it became evident to virtually all world air powers that the primary qualities of a successful fighting airplane were high speed and the ability to operate at high altitudes. Spurred on by a massive war effort, British researchers worked frantically to develop a nitrous-oxide injection system that would allow production war planes to fly high and fast (see Chapter One, Figure 1-2), without seriously impairing engine reliability. Eventually, this development enabled modified high-altitude reconnaissance aircraft to fly with near impunity over Axis territory.

Engineers in the U.S. conducted similar explorations. Records indicate that most of this research was performed with Rolls Royce or Packard-built Merlin V12 engines. Although very few of these nitrous-injected engines were actually used in combat aircraft, they exhibited outstanding performance for the day. Operational altitudes well in excess of 50,000 feet were accredited to some of these planes.

This work was shrouded in heavy secrecy. Obviously the Allied powers did not want the Axis scientists to discover the capabilities of nitrous injection, and there is no indication that these experiments were com-

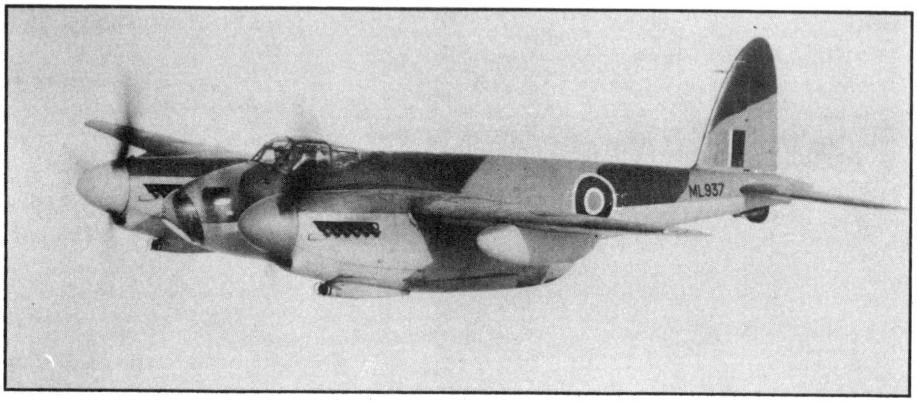

Often known as the "Wooden Wonder," the DeHavilland 98 Mosquito was one of the most successful Allied fighter bombers of World War II. Nitrous-oxide injection was used to boost the performance of certain derivatives that were modified for high-altitude reconnaissance.

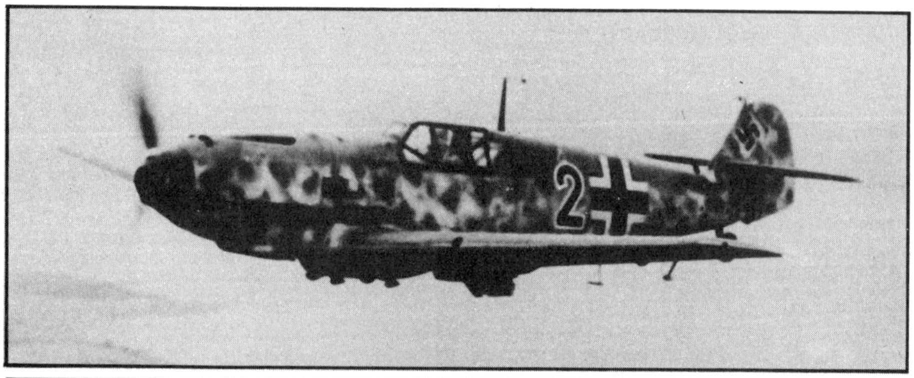

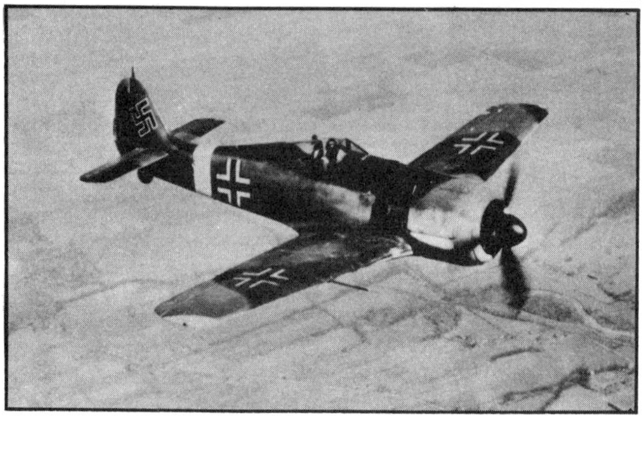

The Messerschmitt BF109 (above) and Fock-Wulf FW 190 (left) were deadly mainstays of the German Air Force during the entire war. Both aircraft made extensive use of the GM1 nitrous-oxide injection system that typically boosted power output by 250 to 300hp.

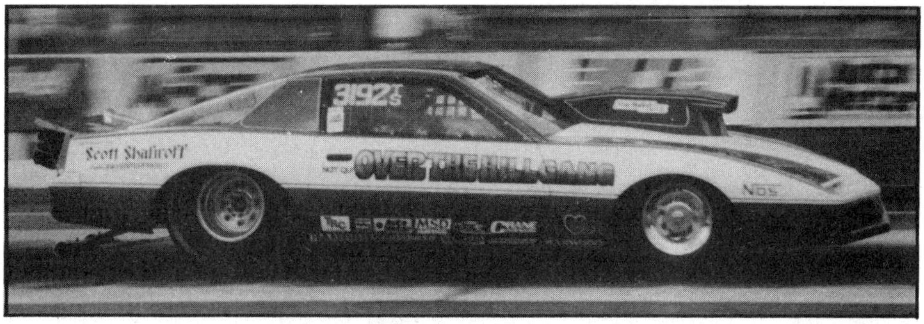

Scott Shafiroff's slick Pontiac Firebird has recorded a best of 7.37/184mph with one four-barrel carb on a 615 cubic inch big block Chevy. This impressive performance is substantially boosted by nitrous-oxide delivered through a multi-stage injection from Nitrous Oxide Systems.

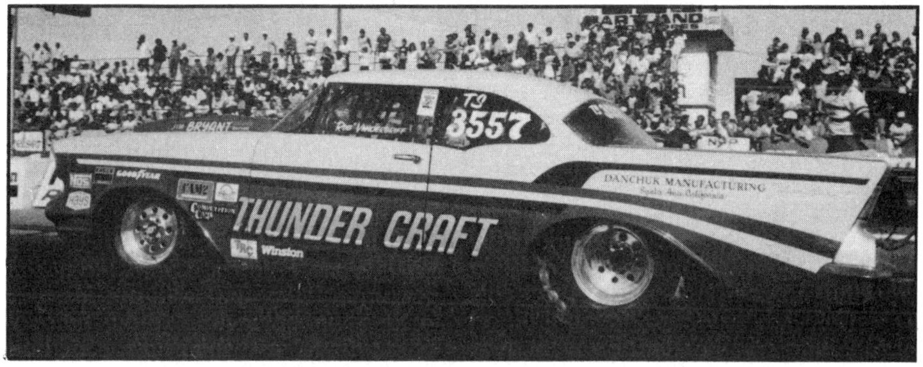

A nitrous-augmented 600 cubic inch Chevy pushes Kenny Hagen's awesome '57 Chevy through the timing lights in 7.31/191mph. This unique race car has a one-of-a-kind, all-fiberglass body over a full Pro Stock chassis.

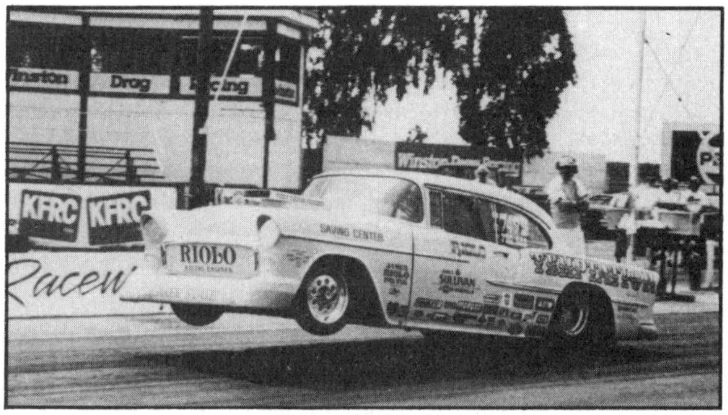

Dave Riolo virtually created "Outlaw Pro Gas" drag racing with his '56 Chevy. A nitrous-injected, 505-inch, all-aluminum Yenko big block has rocketed this missile to a 7.72/176mph time.

promised. In fact, toward the end of the war Axis airmen were openly puzzled by the high-altitude capabilities of certain Allied fighters. Ironically, however, Axis researchers had independently developed a concept for nitrous-oxide injection and believed they were pursuing a unique line of thought.

During the middle and latter years of the war, German engine manufacturers unveiled some very sophisticated aircraft engines. Daimler-Benz performed extensive experiments with derivatives of their DB600 inverted V12 engine. Nitrous injection was reportedly fitted to the 603E version of this impressive engine. The nitrous-oxide was injected into a specially geared supercharger, and the engine supposedly developed full rated horsepower at very high altitudes (in conjunction with other modifications). The system delivered nitrous at the rate of about 12 pounds per minute, boosting the engine output by 350 horsepower. In addition, this system made effective use of the nitrous-oxide, allowing the injection to be used for extended periods--reportedly as long as 20 or 30 minutes.

Had it not been for the advent of jet engines, nitrous-oxide might have remained a closely-held secret for many years. Although the capability of piston engines had been dramatically increased during the frenetic war years, jet propulsion far exceeded the capabilities of piston-driven engines, especially at high altitudes.

During the post-war years nitrous-oxide was virtually forgotten. Eventually, however, a number of astute racing enthusiasts rediscovered the latent potential of the innocuous anesthetic. Indeed, Colin Campbell, the author of "The Sports Car," an early landmark in racing publications, made considerable reference to nitrous-oxide during the late '50s and early '60s.

Nonetheless, the use of nitrous-oxide in automotive engines remained a clandestine matter for many years. Practitioners guarded the secret with a jealousy that exceeded the patriotic verve of WWII, and nitrous augmentation didn't become common knowledge until the early '70s. Indeed, it is amazing that the inside track lasted so long. Early systems were crude, but simple measures effectively camouflaged their existence. When nitrous finally hit the headlines, though, it grayed the hair of more than one tech inspector who had to "hunt the hidden nitrous" at virtually every racing event.

Once the secret was out, entrepreneurs jumped on the bandwagon. Nitrous injection sounded like the answer to a performance enthusiasts' wildest dream: easy to install, simple to maintain and super horsepower. As a result, marketing hypes with limited technical know-how began selling hastily pre-fabricated kits. These systems arrived in public hands long before they were fully developed and tested--the results were predictable (or, depending on your viewpoint, unpredictable).

Shortly after these early kits became available reports of unexplained engine "explosions" began to circulate. These difficulties were generally traced to inadequate engineering or components that were not compatible with the temperature and pressure associated with liquid nitrous-oxide. But as time went by kit manufacturers either went out of business or upgraded their products to achieve high reliability.

Nitrous-oxide injection is currently one of the fastest selling and most popular performance options available. Modern nitrous systems offer tremendous performance potential at a relatively modest cost. In fact, few performance modifications, if any, can match the cost-versus-power ratio of nitrous injection. This is the result of dedicated effort by individuals and companies that have worked to develop reliable nitrous systems. The author hopes the information presented in this book will give the reader technical insight to utilize any high-performance nitrous-oxide injection system safely and to the fullest potential.

CHAPTER 1

NITROUS CHEMICAL PROPERTIES

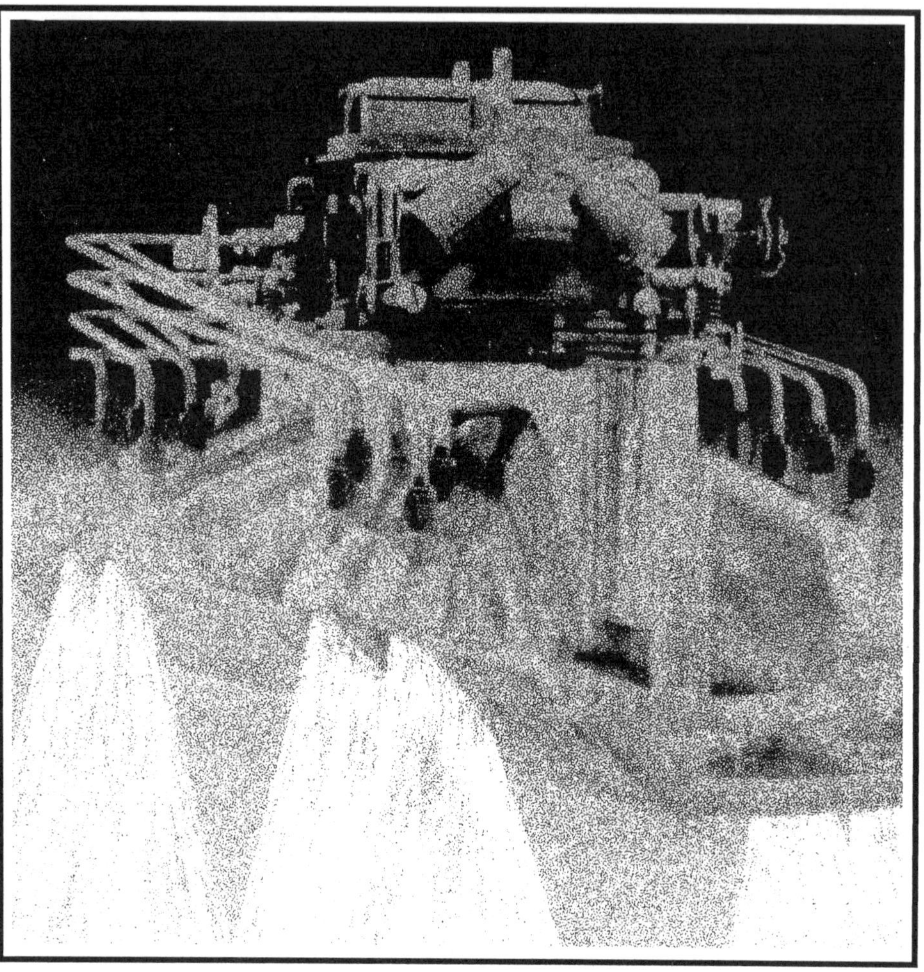

CHEMICAL PROPERTIES

Nitrous-oxide is a colorless, non-flammable gas. The chemical composition is N_2O — two atoms of nitrogen combined with one atom of oxygen—and in suitable concentrations it exhibits a slightly sweet taste and odor. It is non-toxic and non-irritating, and when inhaled in small quantities it can produce mild hysteria and bouts of giggling or laughter. This characteristic eventually caused it to be called "laughing gas."

Early medical experiments resulted in the widespread use of nitrous-oxide as an anesthetic. However, it is not a powerful anesthetic (compared to modern anesthetics), and to have an effect, it must be inhaled in relatively high concentrations together with oxygen. When it is inhaled in pure form it can cause death. This occurs because the nitrous-oxide molecule is strongly bonded, and the single oxygen atom will not readily separate from the two nitrogen atoms. As a result, at standard temperature and pressure, the oxygen atom is not readily available to the body, and breathing pure nitrous-oxide will inevitably lead to asphyxiation.

At standard atmospheric temperature and pressure, nitrous-oxide is a gas; but when the gas is sufficiently compressed, it will transform to a liquid. However, the requisite pressure will depend on the temperature. To convert nitrous-oxide at standard atmospheric pressure of 14.7psi, the temperature must be reduced to -128 degrees Fahrenheit. Conversely, at 70 degrees (F), a pressure of 760psi is required to maintain nitrous-oxide in a liquid form. Therefore, when compressed nitrous-oxide is stored in a closed vessel at standard temperatures, the internal pressure created when a portion of liquid reverts to a gaseous state will create a pressure balance (760psi) that retains the balance of the nitrous as a liquid. The

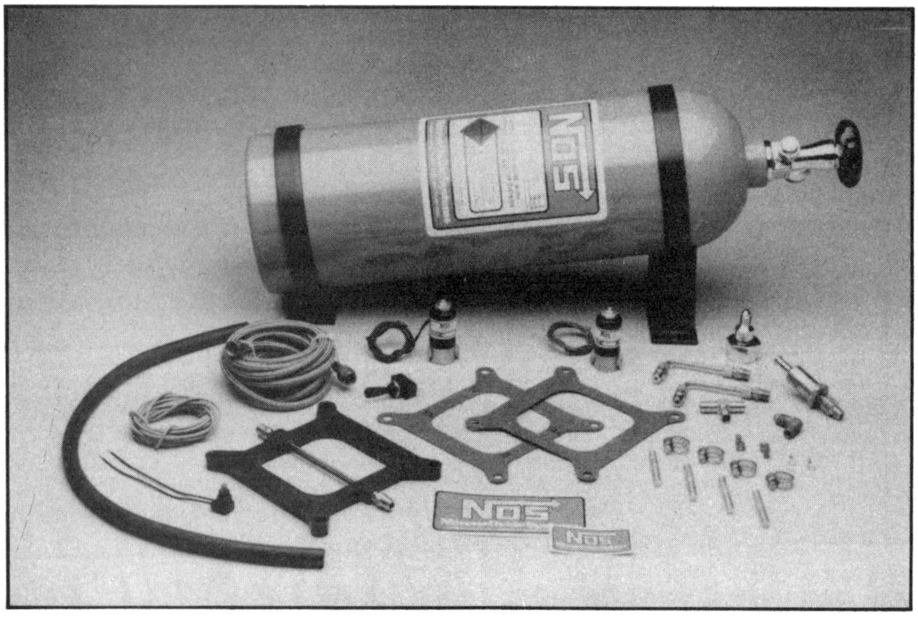

A nitrous-oxide kit looks pretty simple, yet it can pour a lot of power into a typical engine.

FIGURE 1-1

PHYSICAL CONSTANTS	METRIC SYSTEM	US SYSTEM
MOLECULAR WEIGHT	44.013	
VAPOR PRESSURE @ 70°F	52.4 kg/cm^2 gauge	745 PSIg
SPECIFIC VOLUME @ 70°F @ 1 ATMOSPHERE (atm)	543.1 ml/g	8.7 cu.ft/lb
BOILING POINT @ 1 atm.	-89.5°C	-129.1°F
FREEZING POINT @ 1 atm.	-90.84°C	-131.5°F
SPECIFIC GRAVITY, GAS @ 15°C, 1 ATM. (AIR=1)	1.530	
DENSITY, GAS @ 0°C, 1 atm.	1.997 g/l	0.167 lb/US gal
DENSITY, LIQUID @ BOILING POINT	1.266 g/ml	10.56 lb/US gal
CRITICAL TEMPERATURE	36.5°C	97.7°F
CRITICAL PRESSURE	75.1 kg/cm^2 absolute	1069 PSI absolute (72.7 atm)
CRITICAL DENSITY	0.424 g/ml	3.4 lb/US gal
LATENT HEAT OF VAPORIZATION @ BOILING POINT	89.9 cal/g	
LATENT HEAT OF FUSION & MELTING POINT	35.5 cal/g	
SPECIFIC HEAT, GAS @ 25°C, @ 1 atm., AT CONSTANT PRESSURE: AT CONSTANT VOLUME:	0.2098 cal/g 0.1610 cal/g	
SPECIFIC HEAT RATIO, GAS @ 25°C, @ 1 atm., Cp/Cv	1.303	
THERMAL CONDUCTIVITY, GAS @ 0°C	0.0434 cal/0°C	
VISCOSITY, GAS, @ 1 atm. @ 0°C @ 25°C	(°C/cm sec cm^2) 0.01362 centipoise 0.01496 centipoise	
SURFACE TENSION @ -25°C	10.1 dynes/cm	
TROUTON CONSTANT	21.4	
SOLUBILITY IN WATER @ 0°C, @ 1 atm.	1.3 volumes/volume (H_2O)	

FIGURE 1-1: Nitrous-oxide Physical Characteristics

FIGURE 1-2

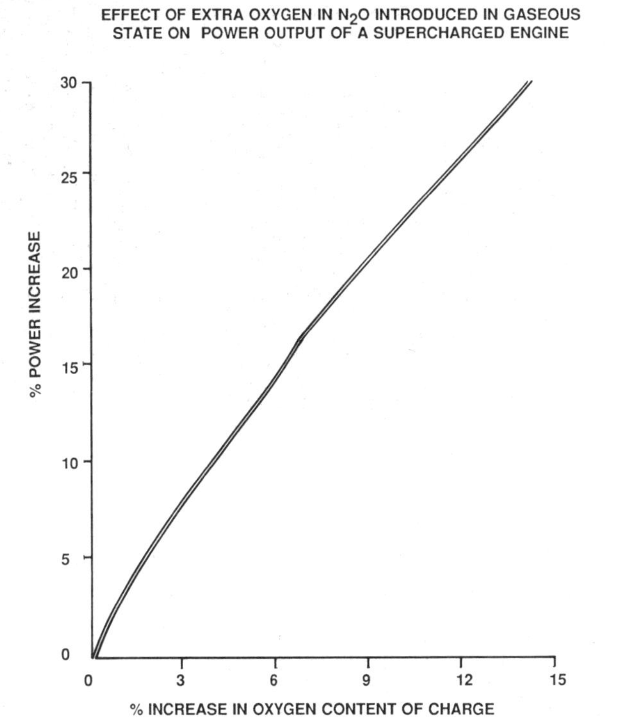

FIGURE 1-2: Potential power gains spurred the development of nitrous-oxide injection for propeller-driven aircraft. Short-duration power boost increased the peak tactical speed of fighter aircraft. Aircraft with larger nitrous tanks demonstrated exceptional high-altitude performance.

pressure generated in this way is known as *vapor pressure.*

The best way to visualize this situation is to first assume that liquid nitrous-oxide exists at a very low temperature. Then, imagine this liquid inside a completely closed storage tank. When the temperature is raised to standard room temperature, the nitrous-oxide tries to convert back to a gas. In other words, it starts to "boil." However, as the liquid nitrous-oxide boils, the pressure of the gas trapped between the surface of the liquid and the inside of the container rises.

(At this point we must recall some basic physics. Experiments readily show that the boiling point of any liquid depends on the pressure to which it is subjected. For instance, at standard pressure, water boils at 212 degrees Fahrenheit; but if the surrounding air pressure is raised by some means to 28.8psi, water will not boil until the temperature is raised to 248 degrees Fahrenheit.)

In our nitrous example, as the temperature rises, the liquid nitrous-oxide continues to convert to a gas until the gas pressure above the liquid nitrous is high enough to prevent further boiling. At this point the contents have reached a stable condition, and the vapor pressure holds the rest of the nitrous-oxide in a liquid form.

As long as the temperature inside the tank rises, the vapor pressure rises, until conditions reach a "critical point." At temperatures above the critical point the vapor pressure can no longer hold the nitrous-oxide in liquid form. The critical point for nitrous-oxide is 97.7 degrees Fahrenheit, which results in an internal pressure of 1069psi. Above 97.7 degrees Fahrenheit the entire contents of the tank become gaseous. Further increases in temperature cause the internal pressure to rise, but all the contents are in gaseous form.

This all sounds pretty simple, but in actual fact the contents of the tank

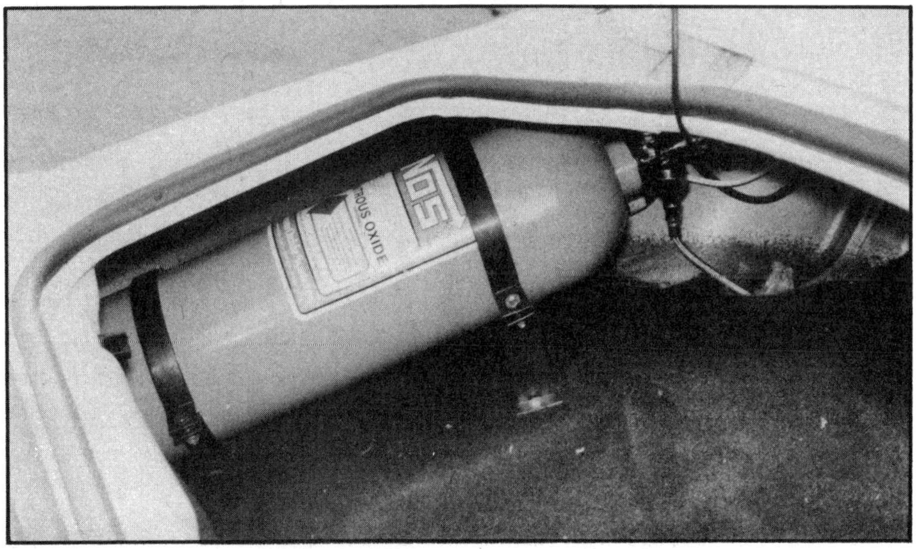

Since the contents of a nitrous bottle are temperature sensitive, the nitrous bottle must be kept out of direct sunlight and as far away as possible from any source of heat.

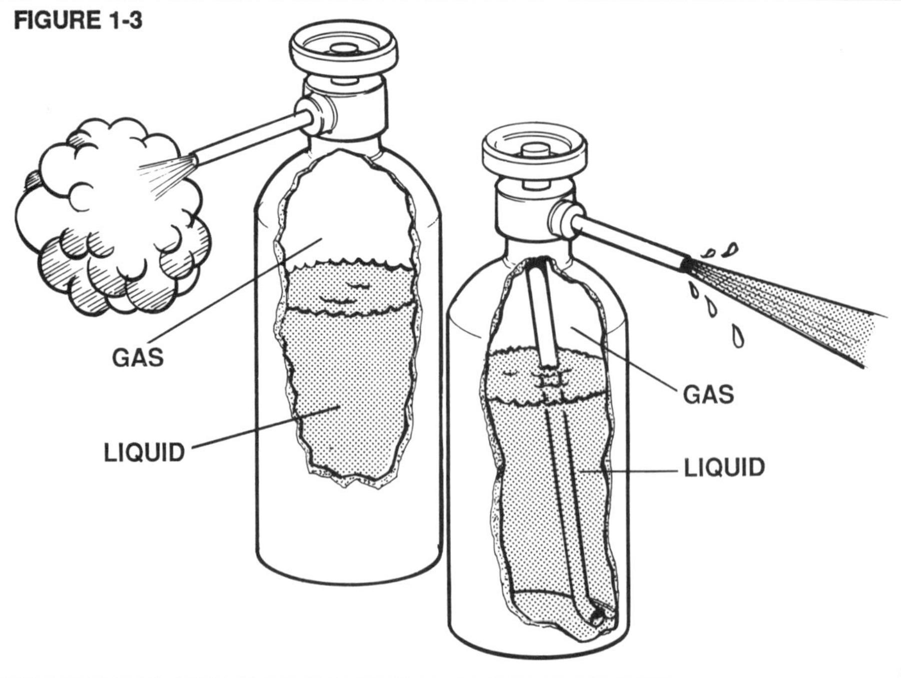

FIGURE 1-3: Because it does not have a syphon tube, the bottle on the left will discharge only gas. The bottle on the right will discharge liquid until almost empty.

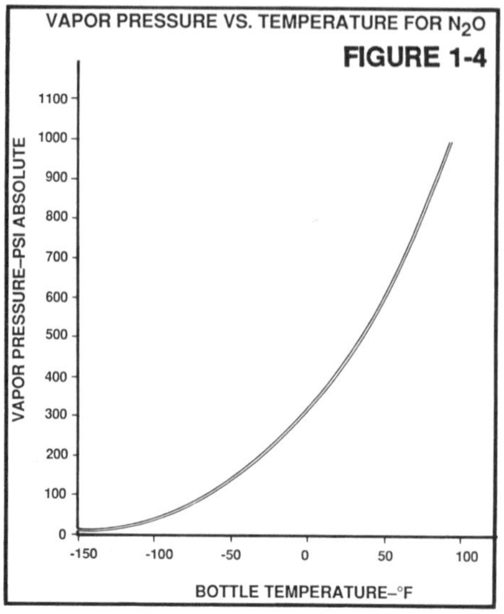

FIGURE 1-4: To find the temperature of the bottle contents, the known vapor pressure (inside the bottle) is extended horizontally until it intersects the curve, then a vertical line is extended down to the temperature scale along the bottom of the graph. The end of the curve indicates the critical pressure and temperature where the entire contents becomes gaseous.

cannot be clearly divided into either a liquid or a gas. At extremely low temperatures, the liquid nitrous-oxide may have a definite surface; but as the temperature varies, the contents undergo a gradual phase change from a liquid to a gas. During this change the interface between the two is probably more like a foaming, boiling fog.

Assuming the temperature of the storage tank is held below the critical temperature of 97.7 degrees Fahrenheit, it is relatively easy to draw nitrous-oxide from the tank in either gaseous or liquid form. Figure 1-3 shows how gaseous nitrous-oxide can be drawn from the tank. As gas is drawn off, the pressure in the gas region is reduced, causing the nitrous-oxide to boil, thus producing more gas until the vapor pressure is restored. To draw liquid nitrous-oxide from the tank, an arrangement as shown in Figure 1-3 can be used. In this instance a pickup tube reaches to the lowermost part of the tank; and when the valve is opened the vapor pressure above the liquid forces the nitrous up the tube and out of the tank. As the volume of liquid nitrous-oxide is reduced the pressure above the liquid declines. This causes liquid nitrous-oxide to boil until the temperature and pressure again reaches equilibrium.

Figure 1-4 shows the temperature and pressure characteristics of nitrous-oxide. At a standard temperature of 70 degrees the vapor pressure is 760psi. When the nitrous-oxide is released in liquid form, it will undergo very rapid expansion—due to the drop from 760psi to 14.7psi (standard atmospheric pressure). This pressure drop will cause the temperature of the escaping nitrous-oxide to decrease. In a similar fashion, pressurized air escaping from the valve of a tire feels very cool. In fact, by comparison with air escaping from a tire, nitrous-oxide becomes "super-cooled." This super-cooling effect will cause any moisture to condense and form frost on and around the discharge nozzle.

Another phenomena often takes place due to the fact that water is slightly soluble in nitrous-oxide: Any water vapor in the air coming into contact with the super-cooled stream of nitrous-oxide will immediately crystalize. Some of this water will also become dissolved in the nitrous-oxide. This produces an ice-nitrous crystalline structure, which can form on any reasonably cold object in the direct path of the discharge nozzle. As we shall see later, this cooling effect can be used to good purpose.

COMBUSTION PROPERTIES

As far as automotive performance is concerned, the oxygen content of nitrous-oxide is the important part. By recalling some high school physics, we can establish the percentage of oxygen, by weight, in each nitrous-oxide molecule. In round numbers, the atomic weight of a nitrogen atom is 14. The atomic weight of an oxygen atom is 16. This means that the nitrogen content of a single molecule (N_2O) represents an atomic weight of 28. Similarly, the weight of the oxygen content is 16. The total atomic weight of each molecule, then, is 44. The weight of the oxygen content can also be easily determined. This is calculated as: 16 divided by 44. The result is 0.3636, which expressed as a percentage, means that nitrous-oxide is 36% oxygen by weight.

As stated earlier, under standard conditions the single oxygen atom is firmly bonded to the two nitrogen atoms. However, as the temperature of nitrous-oxide increases, the bond between the oxygen and nitrogen is more easily broken. At temperatures above 565 degrees Fahrenheit, the chemical bonds readily break down, and the oxygen and nitrogen become separated. Fortunately, this is well below the combustion temperatures inside an engine; so when nitrous is present during ignition, the rapid temperature rise frees the oxygen content, which then becomes available for combustion reaction.

Most performance enthusiasts are aware that oxygen is vital to the operation of a conventional internal-combustion engine. Air is funneled into the engine through the induction system, but the important component within this air is really the oxygen. Oxygen is essential for combustion, and from a performance standpoint, the importance of oxygen is simple:

When more air/oxygen is inducted, the engine can burn more fuel, resulting in more power.

In effect, nitrous-oxide is a form of "liquid oxygen" or, viewed in another sense, it is "liquid supercharging." When nitrous-oxide is fed to the engine the amount of oxygen available to support combustion is dramatically increased. However, *along with this additional oxygen, extra fuel must be added to keep the ratio between the fuel and the oxygen correct for efficient combustion.* As a result, the total fuel-oxygen consumption rate of the engine increases and the power output increases.

In addition to the power boost, the presence of the additional fuel and oxygen will have a pronounced effect on the flame temperatures produced in the combustion chamber. Rich mixtures produce lower combustion temperatures. The excess fuel—which is unable to react because there is not enough available oxygen—soaks up some of the combustion heat. This reduces peak power but generally does not cause engine damage. On the other hand, when the mixture is lean, no excess fuel soaks up heat to reduce the combustion temperatures and detonation can occur sending localized temperatures even higher. These extreme localized temperatures will cause the metal in the combustion chamber, valves and piston to become red hot. The extra oxygen—not reacted during combustion—will attack the ultra-hot components and oxidize them, just like an oxygen-rich acetylene torch burns away metal.

When an engine is operated with lean mixtures, induced by improperly metered nitrous delivery, the damage is swift and catastrophic. In effect, the engine will virtually consume itself. As early experimenters discovered, engines can disintegrate in as little as two or three seconds if too little fuel is delivered along with the nitrous. The lesson here is clear: *lean nitrous-fuel ratios must be avoided at all costs!*

Theoretically, the ideal situation is a "chemically correct" mixture. In this situation all of the available oxygen content in the nitrous combines in proper proportions with the enrichment fuel. In other words, there is just enough fuel to react effectively with the oxygen. In actual practice, however, maximum horsepower is usually developed in a normally-aspirated engine when the fuel-air ratio is about 15% to 20% rich. It is believed that the additional fuel—in excess of the theoretically balanced requirement—aids horsepower by virtue of intake-charge cooling and by the promotion of slightly better combustion characteristics.

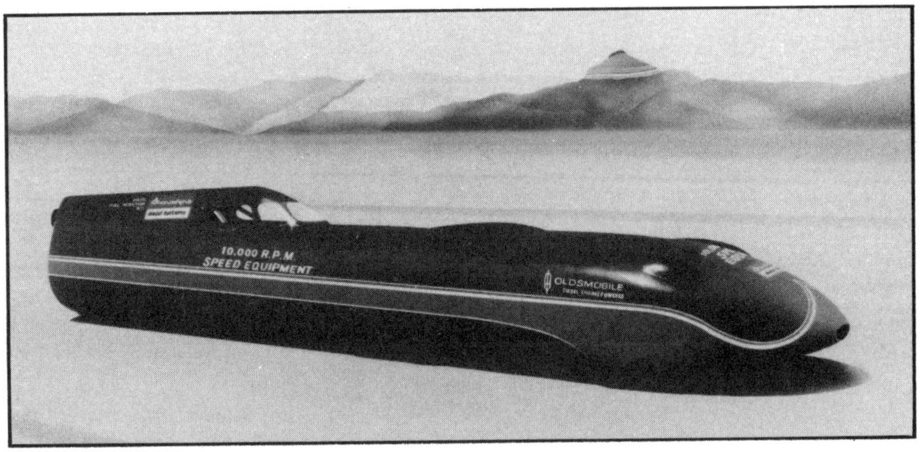

Nitrous-oxide is commonly used as an anesthetic and as a dispensing agent in ice-cream vending machines, but it is also used to boost the horsepower of this Oldsmobile diesel during a land-speed record attempt.

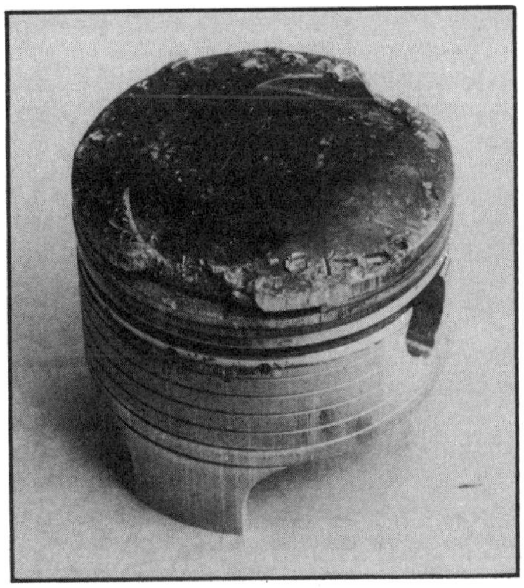

The likelihood of detonation increases as combustion temperature rises. This example shows how detonation can quickly reduce expensive components to scrap value.

Related effects come into play when nitrous is used to boost engine power. Depending on the amount of nitrous injected into the engine—compared with the amount of air and fuel induced—the chemically-correct mixture will cause the combustion temperature to increase simply because the nitrogen content of the induced charge is reduced. This is an important and often overlooked effect of nitrous injection.

Under normal circumstances an engine inducts a charge of air that contains about 23% oxygen (by weight). The rest of the inducted air is composed largely of nitrogen. Nitrogen does not support combustion.

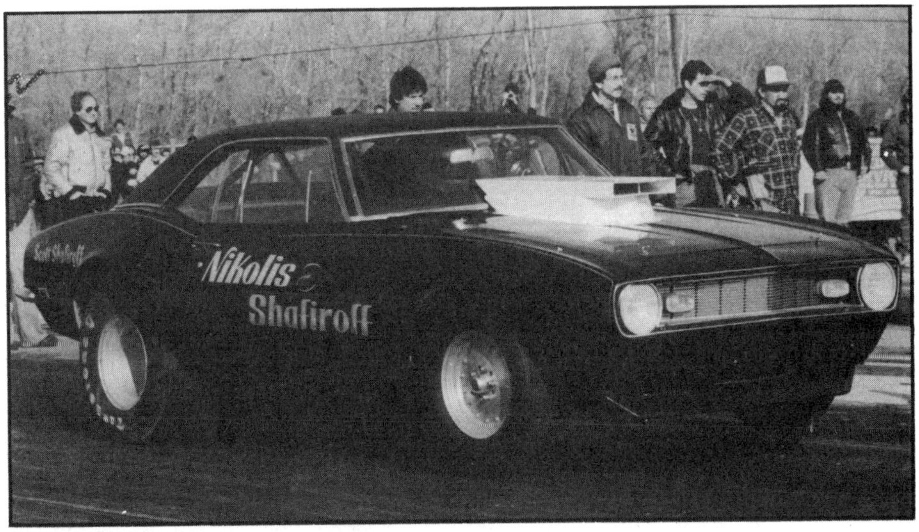

Scott Shafiroff's Camaro runs back-to-back 8.30 elapsed times with the help of nitrous. This killer big-block Chevy records top speeds in excess of 160mph in street trim—with a single 4-barrel!

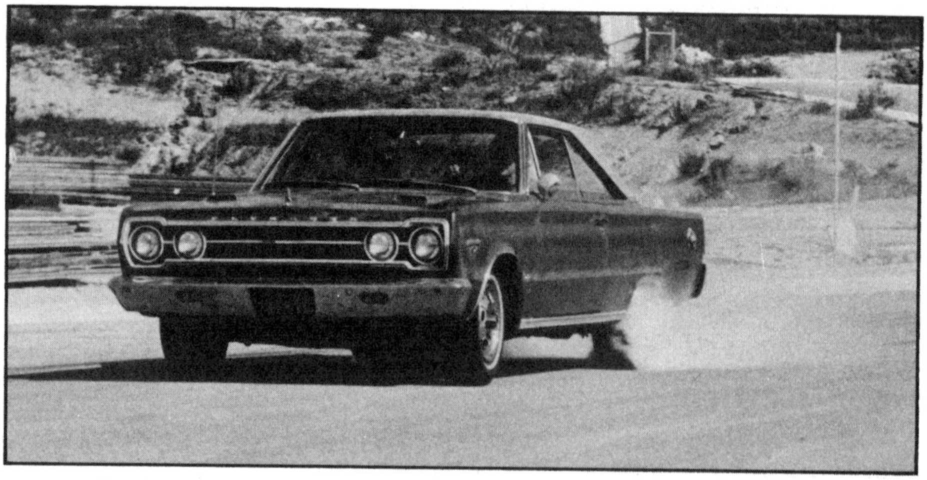

You don't need a high-performance engine to use nitrous, but a heavy-duty engine—built especially for low-speed torque and reliability—and equipped with a street nitrous kit will light the tires of this Plymouth GTX *in any gear.*

Therefore, the nitrogen released during combustion reaction acts as a damper to reduce combustion temperatures. When the proportion of nitrogen in the induced charge is reduced, the dampening effect on combustion temperature is reduced. As a result, the flame temperature and speed increase (of course, within certain defined limits).

Let's examine what happens when nitrous-oxide enters the picture. Our example will be a typical V8 displacing 350 cubic inches and producing about 300 horsepower. At about 5000 rpm this engine will consume approximately 400 cubic feet of air per minute. One cubic foot of air at sea level, under standard conditions, weighs 0.0765 pounds. This means that the engine is inducting 30.61 pounds of air per minute. Of that, 23.6% is oxygen; so the engine is actually inducting 7.224 pounds of oxygen per minute.

Now, let's assume that this engine is fitted with a nitrous system that will deliver—at wide-open throttle—a maximum of about 5.0 pounds of nitrous-oxide per minute. By weight, nitrous contains 36% oxygen; the rest, of course, is nitrogen. This means that of the 5.0 pounds, 1.8 pounds will be oxygen and 3.2 pounds will be nitrogen. Adding the oxygen content of the nitrous to the oxygen content of the induced air charge, we have a total oxygen charge weight of 9.024 pounds and a total nitrogen charge weight of 26.586 pounds. This gives a total combined charge weight of 35.61 pounds. The percentage of oxygen in this total charge will now be equal to 9.024 divided by 35.61. Calculating this as a percentage, we find that 25.34% of the inducted charge is oxygen and 74.66% is nitrogen. This means that the oxygen content, as a proportion of the whole inducted charge, has been increased by 7.3%, while the nitrogen proportion has been reduced by 1.3%.

The foregoing discussion assumes that the nitrous-oxide is being injected as a liquid. If the nitrous is injected as a gas, for a given horsepower increase *the combustion temperature increase is greater.* This is because the gaseous nitrous displaces a larger proportion of the inducted air and fuel.

In addition, the power that would have been produced by the *displaced air and fuel* is no longer available. We must remember, though, that air contains 23.6% oxygen (by weight) and nitrous contains 36% oxygen (by weight). We are still on the winning side, however, because the displaced air is replaced by oxygen-rich nitrous-oxide. Moreover, recent experiments have indicated that the ratio of oxygen to nitrogen increases more rapidly when gaseous nitrous-oxide is injected into the intake tract. Because of this, flame temperatures can be expected to climb more rapidly by gas injection than by liquid injection—for a given power increase from the engine.

Some experiments with nitrous injection have indicated that flame temperatures rise as fast as, if not faster than, the increased percentage of oxygen taken into the engine. In other words, in our example here, *if no steps are taken to cool the combustion mass,* the flame temperatures could easily increase as much as 15% to 20%!

This means that in practical situations, *the chemically-correct mixture is not the ideal practical mixture.* It may be best for horsepower but will almost certainly cause overheating difficulties. So for all practical purposes, rich fuel-to-nitrous mixtures have to be used in order to cool the combustion temperatures to a safe level.

The relatively rich mixture required for peak engine performance can be described, for lack of a better term, as the "excess fuel factor" (EFF), because it is fuel in excess of what is required for the theoretically optimum chemical reaction with a given amount of oxygen. In our future discussions the term *excess fuel factor* will refer to the relative quality of the fuel-nitrous mix delivered to the engine.

NITROUS-TO-FUEL RATIO

The most important factor for successful operation is the ratio between

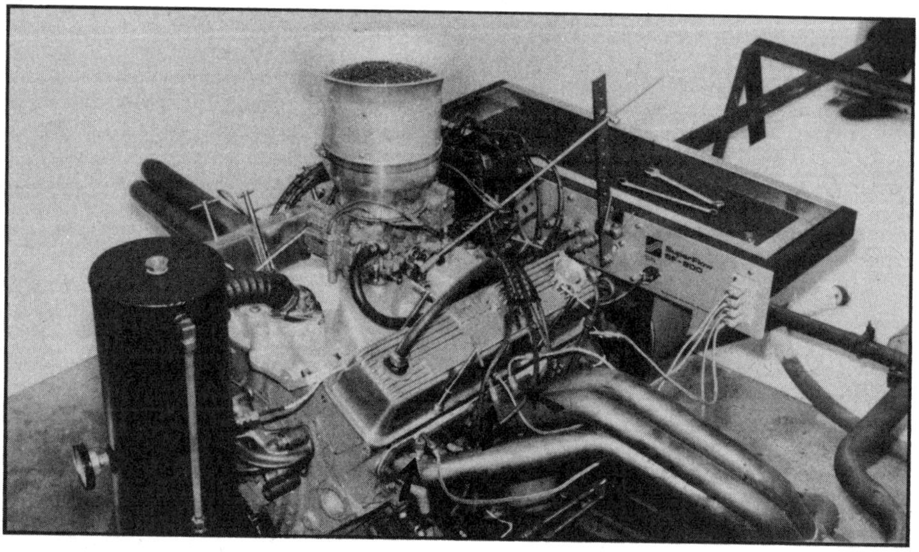

If a conventional spark-plug thermocouple is not available, combustion temperatures can be inferred by measuring the temperature of the exhaust at the port exit into the header. Any time the fuel-to-nitrous mixture approaches the "chemically correct" balance the exhaust temperature rises dramatically.

the nitrous-oxide and the enrichment fuel. This ratio is not the same for each and every engine or application, therefore, it is helpful to understand how this all-important factor is derived.

With a modest knowledge of chemistry and the chemical makeup of common motor fuels the nitrous-to-fuel ratio can be calculated fairly accurately. The best place to start, from a theoretical standpoint, is with the chemically-correct mixture ratio. The calculations are relatively straightforward, but in actual practice there are some problems.

The first difficulty is that the typical gasoline sold at the corner service station is anything but "typical." Currently many different additives are blended into motor gasolines to modify the characteristics for different applications and for sale in different locales and during various seasons of the year. As a result, the actual makeup of pump gasoline is complex and somewhat indefinite.

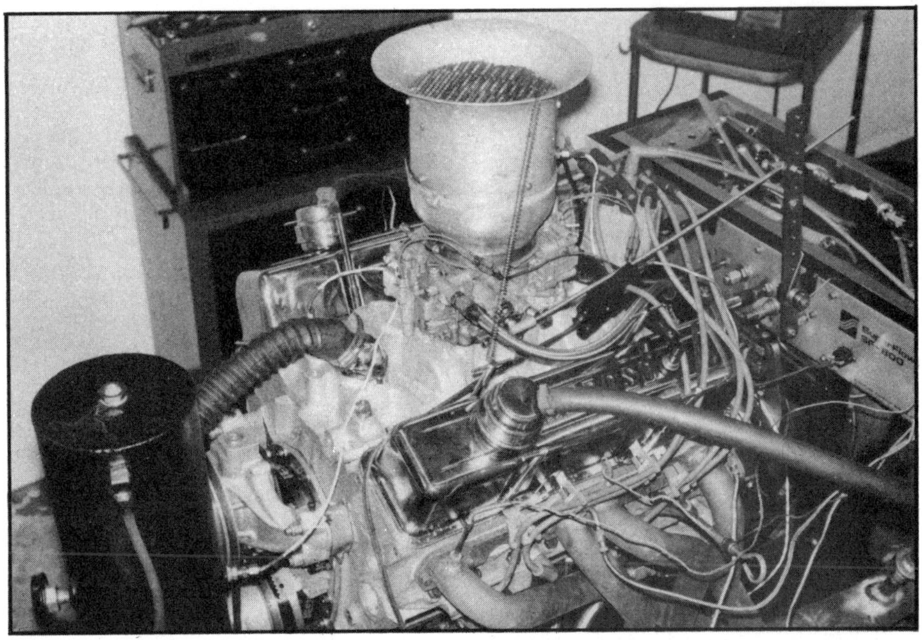

This engine was built by the author to compare the power output produced by various fuels. The engine has high volumetric efficiency, 14.7:1 compression, short duration camshaft and variable ignition. Testing indicated that high octane does not always ensure best performance. However, results consistently indicated that low intake charge temperatures significantly reduce detonation.

There is no way to totally account for these variations, but for most experimental purposes—and for our purposes here—a fuel compound called iso-octane is commonly used. Iso-octane is a single component fuel that is often used for critical laboratory testing and it is not commonly available. Nonetheless, for lack of a better standard, we will use iso-octane in the chemical equations presented here. For all practical purposes the derived results will be reasonably accurate and representative.

The chemical formula for iso-octane is C_8H_{18}. It has a specific gravity of 0.702 (at 60 degrees F), and it belongs to the paraffin/hydro-carbon series. The basic calculations for deriving the nitrous-to-fuel ratio with gasoline (iso-octane) are presented in Figure 1-5. As shown there, the theoretical ratio for a chemically-correct mixture—when the fuel is gasoline—is 9.649:1.

If the base fuel is something other than gasoline this mixture ratio will not be valid. For any given fuel the calculation can be performed in a similar manner. The results for a range of common fuels are shown in Figure 1-6.

FIGURE 1-5

EQUATIONS FOR CHEMICALLY CORRECT FUEL TO N_2O RATIOS USING VARIOUS COMMON FUELS

The atoms of carbon and hydrogen will, when combined with oxygen (during combustion), form carbon dioxide (CO_2) and water (H_2O). The balanced chemical equation looks like this:

Equation 1:
Fuel Nitrous Oxide

$$C_8H_{18} + 25\,N_2O = 8\,CO_2 + 9H_2O + 25\,N_2$$

In other words, the hydrocarbon fuel (in this case iso-octane, a chemically-pure gasoline) combines with the oxygen content of nitrous oxide and forms 8 molecules of carbon dioxide and 9 molecules of water plus 25 diatomic molecules (two atoms per molecule) of nitrogen (N_2).

The atomic weights of the above elements are:

Hydrogen–1
Carbon–12
Nitrogen–14
Oxygen–16

OPTIMUM N_2O/GASOLINE RATIOS

N_2O to fuel ratio by weight can be determined by dividing the mass of the oxidant by the mass of the fuel:

Equation 2:

$$\frac{\underset{\text{(Nitrogen)}}{(25 \times 14 \times 2)} + \underset{\text{(Oxygen)}}{(25 \times 16)}}{\underset{\text{(Carbon)}}{(8 \times 12)} + \underset{\text{(Hydrogen)}}{(18 \times 1)}} =$$

These values were obtained from equation 1 (above); for example, the 25 molecules of nitrogen in the nitrous oxide are multiplied by the atomic weight of nitrogen (14) and that is multiplied by 2 since the diatomic molecule of nitrogen (N_2) contains two atoms of nitrogen. Proceeding with the calculation:

$$\frac{700 + 400}{114} = \frac{1100}{114} = 9.649$$

What does this ratio mean? Because the values for the number of molecules were obtained from the balanced chemical equation (meaning that complete combustion will "use up" all of the molecules called for in the equation), the mass figure ratio gives us a relation (by mass, i.e., weight) how much of the fuel must be combined with the oxidant (nitrous oxide) to obtain complete combustion. Therefore the above value of 9.649 indicates that 9.649 pounds of nitrous oxide is needed to combust 1 pound of gasoline.

This same relationship can be applied to other fuels, as shown below.

OPTIMUM N_2O/PROPANE RATIO

The chemical formula for propane is C_3H_8, and the new balanced equation is:

Equation 3:
Fuel Nitrous Oxide

$$C_3H_8 + 10\,N_2O = 3\,CO_2 + 4H_2O + 10\,N_2$$

Therefore:

Equation 4:

$$\frac{\underset{\text{(Nitrogen)}}{(10 \times 14 \times 2)} + \underset{\text{(Oxygen)}}{(10 \times 16)}}{\underset{\text{(Carbon)}}{(3 \times 12)} + \underset{\text{(Hydrogen)}}{(8 \times 1)}} = \frac{440}{44} = 10$$

This ratio indicates that 10 pounds of N_2O will be required for each pound of propane.

OPTIMUM N_2O/METHANOL RATIO

The chemical formula for methanol is CH_3OH, therefore:

Equation 5:
Fuel Nitrous Oxide

$$CH_3OH + 3\,N_2O = CO_2 + 2H_2O + 3\,N_2$$

Therefore:

Equation 6:

$$\frac{\underset{\text{(Nitrogen)}}{(3 \times 14 \times 2)} + \underset{\text{(Oxygen)}}{(3 \times 16)}}{\underset{\text{(Carbon)}}{(1 \times 12)} + \underset{\text{(Hydrogen)}}{(4 \times 1)} + \underset{\text{(Oxygen)}}{(1 \times 16)}} = \frac{132}{32} = 4.13$$

4.13 pounds of N_2O are needed to fully burn 1 pound of methanol.

OPTIMUM N_2O/ETHANOL RATIO

The chemical formula for ethanol is C_2H_5OH, therefore:

Equation 7:
Fuel Nitrous Oxide

$$C_2H_5OH + 6\,N_2O = 2\,CO_2 + 3\,H_2O + 6\,N_2$$

Therefore:

Equation 8:

$$\frac{\underset{\text{(Nitrogen)}}{(6 \times 14 \times 2)} + \underset{\text{(Oxygen)}}{(6 \times 16)}}{\underset{\text{(Carbon)}}{(2 \times 12)} + \underset{\text{(Hydrogen)}}{(6 \times 1)} + \underset{\text{(Oxygen)}}{(1 \times 16)}} = \frac{264}{46} = 5.74$$

5.74 pounds of N_2O are needed to completely burn 1 pound of ethanol.

FUEL	LBS N2O/LB FUEL
GASOLINE	9.649
METHANOL	4.130
ETHANOL	5.740
PROPANE	10.00
BUTANE	9.930
NITROMETHANE	1.090

FIGURE 1-6: Chemically Correct Mixture Ratios of Nitrous and Base Fuels

FUEL CHARACTERISTICS

Gasoline

The combustion characteristics that we have considered so far are primarily applicable to gasoline fuels. Nonetheless, the characteristics are very similar when other types of fuels are considered. In general we can say that whatever undesirable characteristics any other fuel may have will be exaggerated when the fuel is used with nitrous injection, unless steps are taken to counteract them.

Considering gasoline for a little longer, the biggest problem with currently available gasolines is the low octane value. If a particular gasoline-fueled engine is prone to detonation without nitrous, the engine will be even more prone to detonation when nitrous is used. As has been discussed before, the only means to prevent this is to provide some method to lower the combustion temperature. The most common solution to this problem is to richen the mixture (add more fuel).

Methanol

When we consider other fuels, the game is the same, but the rules are a little different. A good example is methanol. If the mixture is chemically-correct the detonation limit of methanol is actually lowered when nitrous is added. However, methanol fuels are rarely used at chemically-correct mixtures. Methanol has tremendous cooling properties when used in a fuel-rich mixture. This cooling effect can be used to reduce intake charge temperature (increase charge density) and to suppress detonation. Fuel-rich methanol or ethanol mixtures have much the same effect on the combustion processes as rich gasoline mixtures, but the effects are more pronounced.

A factor often overlooked with alcohol-type fuels is that they are more prone to pre-ignition than gasoline fuels, and the addition of nitrous seems to further promote this difficulty. For example, if pre-ignition is about to occur because of a localized hot spot in the chamber—but the spot is not quite hot enough to prematurely ignite the mixture—then injecting nitrous will immediately raise the localized temperature sufficiently to cause the onset of pre-ignition.

Nitromethane

The destructive potential of nitromethane is well known to most racers. This is due to the fact that nitro is sensitive to detonation. In this respect, it is a bad choice for a racing fuel. (Nitro does have an overwhelming virtue: it is almost 53% oxygen by weight. In fact, a careful analysis of nitromethane reveals that this is its only virtue.) The use of nitrous-oxide with a nitro-blended fuel will only increase the inherently bad detonation characteristics to the point where this tendency can reach unacceptable limits.

This doesn't mean that nitrous-oxide and nitromethane are not compatible. It does mean that the difference between the engine detonating itself to pieces in a matter of seconds or holding together long enough to finish a race may be very small, indeed, unless radical steps are taken to reduce the onset of detonation. The key, of course, is the nitrous-to-fuel ratio, but in this case there is another factor: the ratio between the nitromethane and alcohol. In most cases nitromethane is not used in pure form. It is blended with an alcohol-base fuel, and the resulting mixture will have considerably different combustion and detonation characteristics, depending upon the proportion of nitro used in the blend.

It is difficult to predict, therefore, the specific effect nitrous will have with a nitro-alcohol blend. This is a complicated balancing act—only a few professional drag racers have acquired enough experience to play this game with anything even remotely resembling reliability—but there are some interesting questions involved. From a reliability point of view, as speculation, it may be wiser to use a greater amount of nitrous and a fuel blend with a substantially smaller proportion of nitromethane. This arrangement would rely on the oxygen content of the nitrous, not the oxygen content of the nitromethane. Considering the higher power output (per pound) of methanol, the result should be equal or better power figures than a nitro-rich blend without nitrous-oxide.

Under-the-blower nitrous installations, like the one shown here, have been tried on leading Top Fuel engines. However, success has been limited, primarily because nitrous increases the detonation characteristics of nitromethane.

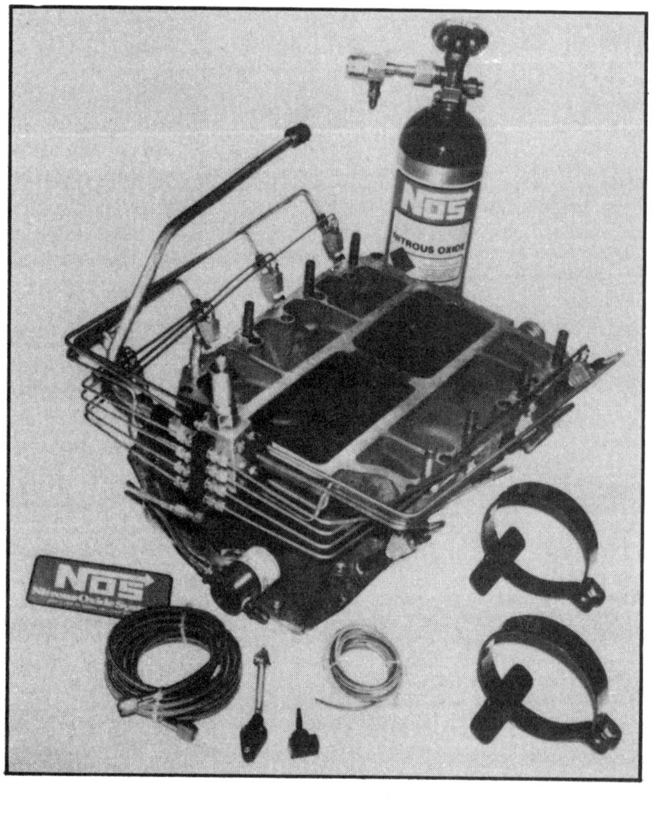

Gaseous Fuels

In an effort to reduce operating costs and circumvent emission difficulties, some fleet operators and performance enthusiasts have turned to gaseous fuels, such as propane and butane. These fuels can be used with nitrous-oxide, but they do have certain disadvantages. Because the fuels are gaseous, the enrichment fuel added with the nitrous will have *little or no cooling effect on combustion.* This means that the combustion temperature will rise considerably. The redeeming factor is that both propane and butane have high octane values and are highly resistant to detonation. Nonetheless, although propane or butane may be suitable for nitrous injection, the engine components may not be able to withstand the extreme heat generated during combustion. Without some means to reduce the combustion temperatures, the amount of power that can be safely developed by a gaseous fuel-nitrous mix is much less than can be achieved by a comparable mix with liquid fuels.

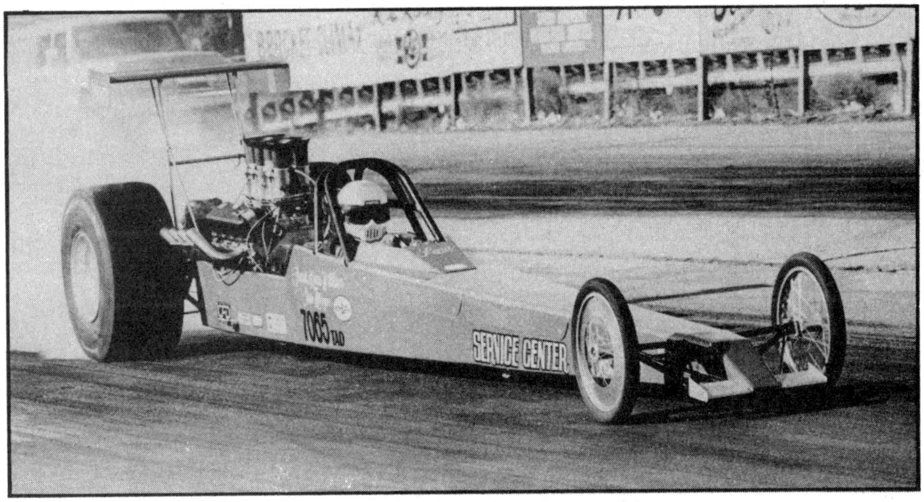

Though the engine is not exotic by present standards, this nitrous-boosted big-block Chevy dragster consistently runs near the 200mph mark.

DETONATION

We are all aware that detonation can destroy an engine in a very short time. With a normally-aspirated engine, the steps to avoid detonation are simple: reduce ignition timing, reduce the compression ratio, or increase the fuel octane.

So much is known about the relationship between compression ratio and a given fuel octane that there's really no mystery to it anymore. But when nitrous is added into the equation, everything changes. The results are quite similar to the effects of a mechanical supercharger. The end function of a supercharger is, of course, to pack more and more oxygen into the cylinders. Consequently, it has a dramatic effect on just how much octane and/or compression ratio is possible before detonation occurs.

Once the compression ratio of a naturally-aspirated engine has been optimized to avoid detonation with a specific fuel, the problem is solved. On the other hand, with a supercharged engine—especially a turbocharged engine—it is possible to gradually raise the boost pressure and boost the power output. At some point, however, the engine will begin to detonate, and for all practical purposes, this will determine the absolute peak power available from the engine (unless additional steps are taken to stave off the detonation). In many respects, nitrous-oxide is like supercharging. It is possible to keep adding more and more nitrous and fuel until detonation ultimately, and firmly, limits the power output.

The effects of nitrous-oxide on the detonation threshold are well known. As early as World War II, nitrous-oxide was studied extensively for use in high-altitude fighters. An early test performed by NACA (National Advisory Committee for Aeronautics, precursor of the current NASA organization) on one cylinder of a 1710 cubic inch Allison aircraft engine is very revealing.

(This engine was chosen as an alternative to the 1650 cubic inch Rolls Royce Merlin engine. The two engines are relatively similar in configuration, except that the Merlin engine is supercharged. To more nearly duplicate the Merlin engine configuration, supercharging was added to the test engine. So in essence, the test engine was a 142 cubic inch supercharged engine with an aluminum head, four valves per cylinder and a bore of about 5.50 inches. Although this engine functions in much the same way as all internal-combustion engines, it is different in many ways from the typical late-model V8 automotive engine. We need to bear this in mind when considering the results of the NACA tests, because these differences may have a significance when we relate the results to modern automotive engines.)

The NACA tests were all performed with gaseous nitrous-oxide (as opposed to liquid nitrous). This means that any charge cooling that may have been available due to injecting liquid nitrous into the engine or supercharger was lost. In spite of this, it was found that if the engine was already on the detonation threshold, replacing 10% of the induced air charge with gaseous nitrous-oxide resulted in a 9% increase in horsepower before detonation became a limiting factor.

This 9% increase in horsepower occurred with 2% less supercharged boost. When the nitrous content was increased 20%, the detonation-limited power output increased to 17% more power with 4% less boost. Figure 1-7 shows the power-output figures in relation to intake temperatures achieved at two mixture strengths: one with a fuel-oxygenation ratio at 0.410:1 and the other at 0.495:1.

There is, in fact, some relevance in these results because the fuel-oxygen ratios are relatively rich with fuel. A fuel-oxygen ratio—irrespective of where the oxygen is derived (ambient air or nitrous-oxide)—of about 0.29 to 0.32:1 represents a chemically-correct mixture for gasoline. At this point, however, we're only considering the oxygen aspect of the charge because the nitrogen doesn't affect the power equation (except when dissociation occurs, but we'll ignore this for the moment).

The important point is that the detonation level of the engine was moved

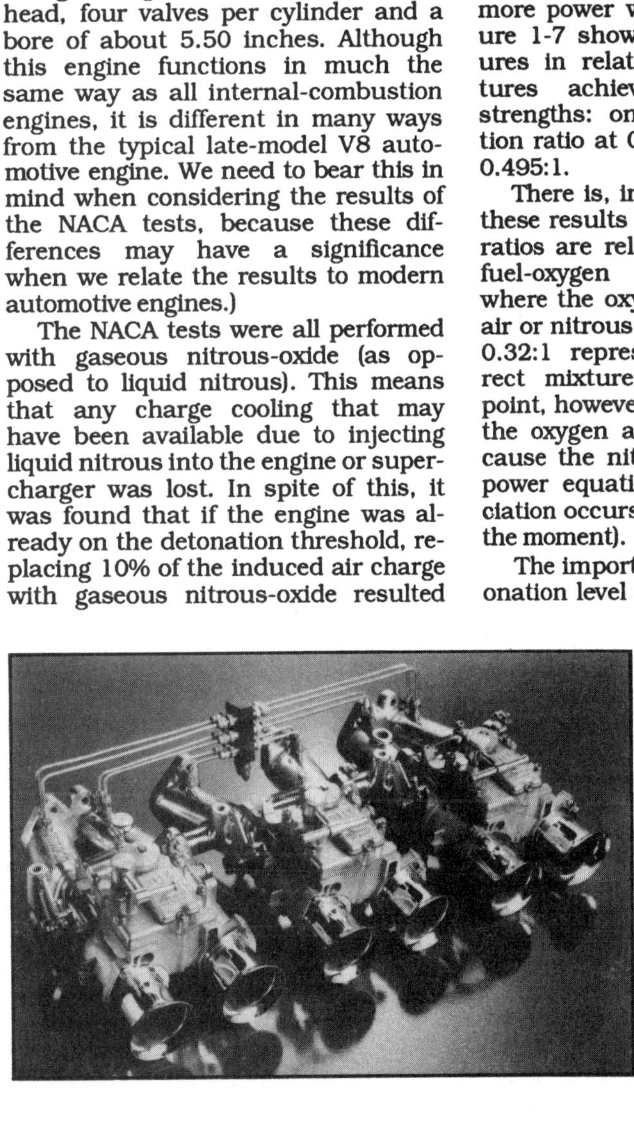

Port injection ensures even distribution and maximizes the amount of liquid nitrous entering the engine. Here a 6-port nitrous system is used with three Solex side-draft carburetors, a complex but effective setup that is suited for racing or "serious" performance.

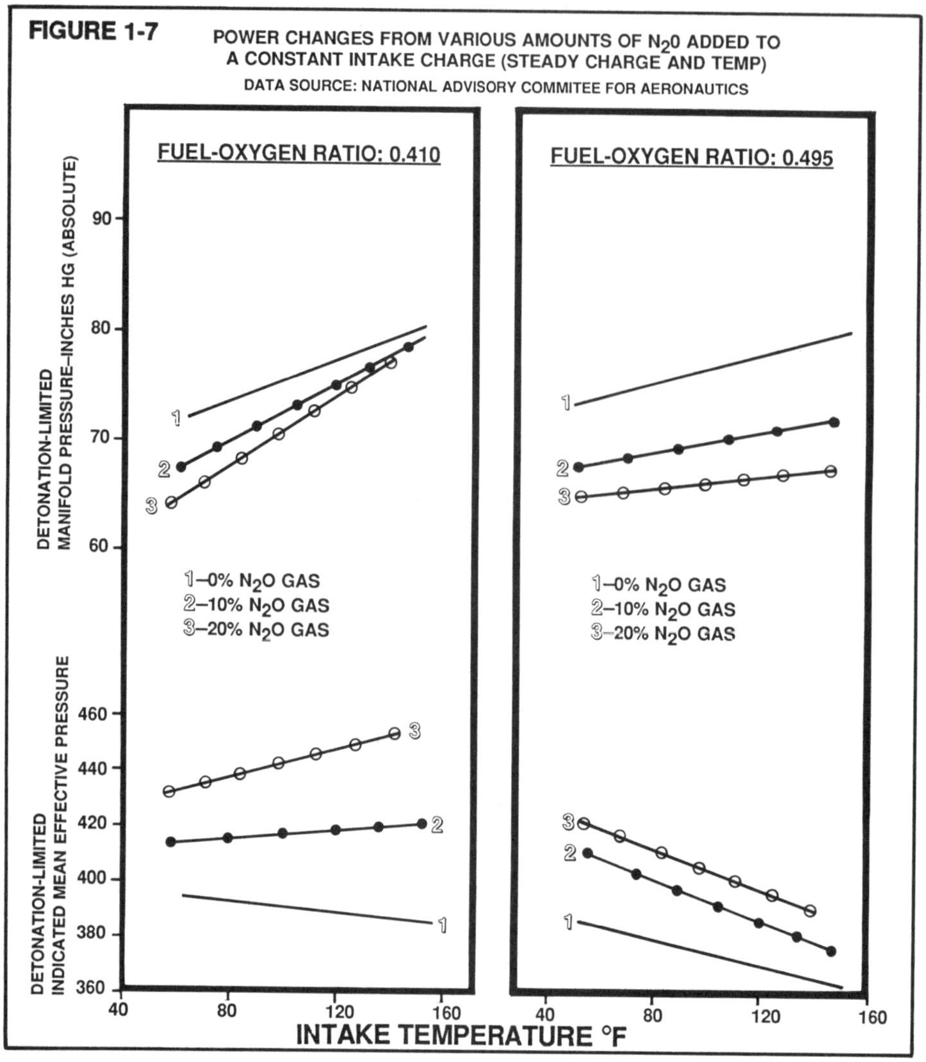

FIGURE 1-7: This may seem confusing; but the graph shows that when nitrous is used there is less tendency to detonate with richer mixtures.

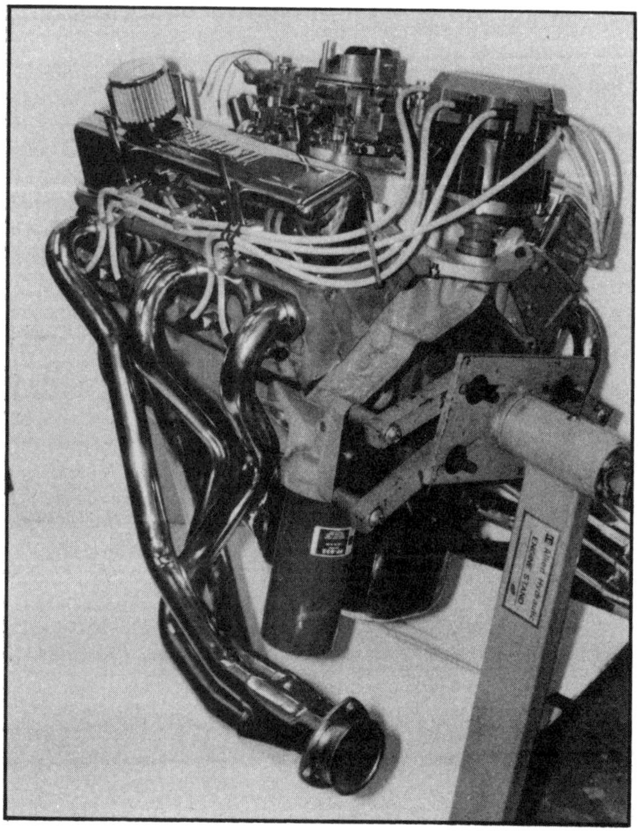

This particular engine was built by the author to test the effect of small amounts of nitrous—delivered both as a gas and a liquid—on flame temperatures and detonation. For a given power increase, liquid nitrous prevented detonation more effectively than gaseous nitrous.

higher, resulting in an increased power output. However, it is likely that this was caused by the excess fuel factor and was *not* necessarily caused by any detonation-inhibiting qualities that the nitrous-oxide may have. Also, we must remember that some of the power increase in the NACA test was undoubtedly due to the fact that less boost was needed to get the same or more oxygen into the engine. Hence, less power was absorbed by the supercharger.

With this in mind, though, it is nonetheless interesting to note that some researchers have verified that at small gross power levels the detonation limit of the engine is raised slightly. This suggests that in the initial stages of injection (i.e., when small quantities of nitrous are used), the nitrous-oxide may suppress detonation.

This is probably not significant in high-performance automotive engines because large amounts of nitrous are required. Power boosts ranging from 75 to 150 horsepower are very common in typical V8 engines, and these power levels require a lot more than "small amounts" of nitrous-oxide.

EXCESS HEAT

We've already looked at the excess fuel factor as a means of reducing detonation difficulties, but we need to examine more closely another property of nitrous that is closely tied to detonation difficulties: the extra heat generated during combustion.

The key to avoiding heat problems is to use some sort of "combustion coolant." We have, of course, already discussed one form of combustion coolant: the excess enrichment fuel injected with the nitrous-oxide. As we stated earlier, this excess fuel suppresses detonation and cools the surfaces of the combustion chambers. The "coolant fuel" is used as a matter of convenience—primarily, because it is relatively easy to enrich the fuel delivery beyond that required for optimum power—but it isn't absolutely necessary to use excess fuel as the primary means to reduce combustion temperatures.

My own experiments with water injection indicate that *water or a water/alcohol mix is a better combustion coolant.* Although it's not generally realized, injecting an auxiliary coolant into a high-compression engine (where the coolant is used solely to reduce detonation) normally results in less power than if the same engine was operated on gasoline of sufficiently high octane. In other words, contrary to popular opinion, water or water-alcohol injection will reduce, not increase, horsepower.

FIGURE 1-8

THE EFFECT OF WATER INJECTION ON POWER OUTPUT

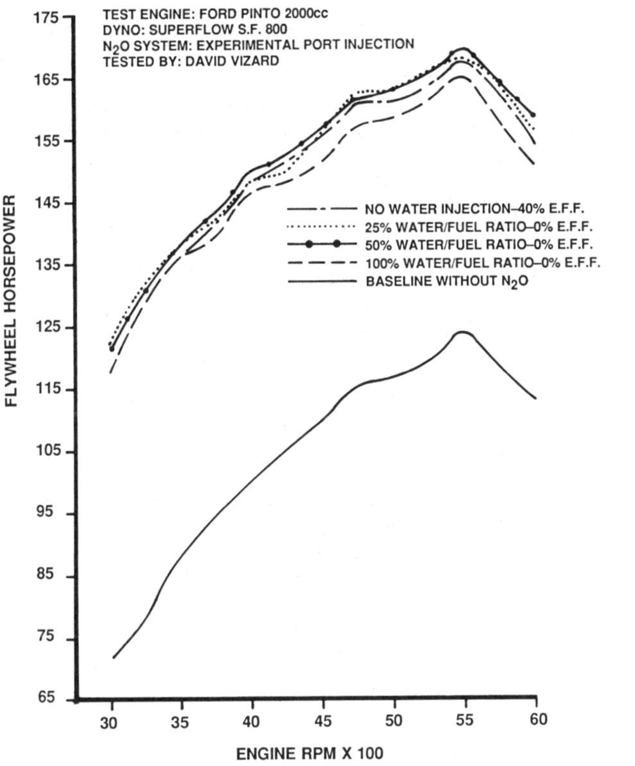

FIGURE 1-8: Water injection will reduce combustion temperature, allow leaner fuel-to-nitrous ratios, and increase power.

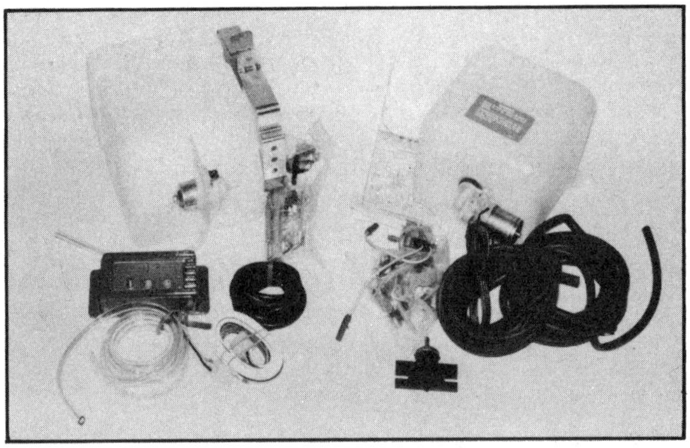

Water injection will significantly enhance the power and reliability of a nitrous engine. Suitable water injectors are produced by Holley, Spearco, and Edelbrock.

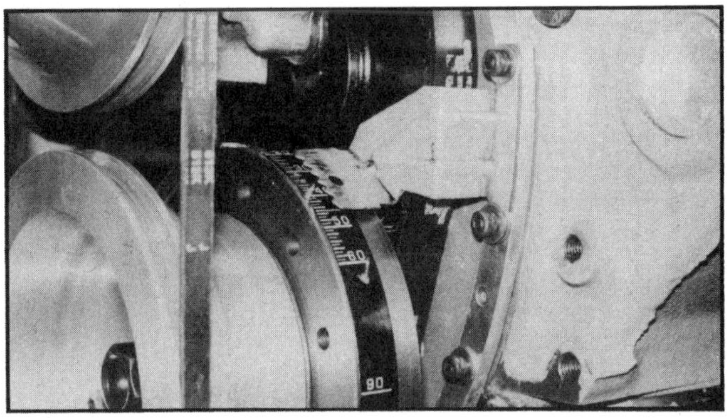

Ignition timing is important if detonation is to be avoided with any high-performance engine. Timing is especially crucial on a nitrous engine because even a little too much advance can destroy the engine very quickly. Also make sure the timing marks on the dampener are properly indexed to crank/piston position.

It is not necessary to inject very much water into an engine before a noticeable power drop is recorded. On the other hand, if a moderate quantity of combustion coolant is used along with nitrous-oxide, some *small* power gains are possible (see Figure 1-8). In addition, I have noted that *substantial quantities of coolant can be injected before any noticeable power drop is observed.* This concurs with the NACA tests cited earlier, which showed that water or a 50/50 water-alcohol mix produced small increases in horsepower, rather than the small power decrease usually experienced when gasoline is used as the primary combustion coolant.

Using an auxiliary combustion coolant with nitrous-oxide has two intrinsic advantages: (1) the high cooling properties of water or water-alcohol can greatly reduce the chances of engine damage caused by overheating, and (2) water or water-alcohol has the effect of raising the octane level of the fuel, which further raises the detonation threshold.

When water or water-alcohol is used as a combustion coolant it is possible to run a chemically-correct or very nearly correct nitrous-to-fuel ratio. The primary limitation with such a system is the amount of available coolant (water or water-alcohol). If the coolant injection fails or the coolant reservoir runs dry, the combustion temperatures will become excessive when the nitrous-oxide and fuel are injected. This will almost certainly result in component or complete engine failure. If this approach is taken, it is highly recommended that the nitrous injection be monitored by a mechanical override in the coolant reservoir. When the coolant level drops below a prescribed limit, the override should automatically deactivate the nitrous-oxide system. If such a fail-safe is not used, the nitrous-oxide system is likely to "deactivate" the engine in a very expensive manner.

Just to make certain there is no misunderstanding, I want to repeat this point: there is no need to use both an excessively rich fuel enrichment and a combustion coolant. The coolant injection serves only to combat a detonation and/or heating problem. If a rich fuel system is already eliminating this difficulty, coolant injection will serve no useful purpose, other than to possibly cool some of the internal components to a safer level. (For instance, the spark plug electrodes may last longer.)

Extra care must be taken if the engine is equipped with aluminum cylinder heads. Aluminum conducts heat more efficiently than cast iron. As a result, the extra heat generated by the nitrous-oxide is more easily conducted to the engine water jacket and carried away by the engine coolant. On the other hand, the amount of temperature overload that the aluminum can tolerate is less than cast iron. If for any reason, the combustion temperature exceeds the critical level, pitting and localized melting will result. The most likely place for this to happen is in the vicinity of the exhaust valve. If overheating occurs there is also a real possibility that the exhaust-valve seat insert may come out of the cylinder head.

CHAPTER 2

NITROUS PERFORMANCE POTENTIAL

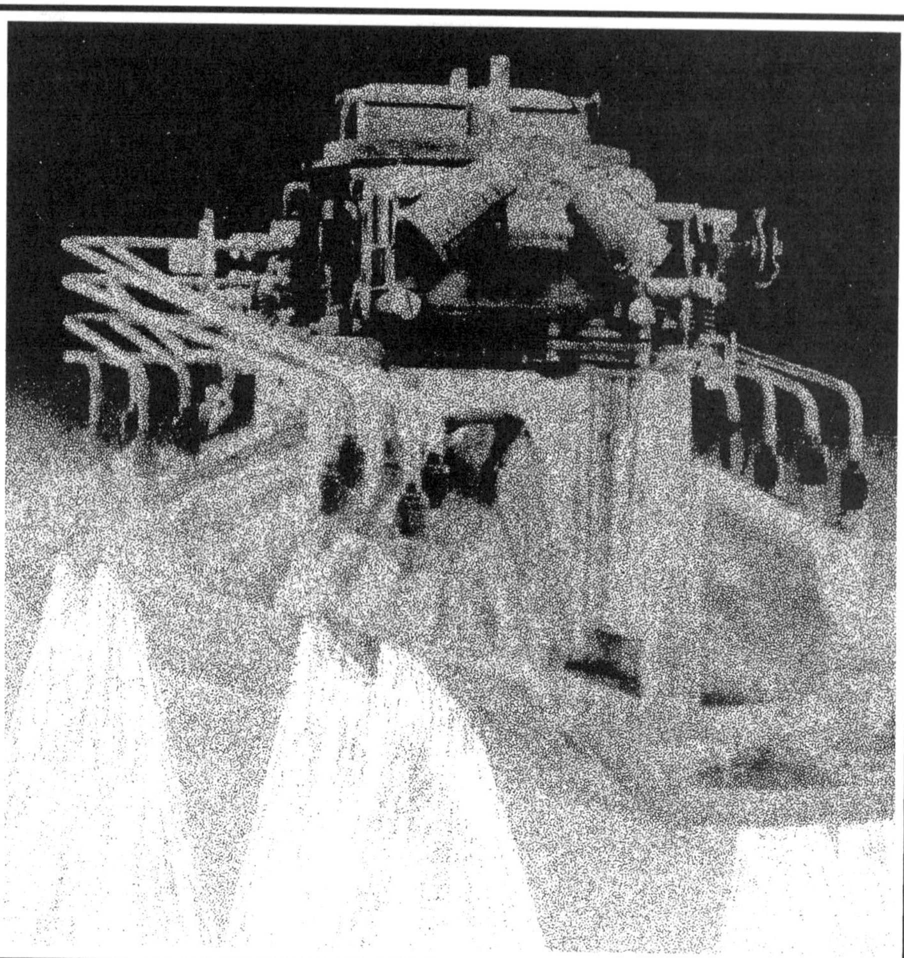

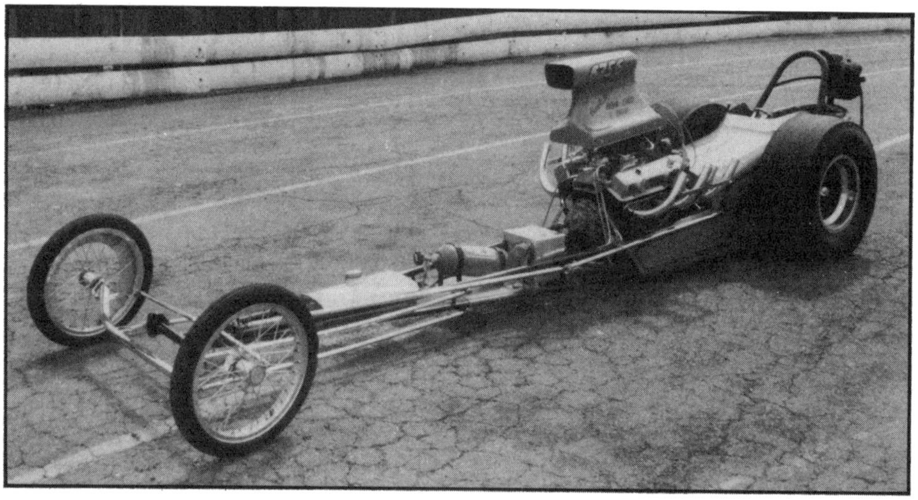

There is little doubt that speed costs money, and going twice as fast usually costs more than twice as much. Nitrous, however, can significantly reduce this trend. Though relatively inexpensive, this nitrous-boosted dragster is fast and reliable.

POTENTIAL

When performance enthusiasts talk about nitrous-oxide, the question of "ultimate power" inevitably dominates the conversation. And of course, speculation is sometimes far removed from hard reality. If we judge the potential simply by the lofty allegations bantered about in magazine advertising, it would seem that nitrous injection is too good to be true. In fact, while large power increases are almost always proclaimed, only small amounts of extra power are actually achieved in some cases. There are many reasons for this disparity (which we will soon examine in greater detail); but nitrous is, unquestionably, one of the fastest routes to high horsepower. The key is a correctly designed system, and at this point, I will attempt to put nitrous power into proper perspective.

NITROUS DELIVERY

As of this writing, virtually all N_2O systems are of the constant-flow, constant-rate type. This means that once activated, the flow is continuous (as opposed to the intermittent flow provided by timed injection) and the rate at which fuel and nitrous are put into the engine is constant, irrespective of engine speed (rpm). This means that the amount of nitrous-oxide delivered to the engine is *fixed* and is not related to engine speed or load. This may seem insignificant, nonetheless it has a direct bearing on the power curve. To get a clear picture of what is happening, we need to analyze not only how nitrous increases the power output but also what effect the delivery system has on overall engine operation.

As we discovered earlier, the power increase is brought about primarily by the oxygen content of the nitrous. We have seen that N_2O is loaded with oxygen; and when this extra oxygen is inducted to the engine, extra fuel must also be added to provide for proper combustion. This extra oxygen and fuel react to produce higher cylinder pressure, which leads directly to increased power.

Whenever nitrous-oxide is injected into an engine as a gas, it displaces air that is normally inducted by the engine during normal functioning. This means that if we inject one cubic foot of gaseous nitrous-oxide into the intake manifold, one cubic foot less of ambient air is going to be drawn in through the carburetor. In other words, *gaseous nitrous is being injected at the expense of induced air.*

For our purposes, I call this the displaced-charge factor (DCF). In a simple way, we can visualize this situation with a simple weight scale. On one side of the scale, we have nitrous-oxide; on the other side, we have the oxygen contained in the normal atmospheric charge. For every cubic foot of nitrous we place on one side of the scale, we have to remove a cubic foot of induced charge on the opposite side. Because nitrous-oxide is 36% oxygen (by weight) and air is 23% oxygen (by weight), we have a good tradeoff. However, these numbers don't tell the whole story. When compared at the same temperatures, nitrous-oxide is 50% *denser* than air. This means that for each comparable cubic foot of gas entering the engine, nitrous-oxide contains 2.3 times the amount of oxygen that the ambient air contains!

Based on oxygen content alone, this means that if the engine was fed pure gaseous nitrous-oxide and suitable fuel, it would produce approximately 230% more power than an engine running on air. Figure 2-1 shows the theoretical power increase available from pure nitrous-oxide (ignoring all factors other than the increased oxygen content of gaseous N_2O).

The gains look impressive, but the question is: Can they be achieved in practice? Surprisingly, the power outputs achieved in actual engine tests exceed the theoretical numbers, *if we take into account only the extra oxygen.* Again, Figure 2-1 shows how much actual power is gained on a typical test engine when nitrous-oxide is fed into the intake airstream. As can be seen, when 10% of the induced charge is made up of nitrous-oxide, the power increase is an impressive 20%!

An immediate question springs to mind: Where does the additional power come from? If we look at the situation in detail, we can see that several things happen at once, and a combination of factors is leading to additional power.

First, the fact that we have reduced the nitrogen content of the total charge means that the flame front, once initiated, propagates quicker and burns faster. This means more

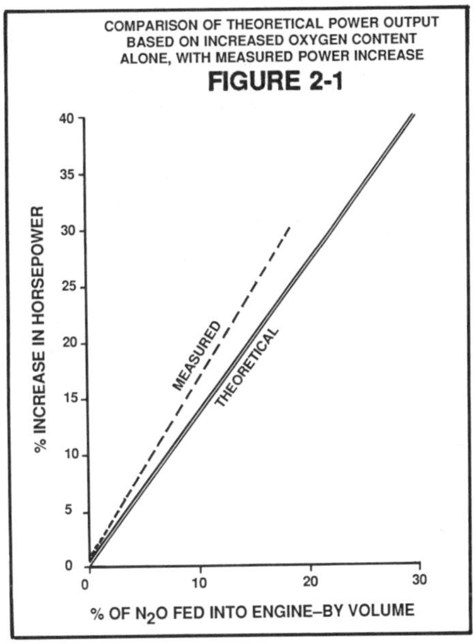

FIGURE 2-1: This theoretical presentation is based on oxygen content alone, but in real life other factors come into play. The measured output of a nitrous-injected engine tends to exceed the "simplified" predictions here.

efficient combustion. Second, the temperature of combustion is higher, which results in greater thermal efficiency. Third, we have to take into account the fact that when nitrous-oxide breaks down into the chemical constituents of nitrogen and oxygen, it does so in the form of an exo-thermic reaction. In other words, the simple reduction of the N_2O produces heat. This means that, apart from the heat of combustion, additional heat is produced by the breakdown of nitrous-oxide. All these factors combine to produce more power.

The amount of extra power produced also depends on the engine type and configuration. The data obtained for Figure 2-1 was developed from a low-compression engine operating at 3000rpm. In high-compression racing engines, where the flame front is already traveling fairly quickly, speeding up the flame front may have a significant, but different, effect. A high-compression, racing-type engine in a competition state of tune will already be operating very near the detonation threshold; and when flame speed is increased further through the addition of nitrous, severe detonation may result. To avoid this difficulty, it may be necessary to retard the ignition, add extra enrichment fuel, or take other measures (or combination of measures) that will eliminate the detonation difficulties.

When gaseous N_2O is inducted, most engines should fall between the theoretical and measured line on Figure 2-1. Under these conditions, the problems of fuel and N_2O distribution are minimized. If N_2O is introduced at some central point (where all cylinders have equal access to the nitrous), the N_2O distribution should be no better or no worse than the air distribution. For instance, a simple point of access is the plenum of a single-plane intake manifold. If nitrous-oxide gas is injected in the center of the plenum, it is likely to be distributed fairly evenly between cylinders.

The distribution of enrichment fuel is equally important. The simplest method is to deliver the fuel in a manner similar to the nitrous injection—with some sort of nozzle or spray bar positioned in the center of the plenum.

An additional factor that must be taken into account is the effect of fuel atomization at the point of injection. If the fuel droplets injected into the airstream are too large, they may not be evenly distributed to the cylinders. Although the overall nitrous-to-fuel ratio may be right, individual cylinders may run either rich or lean. To reduce these distribution problems, it is essential that adequate fuel atomization takes place, especially if a simple spray bar is used.

(A more satisfactory injection method is to meter a specific quantity of fuel directly into each port runner in the manifold. Modern direct-port fuel-injection systems use this method—along with sophisticated electronic monitoring and metering control—to produce accurate cylinder-to-cylinder fuel distribution, resulting in greater fuel economy and reduced emissions. However, this type of system is usually too complex and expensive for the average nitrous user.)

In addition, if the nitrous-oxide gas is not evenly distributed, there will still be an imbalance between the amount of nitrous and enrichment fuel delivered to each cylinder. One way of overcoming this is to attempt to mix the nitrous-oxide and fuel before they are delivered to the intake. This can be accomplished, in a limited way, by aiming a stream of nitrous-oxide gas directly toward the enrichment-fuel delivery nozzle. Some manufacturers, in fact, use this technique. However, at this point, another question arises: Would it not be better to inject *liquid* nitrous-oxide into the stream of fuel and thereby create a more homogeneous mixture and better distribution?

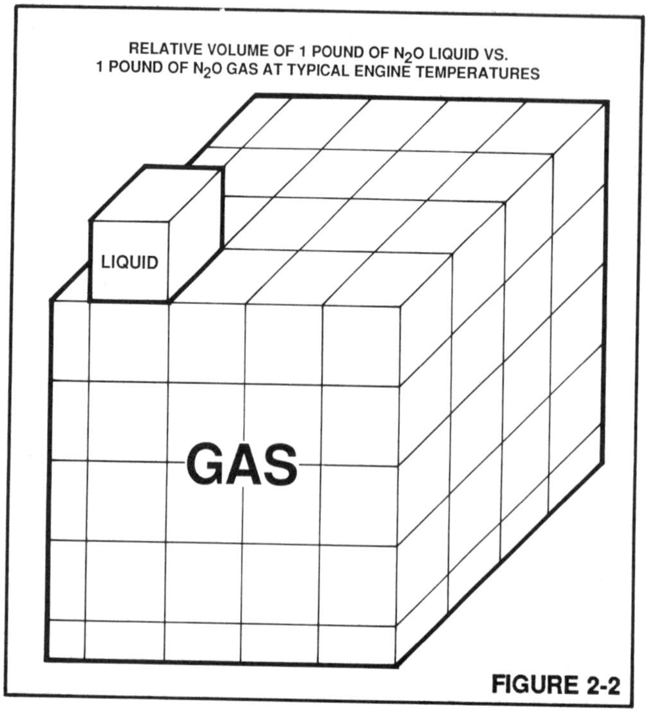

FIGURE 2-2

FIGURE 2-2: Liquid nitrous produces a greater "boost effect" than gaseous nitrous. If the nitrous is injected as a liquid, more oxygen and substantial cooling of the inducted charge (from nitrous evaporation) produce more power.

GAS VERSUS LIQUID

When a cubic foot of nitrous-oxide gas is induced into an engine, it does so at the expense of a cubic foot of atmospheric air. On the other hand, the same amount of N_2O, if retained in liquid form, occupies a far smaller volume, as shown in Figure 2-2. This shows that the displaced-charge factor is substantially reduced if we assume that the liquid nitrous-oxide remains liquid all the way into the cylinder. In actual practice, this won't be the case. Some of the N_2O will convert to a gas in the induction system; but in doing so, it will cause a substantial drop in the intake-charge temperature. This means that as some of the liquid nitrous expands and converts to a gaseous state, the inducted volume in the intake manifold *contracts* (compared to the volume during gaseous-only induction). The result is a denser, more highly oxygen-laden charge.

Tests indicate that on a typical engine the cooling of the intake charge can reduce the overall volume as much, and sometimes more, than the volume increase created as the nitrous converts and expands into a gas. Theoretically, this differential during typical operation—when power is boosted by about 25 to 30%—increases the volumetric efficiency of the engine by as much as 10%. In other words, the engine should be able to draw about 10% more air through the induction system. However, the key to obtaining this gain seems to lie in finding the optimum point of injection along the intake tract.

Under ideal circumstances, the amount of oxygen taken into the engine may increase, even though the mass flow of nitrous-oxide remains the same. Figure 2-3 shows the amount of oxygen inducted to the engine when a specific amount of nitrous-oxide is injected in either gaseous or liquid form. As can be seen, when the nitrous is delivered in liquid form, the engine inducts greater charge weights of oxygen. As expected, engine power should be affected by these conditions, and the comparable power plot in Figure 2-4 indicates this difference. Remember, in both instances, the same maximum amount of nitrous-oxide is being injected.

However, airflow measurements performed by myself during engine tests of currently available nitrous systems reveal that in many instances this extra airflow does not occur. A lot of time and effort has been expended to determine why this is so (details are included in a later chapter). Nonetheless, I feel that the displaced-charge effect for liquid nitrous-oxide injection is usually an uncertain factor.

LIMITATIONS

Since liquid nitrous-oxide can be injected into the engine at little or no expense to the air normally inducted, it would seem that there is almost no limit to the power boost available. If we consider the actual physical re-

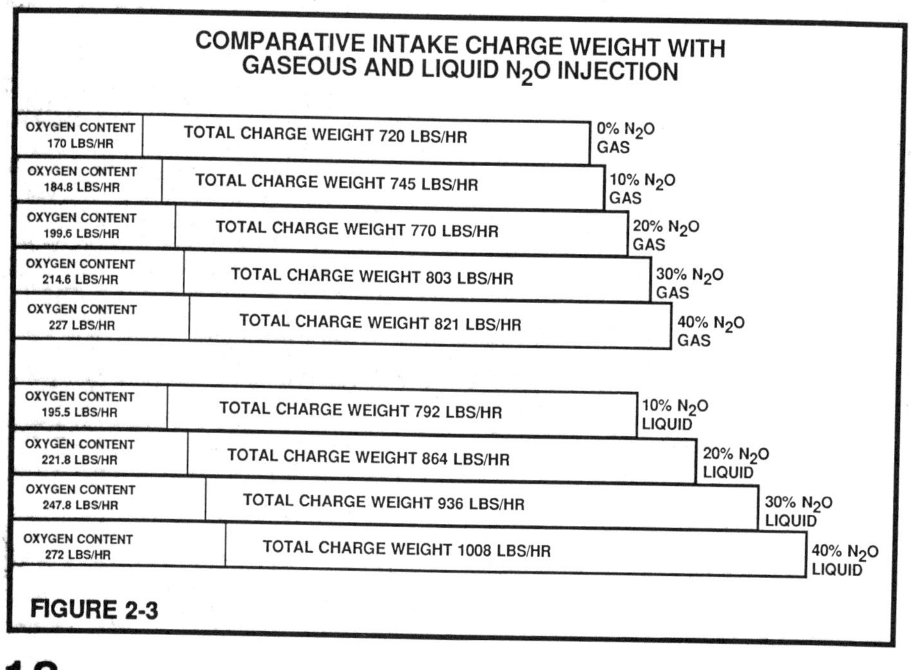

FIGURE 2-3

FIGURE 2-3: Shown here are the computed effects of various nitrous mixtures on the inducted charge weight. Without any nitrous injection, the 2-liter Pinto test engine inducted 720 pounds of air (per hour), with an oxygen content of 170 pounds. When some of the charge is replaced with nitrous, the total charge weight increases due to the relative density difference between nitrous and air. The comparison of oxygen content is interesting. Note that a 20% mix of liquid nitrous has almost the same oxygen content as a 40% gaseous mix. Injection of liquid nitrous will increase the total charge weight beyond the level shown here due to the cooling effect as the nitrous converts to a gaseous form.

quirements for injecting the nitrous-oxide, this appears to be the case. The parts and pieces required to deliver enough nitrous and enrichment fuel for a power increase of 1000 horsepower can be fabricated with little trouble. In actual fact, it is difficult to effectively convert this much nitrous-oxide into usable power.

The practical power limit of a nitrous-boosted engine is generally governed by two factors: the mechanical integrity of the engine and the detonation limit of the engine. These limitations must be considered before a nitrous system is installed and during any subsequent "tuning" efforts.

When nitrous is injected into the engine, it produces additional power by virtue of higher cylinder pressure—which results in extra torque. The higher the cylinder pressure, the nearer the engine is to the detonation threshold, regardless of the fuel used. Also, high pressures will impose greater mechanical loads on the pistons, rings, connecting rods, and crankshaft.

The forces acting on these mechanical components comprise two separate entities. The first is the load brought about by the reciprocating masses; the second is the load brought about by gas pressures generated during the combustion and expansion cycle. By far the most important to consider at the moment are the gas pressure forces.

With a conventional nitrous-oxide injection system, the mass flow of nitrous oxide is constant. In other words, a certain quantity of nitrous is injected into the engine in a given time, irrespective of engine speed (rpm). This has a distinct effect on the power curve of the engine; and, of course, the power curve is directly related to the gas pressures in the cylinders. With a constant rate of injection, the cylinder pressures *increase* as the engine speed is *reduced.* This results in increased torque output as the engine speed is reduced.

This occurs only because of a constant injection rate. At low engine speeds, each induction stroke receives a larger quantity of nitrous-oxide, comparatively, than it does at higher engine speeds. The result is that igniting this "heavier load" of nitrous causes greater pressure build-up in the cylinder, which directly translates to more torque. As engine speed is further reduced, the charge (mass) of nitrous passing into each cylinder may become too great. At this point, the cylinder will either detonate or a mechanical failure will occur.

In most cases, severe detonation will be the first indication that the quantity of nitrous per induction cycle is too high. For this reason kit manufacturers usually recommend that a nitrous system not be activated below a certain specified engine speed, typically about 2500 to 3000 rpm. (Sophisticated two-stage systems can overcome this limitation to some extent, but we will discuss this type of system in a later chapter).

The question is: How much is too much? Basically, it boils down to the specific engine design, gasket capability, the strength of the pistons and, to a lesser degree, the rods and crank. But with nitrous injection, as

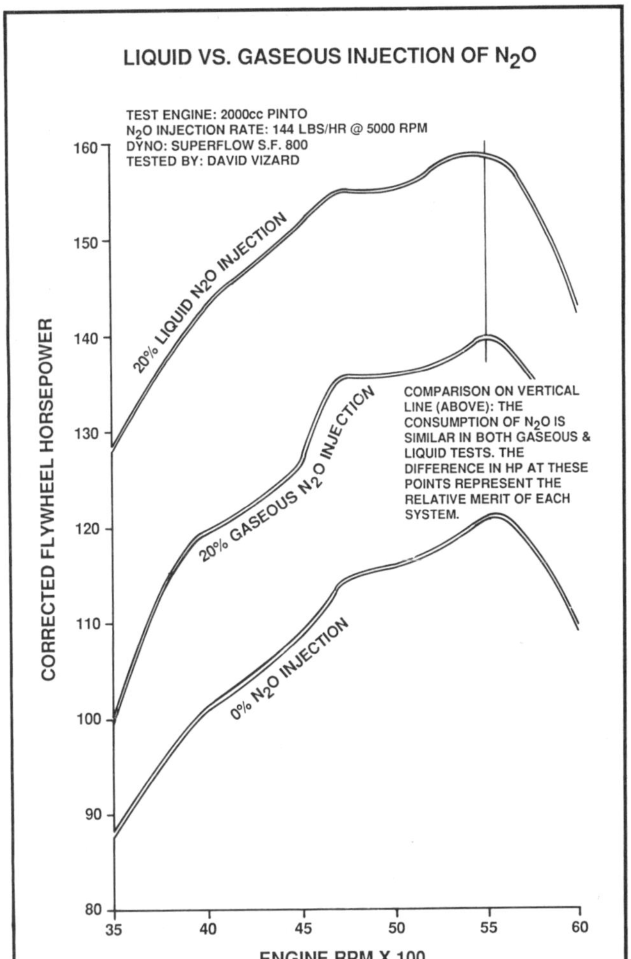

FIGURE 2-4

FIGURE 2-4: The theoretical advantage of liquid nitrous is demonstrated by the test results shown here. For the same rate of delivery (mass/minute), liquid nitrous produces considerably more horsepower than gaseous nitrous.

The results in Figure 2-4 were produced by injecting gaseous nitrous with a calibratable port-injection system. In order to minimize variations from intake charge cooling and to ensure that only gas (no liquid) nitrous was injected, the gas-injection temperature was raised to about 70 degrees by passing it through heated coils.

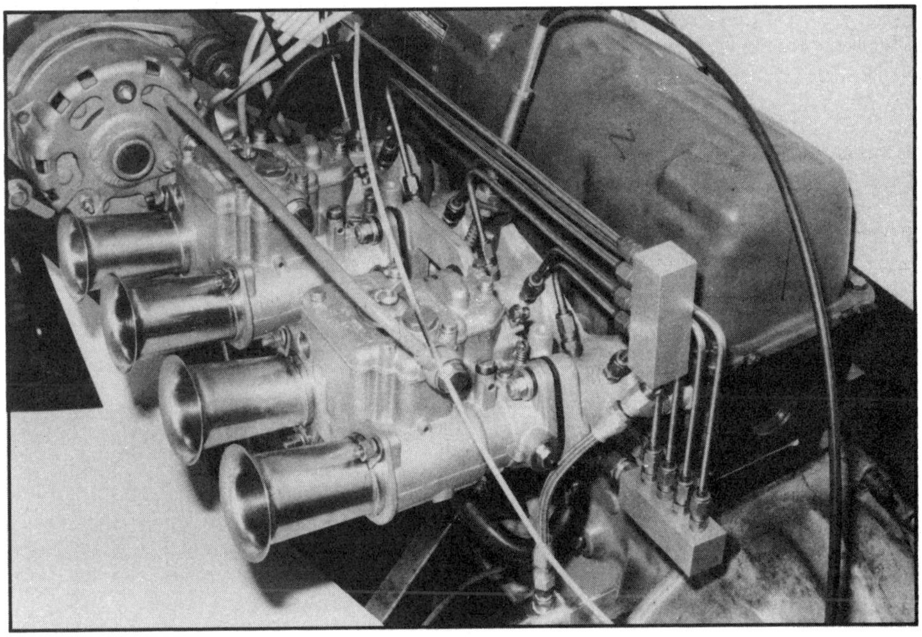

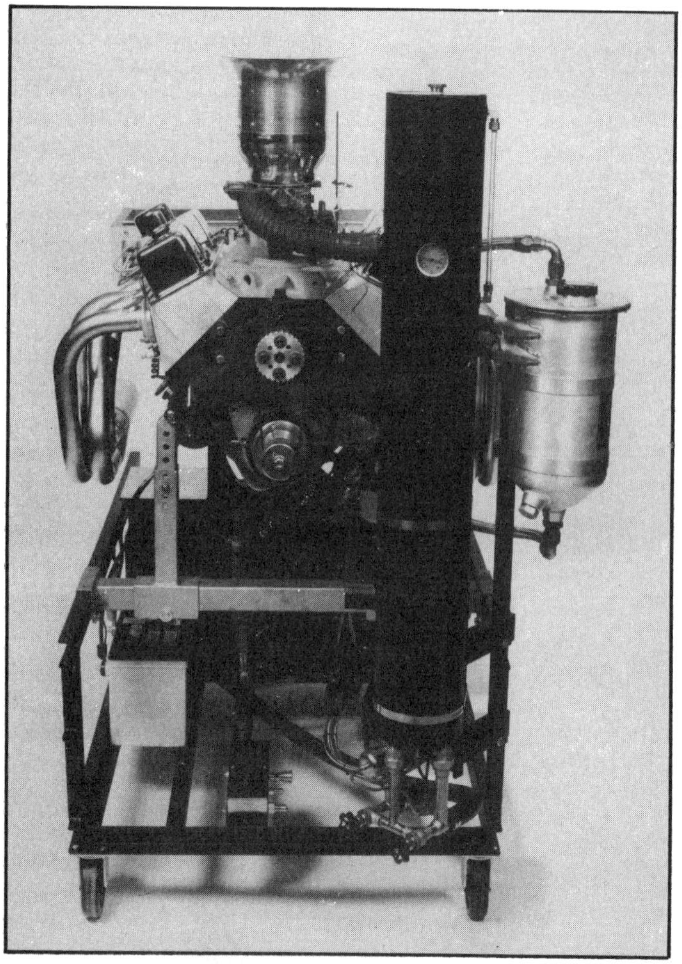

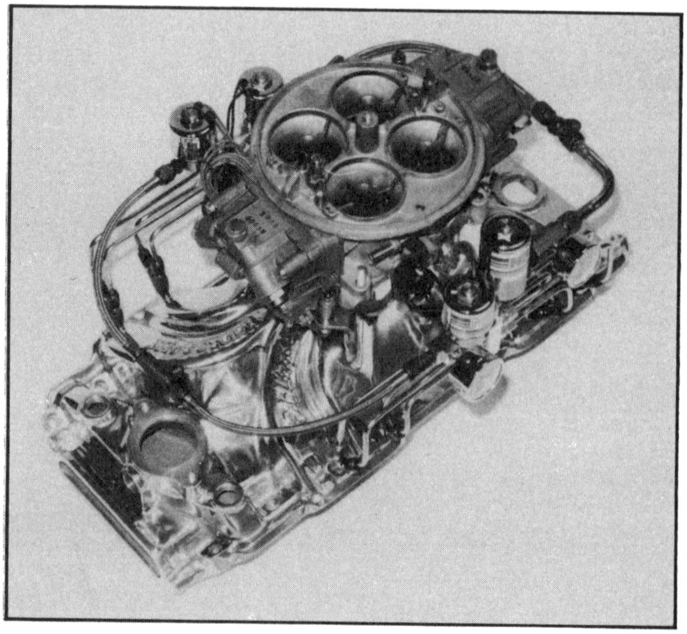

Nitrous produces an "instant" boost in low-speed torque. It is possible, therefore, to use a large carburetor and let the nitrous cover up a "hesitation" if the throttle is snapped open at low speed. A Holley Dominator is used on this small-block to enhance high-rpm breathing and power.

The research for this book required a lot of time and effort. Much of the information was gathered during test sessions on the author's dynamometer.

in all things, there will always be some notable exceptions to the accepted generalizations.

In engineering terms, brake-mean effective pressures (BMEP) within the cylinder of about 460 to 500psi are the practical limit for conventional automotive engines. If alternative fuels (such as alcohols) are used, under the right circumstances, this limit could be pushed to as high as 700psi—provided, of course, the engine could withstand this much internal pressure. Genuine racing engines with premium components will withstand this sort of pressure, but the fuel will reach the detonation limit before mean-effective pressures as high as this are achieved.

If the engine in question can withstand the mechanical stress and if detonation can be suppressed, power levels produced by nitrous-augmentation can be extremely high. On gasoline, 2.0 to 2.5 foot pounds of torque per cubic inch can be achieved; and with alcohol/gasoline-mix fuels, this number could go as high as 3.5 to 4.0 foot pounds per cubic inch. As far as power is concerned, 4.0 horsepower per cubic inch, with a suitable fuel, is a distinct possibility. But for normal street applications, these numbers are *meaningless*. They refer to pure-bred engines built for all-out racing, and this type of engine does not have a very long life expectancy.

The object of nitrous-oxide for street applications is to *produce a substantial power increase without incurring any reliability problems.* This inevitably means power has to be reduced to more temperate levels. For street use, a 30 to 50% increase in horsepower will produce an amazing difference in performance without necessarily incurring any gross reliability problems.

Most street nitrous kits are calibrated to give about this much power boost; and although it doesn't sound like much when compared with the power output of a racing engine, the power levels achieved with nitrous produce bigger gains in performance than the number suggests. The reason for this is the ability of nitrous augmentation to produce a massive and virtually instantaneous increase in *torque*, especially at the lower engine speeds where most street engines operate.

This factor is important, especially when the effect is compared to the results of conventional hot-rod modifications. Traditional "speed tuning" techniques—e.g., long-duration cams, multiple carburetors, etc.—inevitably produce increased power output within a narrow band at very high engine speeds. As a consequence, it is necessary to wind the motor higher to realize any real performance gains from these alterations. With nitrous injection, on the other hand, pushing the button instantly increases torque *no matter what the engine speed.* In real life this instant torque feels like a lot more "horsepower" than it actually is.

BOOST POTENTIAL

Performance enthusiasts sometimes make the mistake of comparing the power output of a nitrous-injected engine with that of a non-nitrous engine, and assume that engines producing equal peak power will perform similarly. Such comparisons are a lot less valid than they appear at face value. Testing has shown that an 800-horsepower engine deriving a substantial proportion of the power output from nitrous augmentation will outperform an 800-horsepower normally-aspirated engine by quite a healthy margin. This unusual situation boils down to what can best be described as the average power output.

When a normally-aspirated engine is modified in a conventional manner, the horsepower increase is concentrated in the higher speed (rpm) ranges. No matter what techniques are used, it is quite difficult to increase the torque output of a normally-aspirated engine past a certain level. In real life the output is always limited by the amount of oxygen the engine can induct during one intake stroke. This in turn is dictated by the pressure differential between atmospheric air pressure (14.7psi standard ambient) and the relatively lower pressure created inside the cylinder as the piston moves downward.

A nitrous-augmented engine, on the other hand, is supercharged by virtue of the additional oxygen and fuel contained in the nitrous and the enrichment fuel. To illustrate this point, imagine an engine equipped with a nitrous kit capable of delivering 200 additional horsepower. When the system is actuated, it produces 200 extra horsepower at whatever point in the speed range (rpm) the engine is operating when the nitrous is activated. At lower engine speeds, the nitrous will produce a greater *proportion* of power boost in relation to the non-boosted operation.

For example, consider a drag-race Chevy that may have a usable power band (typically) between 4500 and 7500rpm. The factor that will govern the rate at which the race car accelerates down the strip is the *average power* produced by the engine between 4500 and 7500rpm. Figure 2-5 shows a power curve for a smallblock Chevy V8. The comparison curve is a nitrous-augmented engine producing similar—but slightly lower—maximum output. In spite of the lower peak power, the average power of the nitrous engine—computed throughout the usable power band—is actually higher.

These are actual numbers taken from engines tested by the author. The nitrous-oxide, in actual practice, *produces a greater percentage increase in power in the lower rpm range than in the upper rpm range.* In other words, nitrous has turned the engine into a more effective torque generator; and as veteran racers know, it is torque output that determines how quickly a car accelerates.

This effect on the power output is so unusual that even professional engine builders, experienced at assessing vehicle performance as a product of peak engine power (measured on the dynamometer), can be easily fooled. Anyone who experiences a nitrous-augmented engine for the first time will readily believe that a typical 125-horsepower kit is producing 200 horsepower or more. The seat-of-the-pants impression is very convincing because the engine feels so much stronger as a result of the broad effect that nitrous has on the power output.

STREET POWER

At this point it seems simply a question of injecting the right amount of nitrous-oxide to produce the power desired; and that for a given flow of nitrous, all kits should produce the same power. This line of thought is very reasonable, but in actual testing, things do not work out this way. I tested a number of typical nitrous kits on my dynamometer and the results revealed quite a difference

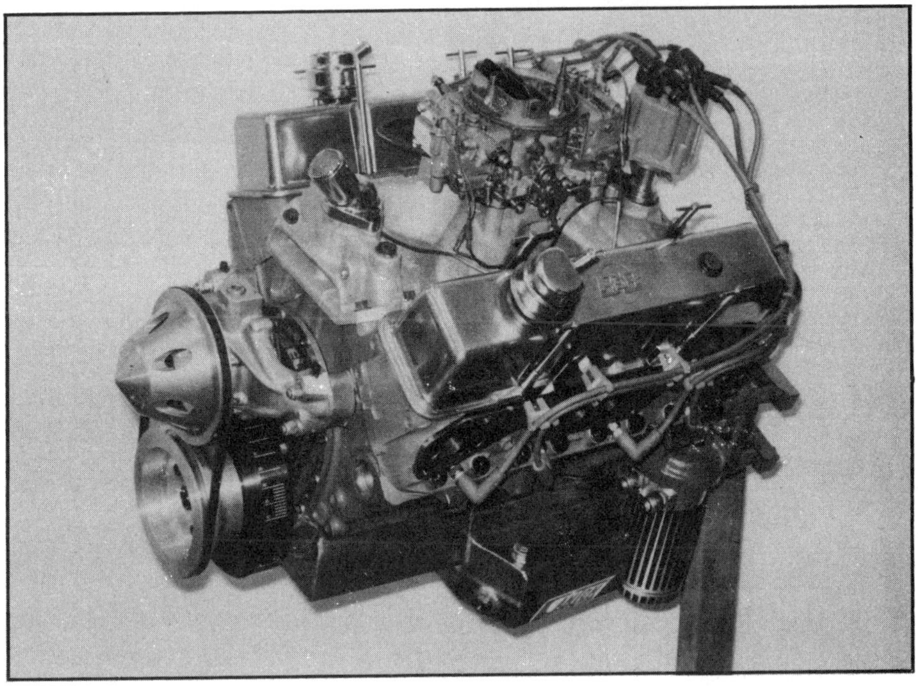

The results shown in Figure 2-5 were gathered with this Chevy dyno engine. It is equipped with a Competition Cams camshaft, steel connecting rods, Sealed Power pistons, and modified big-valve heads. During 12 months of nitrous testing, the only problem was bore wear; three cylinder blocks were used during the testing.

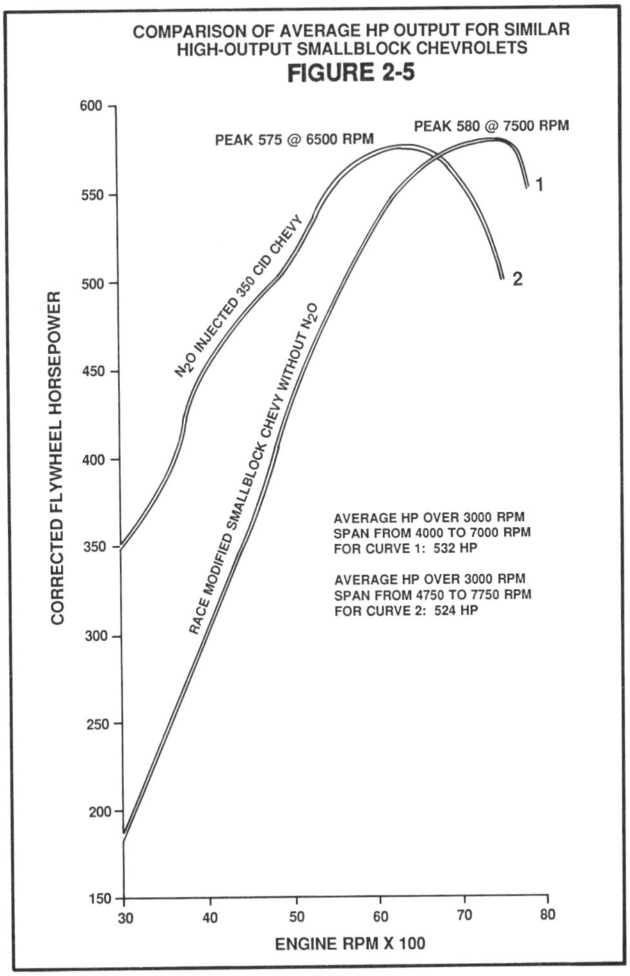

FIGURE 2-5: Peak horsepower is a misleading number. Acceleration depends on "average horsepower throughout the usable rpm range." Horsepower is a function of engine revolutions and torque, so torque becomes the predominant factor. Nitrous often produces torque that exceeds the capabilities of conventional supercharged engines.

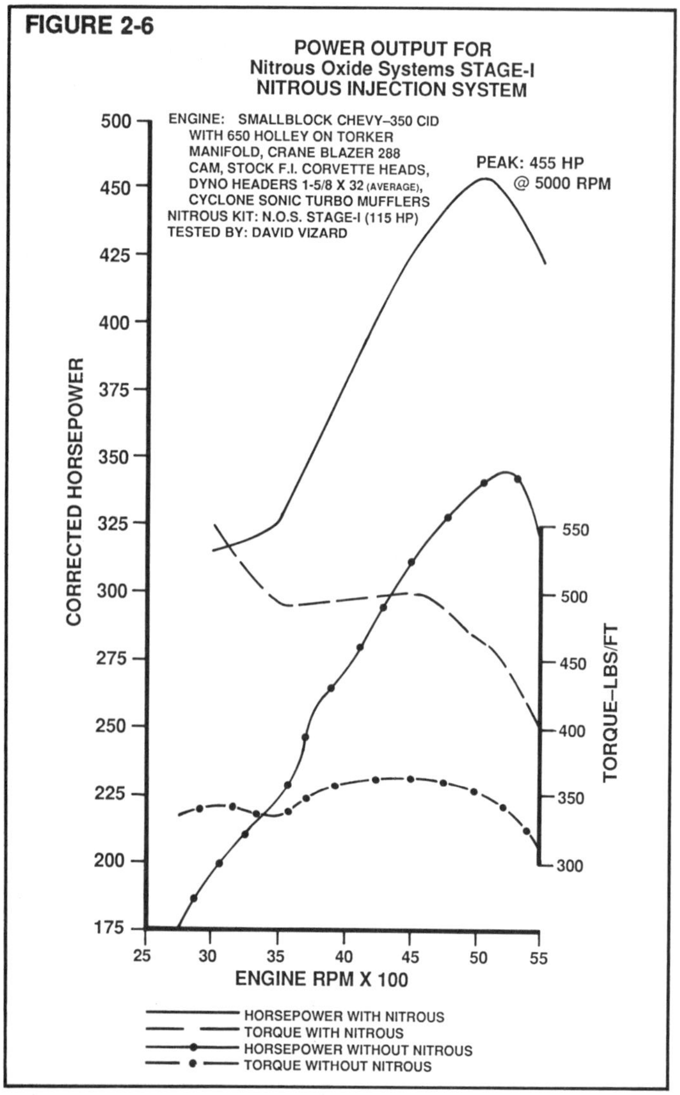

FIGURE 2-6: Power Produced by NOS Stage-I System

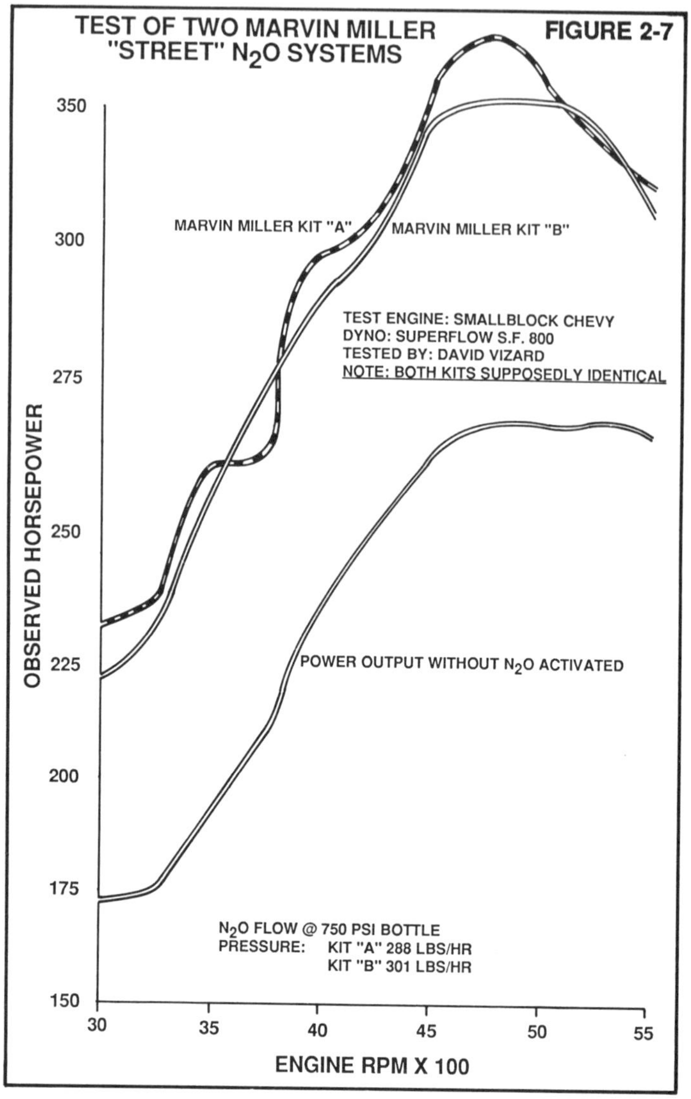

FIGURE 2-7: Power Produced by two Marvin Miller Systems

between kits that appeared to be very similar.

The emphasis was on typical street-type engines, not racing engines, and the kits tested were supposed to produce power increases of about 115 to 200 horsepower. Some produced the claimed increase in output; others did not.

Figure 2-6 and 2-7 graphically compare the power increases given by various examples of basic street-oriented nitrous kits. In one typical situation the horsepower output was increased by 115 and torque was increased by approximately 160 foot-pounds. Similar increases were given by two other kits. However, note that one kit produced 87 horsepower and another kit—supposedly identical—produced only 74 horsepower.

The amounts of nitrous-oxide being injected by these various kits were about the same. The surprising difference in power can be attributed to such things as the mixing of the nitrous with the enrichment fuel, nitrous-fuel distribution among the cylinders, unwanted heat input to the nitrous system, and other system variables. Dynamometer tests show that these variables can dramatically affect the amount of power delivered by a system.

The design of the system can also produce a fluctuating power output, as shown in Figure 2-8 When this occurs, engine output surges and the measured power may rise and fall by as much as 30 or 40 horsepower over a short time span—typically as short as 1.0 to 1.5 seconds. This phenomenon seems to be more prevalent with spraybar systems than with nozzle systems.

Most companies use a spraybar to deliver the nitrous and/or enrichment fuel in their street-oriented kits, especially if the kit is intended for V8 applications. However, at least one company uses a twin-nozzle setup for the nitrous fuel and a spraybar for the fuel delivery. The author's testing seemed to indicate that nozzle systems produce a more stable power output, in general, than spraybar systems. The nozzle-type systems also seemed to deliver a rapid power boost; they reached the intended power level quickly (usually within a few tenths of a second); and they held the max-power level fairly consistently. On the other hand, spraybar systems generally seemed to hit softer, sometimes with a delay of 0.5 to 0.75 seconds, and they often fluctuated at maximum power.

As a point of speculation, it is possible that power fluctuation of some spraybar systems may be caused by thermo-hydraulic resonance within the system. Whenever nitrous is trapped, or even partially trapped, within a heated pipe, the nitrous within that pipe—in this instance the spraybar—can turn to a gas; fill up the pipe or spraybar tube; and for a moment, inhibit the flow of liquid nitrous through the system. As soon as the gas is expended through the delivery orifices in the spraybar, the pipe will cool and the flow of liquid nitrous resumes.

If there is a cavity, or anything re-

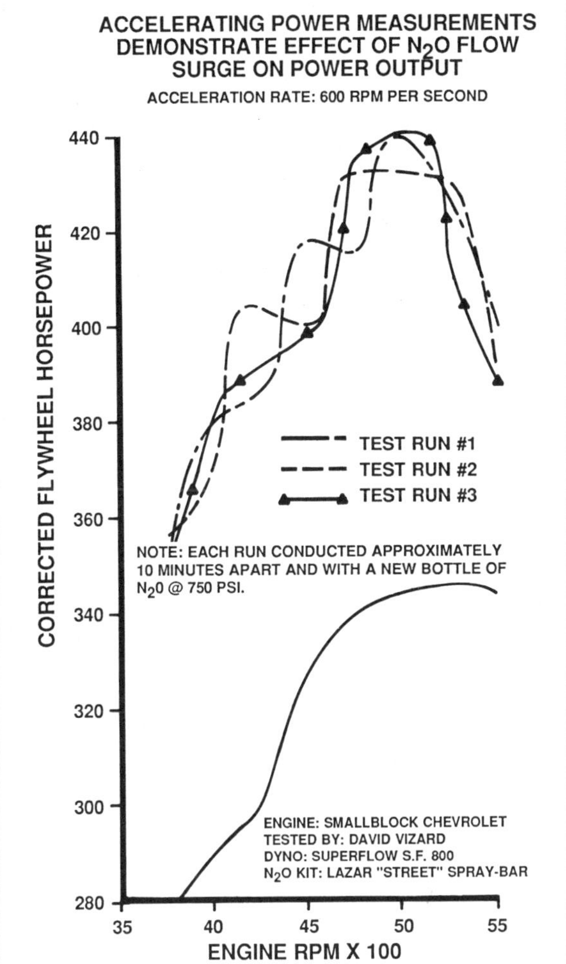

FIGURE 2-8

433 CID BIG-BLOCK CHEVROLET WITH N_2O

RPM	WITHOUT N_2O 32° IGN. ADV. TORQUE	WITHOUT N_2O 32° IGN. ADV. HP	WITHOUT N_2O 28° IGN. ADV. TORQUE	WITHOUT N_2O 28° IGN. ADV. HP	WITH N_2O 28° IGN. ADV. TORQUE	WITH N_2O 28° IGN. ADV. HP
5000	573	546	435	414	–	–
5250	570	570	452	452	–	–
5500	557	583	453	474	–	–
5750	559	512	464	508	–	–
6000	552	631	456	521	760	872
6250	541	644	433	515	717	853
6500	522	646	423	524	680	841
6750	498	640	–	–	661	850

ENGINE: BIG-BLOCK CHEVROLET–433 CID
BUILDER: SCOTT SCHAFIROFF
FUEL: C-12 RACING GASOLINE–5 TO 6 PSI
DYNO: SUPERFLOW S.F. 800
FACILITY: MC BETTS RACING, COPIAGUE, NY

N_2O BOTTLE PRESSURE: 800 PSI
N_2O JETS: 0.055 GASOLINE
0.042 N_2O

FIGURE 2-9

FIGURE 2-8: Power fluctuations are not uncommon in spacer-type systems. These are plots of three consecutive dyno runs using the same plate system. The shapes vary substantially, although the curves are considerably above the output of the stock engine (shown at the bottom).

FIGURE 2-9: Even though the first readings with nitrous were taken at 6000rpm, a reasonable estimate of the torque and horsepower at 5000rpm would be 820lb/ft and 780hp. Optimum total advance during nitrous injection proved to be 28 degrees, and 32 degrees was used when the nitrous was not activated.

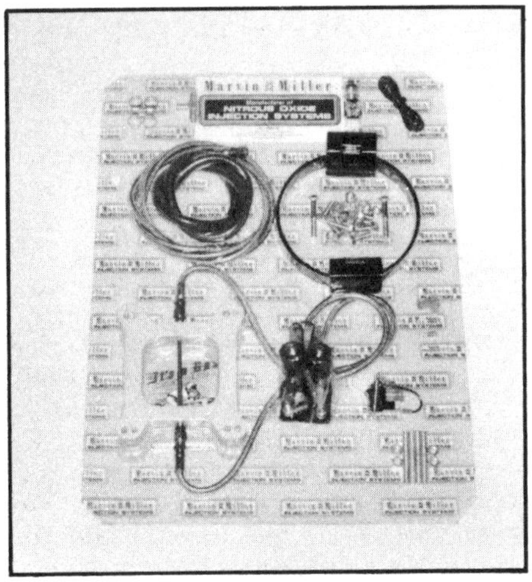

This is one of the nitrous kits that produced the results in Figure 2-7.

sembling a cavity, at the end of the nitrous supply line and a lot of heat is put into this cavity, it seems that the resonant effect will increase. Obviously, if this effect is increased past a certain level, the flow of nitrous can be greatly inhibited, whereas the flow of additional fuel will not. As a result, the nitrous-fuel ratio can change dramatically. In fact, the mixture can become so rich that the amount of horsepower developed is not only reduced because of the falloff in nitrous delivery but also because the oxygen-fuel ratio is now extremely rich in overall fuel content.

A major problem with a system that delivers nitrous from an injection nozzle is that the injection point may be some distance from the point where the enrichment fuel is added. This reduces the amount of mixing between the nitrous and the enrichment fuel. The results may be reduced power output and distribution problems. An imbalance in distribution may cause some cylinders to run lean, and the only way to prevent localized overheating problems is to increase the overall enrichment fuel delivery to compensate for the leanest-running cylinders. As a result, the amount of nitrous used for a given power output can, with such systems, often be greater than with spraybar systems.

Power increases produced by the kits tested here should be considered about the maximum for a typical V8 engine that is in near-stock condition. Most production engines employ cast pistons designed for quiet running and long life. They are not suited for very high cylinder pressures and temperatures. For this reason, nitrous systems for stock-type engines should be limited to a power increase of about 110 or 125 horsepower. If the desired power level is beyond this limit, it will almost certainly be necessary to use either a forged racing piston or a heavy-duty performance piston designed expressly for use with nitrous.

SUPER POWER

Street systems represent only one end of the spectrum. Most manufacturers also offer "high output" nitrous kits that deliver as much as 300 horsepower (claimed). These, for the most part, are very similar to the street kits, but they deliver greater quantities of nitrous and enrichment fuel. However, 300 horsepower is not necessarily the limit of what can be built. It is, nonetheless, considered the practical limit for most engines, unless they are specifically built for use with nitrous-oxide and outright power is more important than total reliability.

The results shown in Figure 2-9 are from an engine used by Scott Shafiroff. The engine was built to a relatively mild specification with off-the-shelf TRW parts and a race cam. The engine produced 646 horsepower when tuned (power timed) for use without nitrous and 550 horsepower when tuned for best results with a nitrous injection system. With the N_2O injection in operation the peak power jumped to 872 horsepower. This represents an increase of 226 horsepower.

If the desired power level is to be increased much above 850 to 875 horsepower—with this type of engine—it will be necessary to custom-build the motor expressly for nitrous. For instance, if the power increase from the nitrous will exceed 400 horses, it may be necessary to have specially-made pistons with the rings—the top rings in particular—further down from the piston deck and a lower compression ratio.

From experience, I feel that it is probably best to consider nitrous-oxide kits that boost output by 300 to 350 horsepower to be more practical for large-displacement, big-block motors, rather than smallblocks. This is not to say that some smallblock engines won't take it; some can (see Figure 2-10). With a heavy-duty block, a specially designed bottom-end and proper assembly techniques, some smallblocks can withstand this much power boost. However, some small engines simply cannot comfortably cope with boost figures approaching 300 horses. For this reason, as a general rule, it is wise to consider the practical power boost for conventional smallblocks to be about 200 to 250 horsepower—where long-term reliability is still an important consideration.

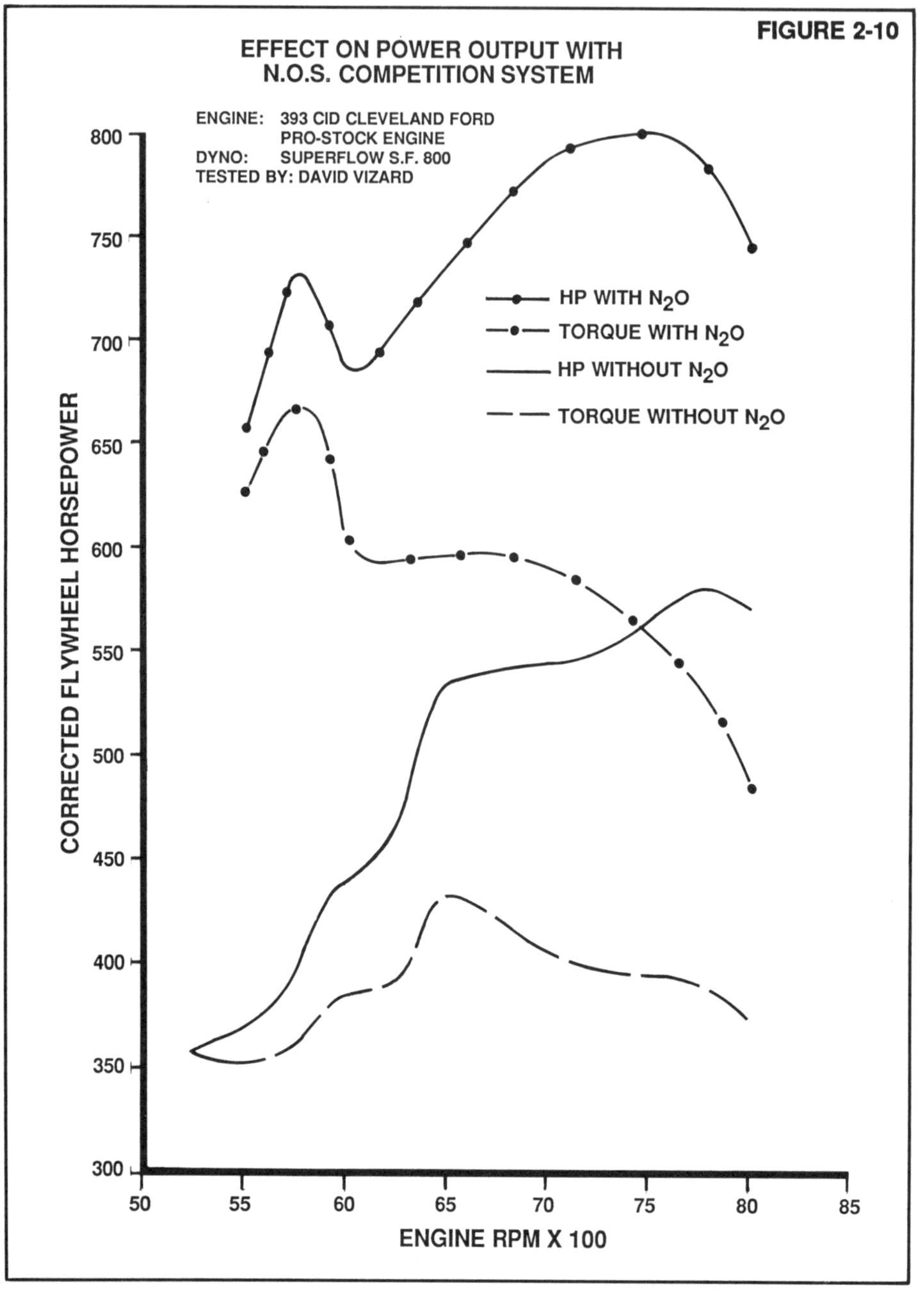

FIGURE 2-10: Comparing the torque curves shows how much the torque has increased in the lower rpm range. To a great extent, it is torque that accelerates a vehicle, and short shifting keeps a nitrous engine within the most favorable part of the torque curve.

When selecting a system, the best advice that I can give for young enthusiasts is to be conservative. To get impressive results, it's just not necessary to risk overkill. *A little nitrous goes a long way, especially in a street engine.*

And this leads to the subject of nitrous consumption. If the system is used on the street, it is necessary to consider how often you have to refill the bottle and whether all the "extra power" will, in fact, be practical in a vehicle that generally has a weak suspension system and relatively narrow tires. A basic rule of thumb is that 1.0 pound of nitrous sent through the engine in 10 seconds will produce a 100hp increase. This means that the typical 120-horsepower kit will operate for about two minutes on a 15-pound bottle.

While on the subject of nitrous consumption, it might be wise to mention fuel economy. Even though performance is the prime goal, most street enthusiasts must be concerned about fuel economy. One of the real beauties of nitrous-oxide injection is that while the system is not in operation, it does not affect the basic economy of the vehicle. When the nitrous system is in operation, of course, the fuel consumption increases dramatically. However, the overall fuel consumption in relation to the maximum horsepower potential is very good with nitrous engines.

Assuming the system is well tuned (properly balanced nitrous-and-fuel delivery rates), the specific consumption figures (i.e., fuel consumed, per horsepower, per hour) can be very good. In fact, the fuel consumption of the vehicle—under full-throttle conditions—is not likely to be any worse than that produced by any other form of modification that would increase engine output by a similar amount.

MAX POWER LEVELS

At this point, let us assume that the engine is designed for absolute maximum horsepower. Under these circumstances, as explained earlier, either the strength of the engine or detonation will ultimately limit the amount of power that can be developed.

Assuming that it has sufficient strength, a conventional race engine, in normally-aspirated form, can usually cope with a power increase between 0.50 and 0.75 horsepower-per-cubic-inch from nitrous-oxide injection. In round terms, you can consider that this power increase will amount to about 200 horsepower for a typical smallblock and 300 horsepower for a big-block.

However, there are some exceptions to this. Some big-block engines such as the 429 and 460 Ford engines may not have sufficient strength in the bottom end to withstand heavy nitrous loads. Of course, here I assume that these big engines have already been modified to develop substantial power outputs with conventional racing modifications. On the other hand, the big-block Chevy, especially with the heavy-duty, 4-bolt main block, can withstand a lot of increased power.

Sometimes the consequences of ignoring the basic strengths, weaknesses and performance capabilities of an engine can be dire. For instance, a friend of mine was determined to run his 460cid Ford jet boat as fast as possible and ordered a 300-horsepower racing nitrous system. After installation, he made a few impressive high-speed passes across the lake. But before the end of the second nitrous bottle, the exceptional stress took its toll on the bottom end: a rod came through the pan and exited through the bottom of the boat. This left the hull less than watertight and resulted in the loss of both engine and the boat in 150 feet of water.

The lesson here is pretty clear. If you intend to build an engine that will produce a lot of horsepower, then it is necessary to utilize heavy-duty components that will withstand the exceptionally high internal pressures and heat. We will discuss the details of engine building for nitrous in other chapters; but for now, let's look at the other major limitation—compression.

When the desired power output is very high, it is generally necessary to reduce the compression ratio in an effort to move the detonation threshold higher in relation to engine output. If 50% of the power output is derived from nitrous/fuel augmentation, the highest practical compression ratio will be around 8.0 to 9.0:1, rather than the 12.5:1 ratio found in most conventional naturally-aspirated racing engines. Unless you are quite certain of the engine combination and application, it is always wiser to select a conservative compression ratio. If you are a little on the low side, it is relatively easy to compensate by increasing the nitrous/fuel concentration. On the other hand, if you select a compression ratio that is too high, you will inevitably spend time searching for the parts that exit through the bottom of the pan.

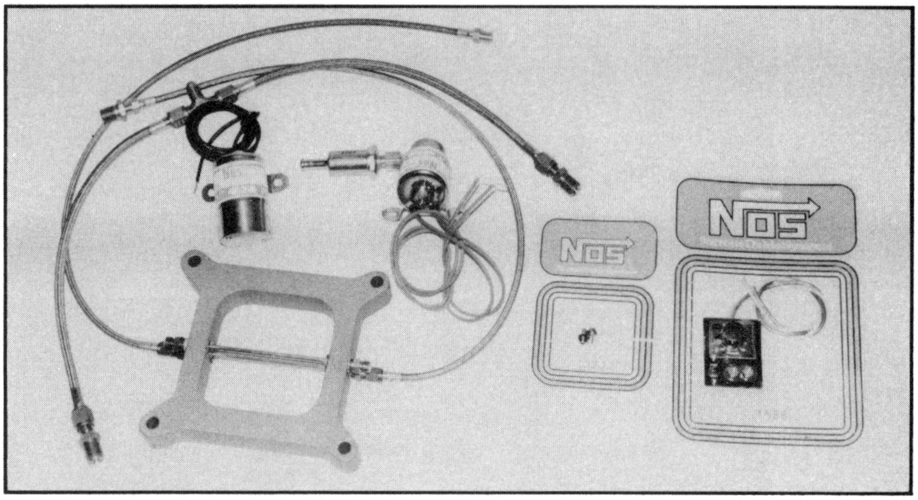

There is more to this nitrous system than meets the eye. It will significantly boost the brake mean-effective pressure (BMEP) throughout the usable engine speed range and, thereby, increase the torque output. A close look at the plate reveals...

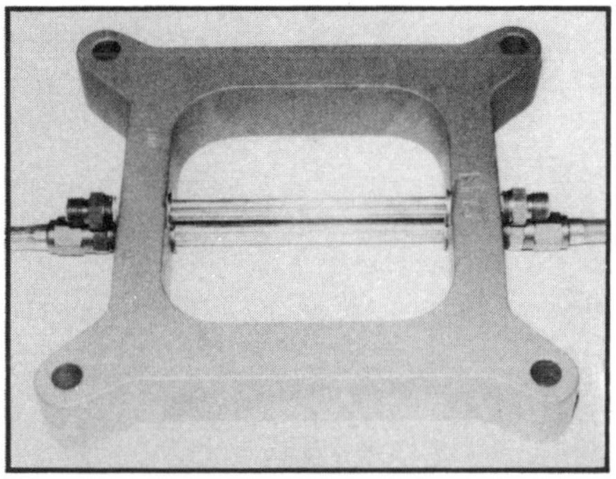

...this is a double-spraybar system that has been set up for three-stage operation. One spraybar is calibrated to deliver a 50hp boost and the other is calibrated for 100hp. Initially, only the 50hp spraybar is activated; at a preset engine speed (rpm) the 50hp spraybar is shut down and the 100hp system is activated; then at a higher speed, the 50hp spraybar is reactivated, providing a total boost of 150 horsepower.

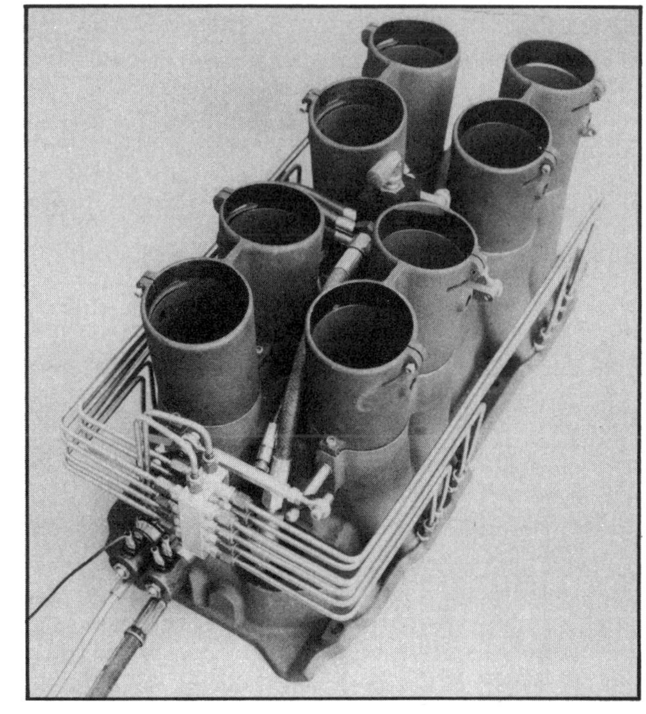

The system on this big block Chevrolet fuel-injection manifold is for all-out racing. The big Chevy cylinder block is extremely strong and rigid. It will endure nitrous boost levels up to 350 horsepower and produce peak power as high as 1000 horsepower.

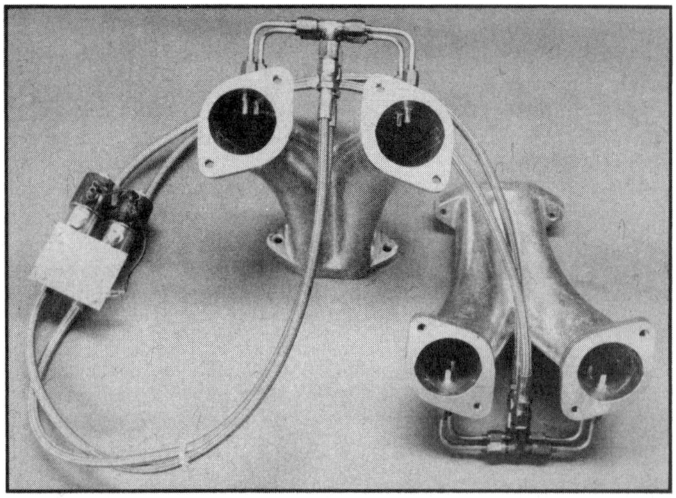

An inspection of these Volkswagen manifolds clearly shows that the nozzles are positioned so injected nitrous "impinges" on the fuel stream.

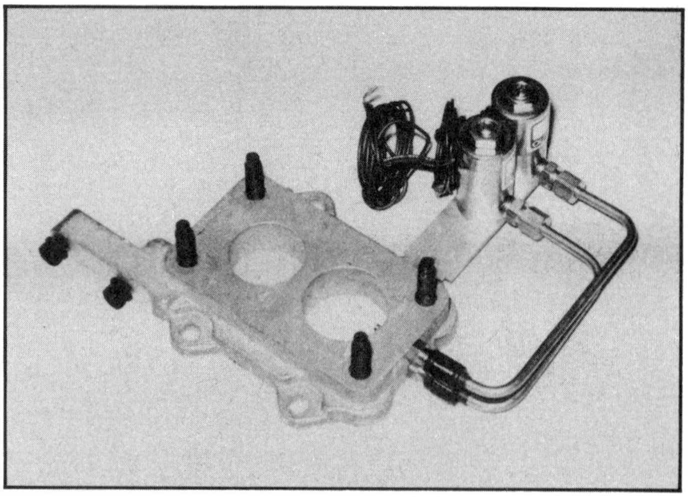

When a manifold with a relatively large plenum is used with a two-barrel carburetor or injection system it is possible to inject both nitrous and fuel at approximately the same point.

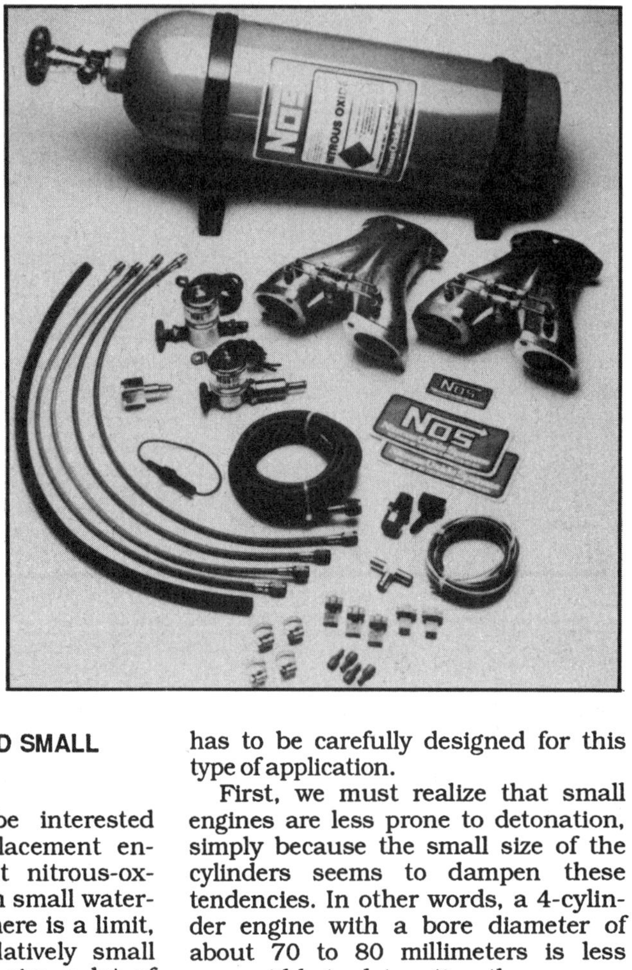

This is a nitrous kit for the Volkswagen air-cooled four-cylinder engine. Most of the nitrous technology discussed so far also applies to air-cooled engines, however the fuel calibration must be relatively rich to ensure reduction of cylinder head and sleeve temperatures.

NITROUS-OXIDE AND SMALL ENGINES

Most readers will be interested primarily in large displacement engines—V6s or V8s—but nitrous-oxide can also be used with small water- or air-cooled engines. There is a limit, however, because a relatively small amount of nitrous will give a lot of boost to a small engine, and it is difficult to successfully meter nitrous through the tiny orifices required for a reasonable amount of boost.

In general, it is not practical to build a nitrous system that will reliably deliver less than 5 horsepower of boost. This doesn't sound like much power, but in a small motorcycle, ATC, ski-jet or similar air-cooled engine, five horsepower could represent a 100% increase in output. Nitrous injection can and has been successfully used in engines displacing as little as 90-100cc, however, the system has to be carefully designed for this type of application.

First, we must realize that small engines are less prone to detonation, simply because the small size of the cylinders seems to dampen these tendencies. In other words, a 4-cylinder engine with a bore diameter of about 70 to 80 millimeters is less susceptible to detonation than an engine with 100-millimeter bores. However, before we go further, we must make a clear distinction between "small" and "large" engines. A 4-cylinder Volkswagen engine can displace 2.8 liters with a bore size around 100 millimeters. However, the venerable smallblock Chevy 4-inch bore also equals approximately 100mm (101.6 mm, actual). Even though the VW engine would seem "small" by comparison to the Chevy, the bore sizes are approximately equal, therefore the VW will react to nitrous (and detonation limitations) much as would the Chevy.

It is also important to realize that air-cooled engines, regardless of displacement, have very little "thermal reserve." In other words, if the combustion temperature increases, the temperature of the heads and barrels will also increase *very* quickly. In the first place, air-cooled engines tend to run hotter than water-cooled engines, and since there is not a large mass of liquid coolant to carry away excess heat, there is far less margin for temperature increase. In practical terms, this means that *even a small imbalance in the nitrous-to-fuel ratio can cause a lot of trouble.* As a result of this idiosyncrasy, the "correct" ratio for an air-cooled engine should be much richer (with fuel) than that normally used for water-cooled engines.

Special care must also be taken with 2-stroke engines. All 2-cycle engines are seemingly prone to piston seizure, and the addition of a lean nitrous mixture will hang a piston in plenty short order (as little as two or three seconds after system activation).

FUEL SUPPLY

As with any nitrous system, the supply of enrichment fuel—both pressure and volume—will be crucial. However, if you are working with small 4- or 6-cylinder engines of European origin, remember that most of these vehicles have fuel pumps that deliver far lower pressure than the typical Detroit product. The normal fuel pressure for a European vehicle is about 3 to 4psi. This is below the level required by most nitrous kits. As a consequence, the nitrous fuel delivery must be recalibrated for the reduced pressure or an auxiliary pump

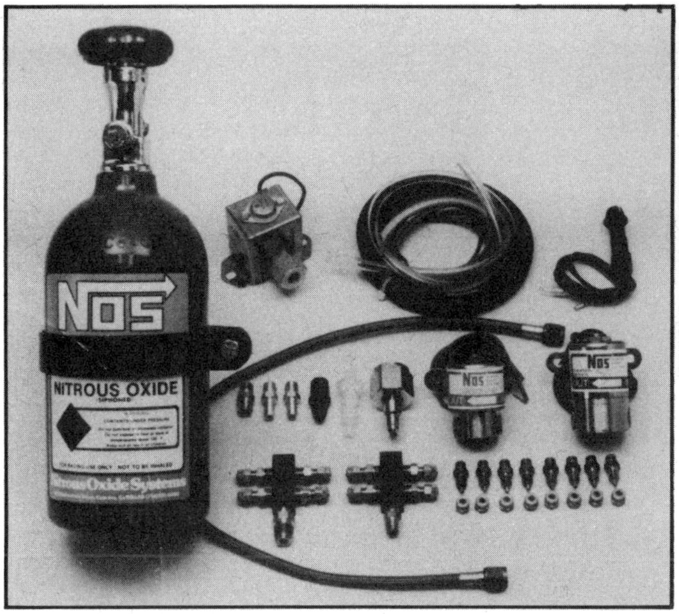

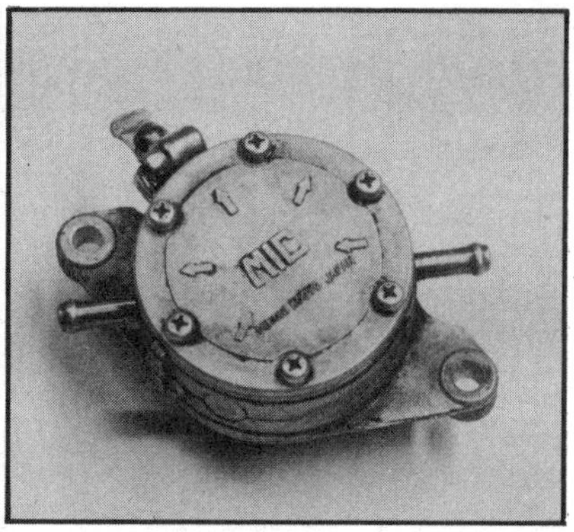

Provisions must be made to ensure adequate fuel flow when nitrous is added to a small engine. The NOS kit (left) utilizes an auxiliary electric pump to deliver enrichment fuel. The crank-mounted Mikuni snowmobile fuel pump (right) can be used on two-stroke engines.

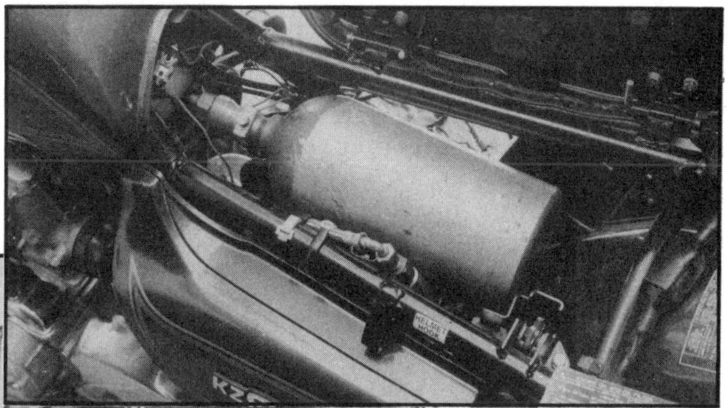

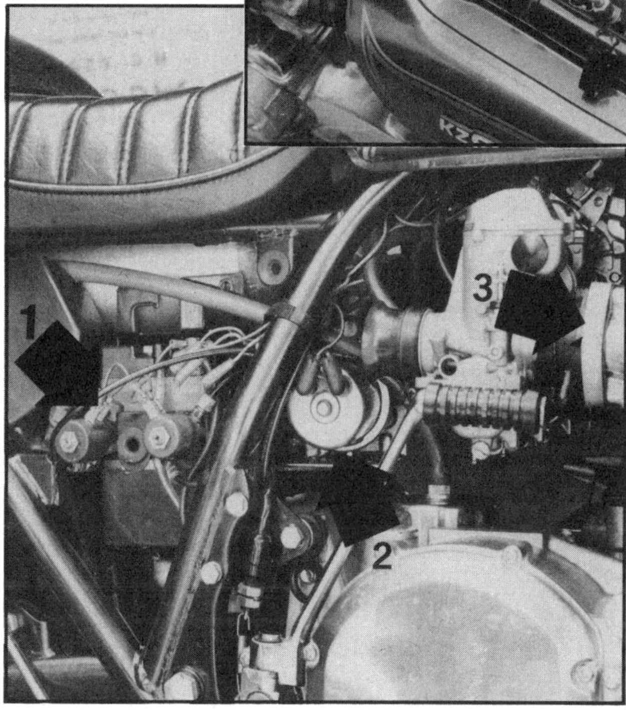

A hidden nitrous system boosts this stock-looking Kawasaki to 11.33/ 121.43 quarters. Most of the system is concealed under the side panels. The nitrous bottle is mounted under the seat. The arrows indicate: 1) solenoids; 2) electric fuel pump (Carter); 3) injector plate.

must be used. If the engine is 2-cycle, an auxiliary fuel pump will be mandatory.

Fuel-injection is very popular on late-model engines, and this will present a unique situation for the nitrous system designer. Usually, fuel-injection systems operate with a lot of fuel pressure, and this pressure is modulated by some form of distribution and/or metering device or by a sequentially "timed" injection directly to the ports. Whichever the case may be, there is usually a fuel line that recirculates excess fuel (the fuel pump always delivers more fuel volume than is required for engine functioning) through the system. It is unwise to utilize this return line as a source of enrichment fuel, because it may alter the calibration of the fuel-injection. However, it is usually possible to tap into the fuel line somewhere on the pressure side, prior to the fuel distribution/metering unit. This fuel can then be routed—through a suitable pressure regulator—to the enrichment side of the nitrous system.

Some fuel-injection systems—especially those models that have been adapted to a wide variety of engines—may *not* have enough capacity to successfully supply the injection system *and* the nitrous enrichment system. In this case, a separate fuel system with a suitable auxiliary pump must be installed.

The point of injection is also important. With many fuel-injection systems, inducted air passes through an airflow-mass sensor before it reaches a throttling air valve. After the flow passes the throttling point, it moves into a plenum, and subsequently, into individual port runners. With this type of fuel-injection, the nitrous must be introduced downstream of the airflow sensor. The best alternatives are to either install a "pseudo-plate" (containing fuel and nitrous injection orifices) between the air valve and the plenum or to use a port-injection system.

Of the two possibilities, the port-injection system generally produces better results because it ensures uniform nitrous/enrichment-fuel distribution among the cylinders. A pseudo-plate system is simpler and will work fine *if the nitrous and fuel are mixed properly*. I use the term "pseudo-plate" because it is often possible to use one large nitrous orifice in this plate. Since all of the cylinders are fed by the air passing through the plenum entrance—and consequently, through the pseudo-plate—one nitrous orifice and one enrichment-fuel orifice will do the job. However, this simple setup will also encourage distribution problems. It is difficult to predict the results, but since the nitrous issues from the orifice at a relatively high speed, there may be sufficient momentum to carry most of the nitrous-fuel mix past the front-most port entrance. This could, as a result, overload the ports (and cylinders) fed from the rear of the plenum. It's essential, therefore, to *check the plugs carefully for indications of uneven heating*. If there are signs of overheating on just one or two plugs, there are distribution difficulties. This can be corrected only by careful experimenting with the design of the injection nozzle or jet and the location or number of injection points.

CHAPTER 3

NITROUS SYSTEM BASICS

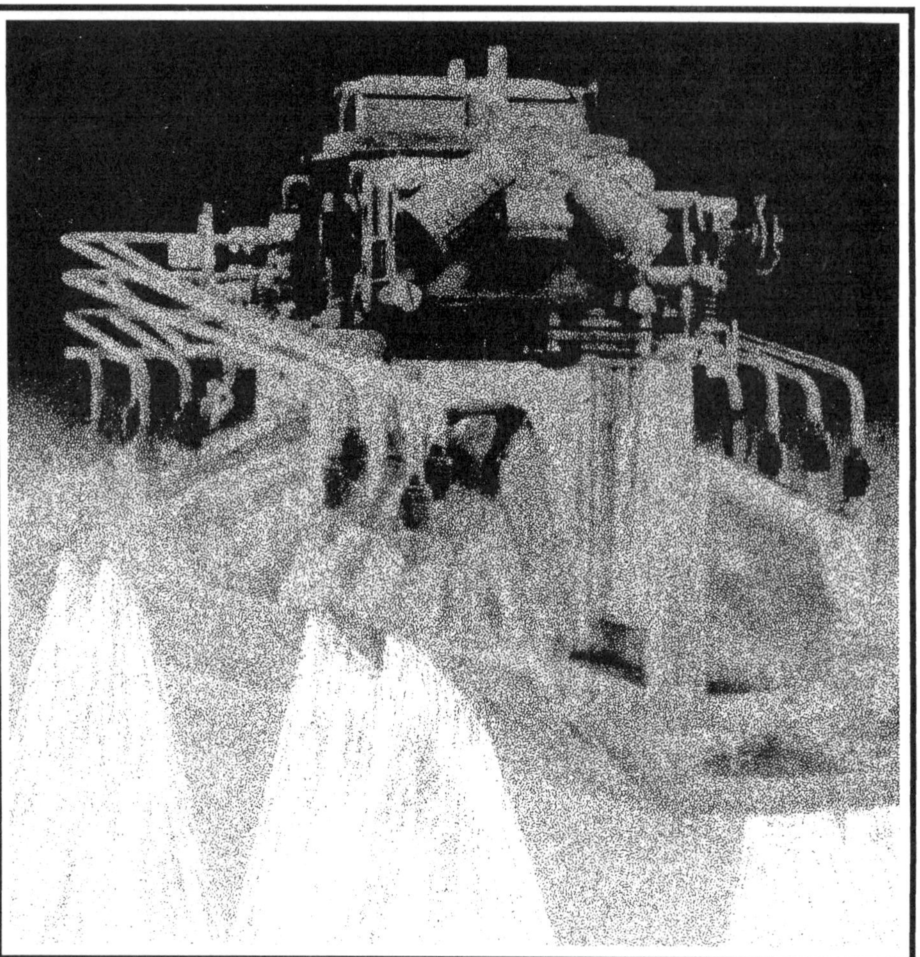

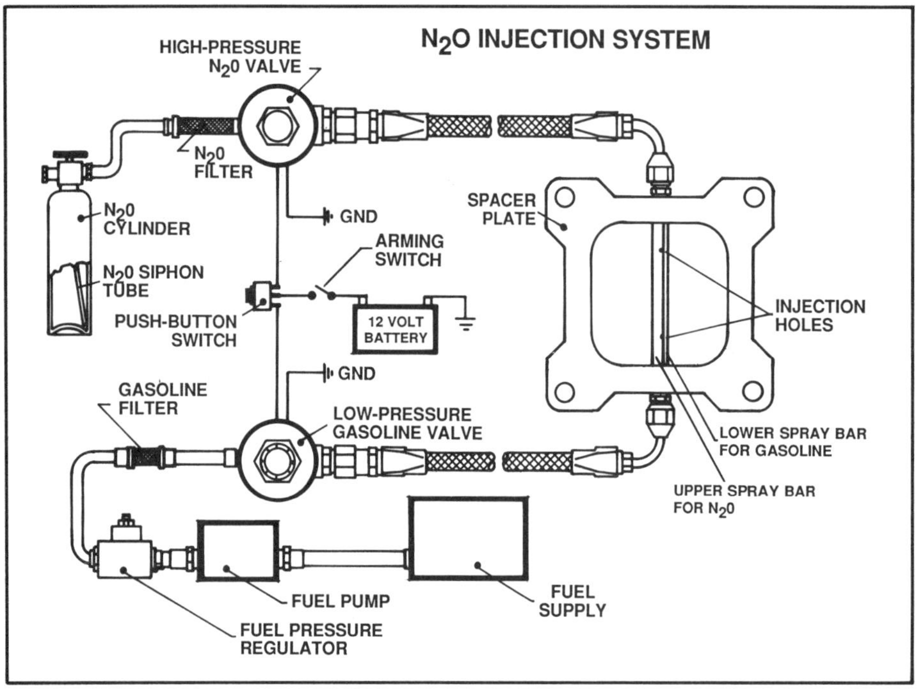

FIGURE 3-1: This is the typical layout of the most popular type of nitrous kit: a plate-mounted spraybar system.

SYSTEM ENGINEERING BASICS

By now most readers will have a basic understanding of the theoretical aspects of nitrous-oxide injection. So at this point it is time to put theory into practice. This chapter examines the practical aspects of nitrous-oxide and fuel-enrichment systems.

Figure 3-1 is a generalized schematic of the most basic and most popular type of system available for a typical V8 engine. Most street-oriented kits are based on this type of system, which utilizes a spacer plate—installed between the carburetor and manifold—to provide a mount for the nitrous and fuel delivery nozzles. It is a simple and reliable system and relatively easy to install in nearly any type of vehicle.

As can be seen in the drawing, the spraybars are situated one above the other in the spacer plate. The nitrous spraybar should always be positioned *above* the fuel spraybar. It is also desirable to have the spray of nitrous impinging upon the spray of fuel so that the *nitrous and fuel mix.*

Apart from the basic necessity of correctly calibrating the delivery volume of both spraybars—an important aspect of any nitrous system—the biggest drawback with this system is distribution eccentricities. Due to the central delivery point for the nitrous and fuel, there will inevitably be some distribution problems, and some cylinders will receive slightly richer or leaner nitrous-fuel mixes. This is a byproduct of the asymmetric flow characteristics within most intake manifolds. However, mixing the nitrous and fuel at the point of delivery will somewhat lessen these difficulties.

If the fuel and nitrous distribution is not fairly consistent, *it will be necessary to deliver extra fuel to counteract the potentially hazardous lean effects that may occur in one or more cylinders.* Though the spraybar system is simple, note that the positioning of the delivery orifices for both the fuel and nitrous will significantly affect engine power and reliability.

SYSTEM OPERATION

The key to the successful operation of the system is, of course, largely dependent upon finding an easy way to turn the flow of nitrous and enrichment fuel on and off. This requires a valve; and in most nitrous systems an electrically actuated, high-pressure valve is generally used. This type of device is commonly called a *solenoid valve.*

In the normal condition—with no electrical potential supplied to it—this solenoid valve is in the "Off" position. This totally blocks flow through the valve. When an electrical potential is applied to the coil in the solenoid, the valve opens, allowing flow. In this "On" position nitrous or fuel, as the case may be, flows through the system and is emitted from the delivery orifice in the spraybar or nozzle.

Since it is electrically activated, this type of valve is readily actuated by a conventional switch. The switch can be either a simple push-button switch, located somewhere handy for the driver to operate, or it can be something a little more sophisticated. In some cases a microswitch is mounted on the throttle linkage of the carburetor. When the throttle reaches wide open (or some preset condition), the microswitch closes, electrical potential is supplied to the solenoid valve, and the valve opens. However, since microswitches can handle only a small amount of current—in most cases too little to successfully activate the solenoid—a relay is also required. Essentially, the microswitch "switches" the relay, which in turn actuates the solenoid valve.

Another method is to place a vacuum switch in the intake manifold. When the throttle opens, the pressure in the intake manifold will rise (vacuum decreases). This will cause the vacuum switch to "close" and turn on the nitrous system. Such a system, though, must be buffered with several safeguards; otherwise, the vacuum system can become unpredictable. For instance, if the engine stalls, the pressure in the intake manifold would rise to atmospheric (zero gauge vacuum). The vacuum switch would mistake this for a full-throttle condition and allow nitrous and fuel to be injected into the stalled engine. This would be very hazardous when the engine was restarted. To prevent this problem, a vacuum-operated system must be overridden by an engine oil-pressure-activated disarming switch connected in series with the vacuum switch. With this setup, as soon as engine oil pressure vanishes, the oil-pressure switch opens the solenoid circuit. This keeps the valves closed, preventing any flow of nitrous or fuel whenever the engine is not operating.

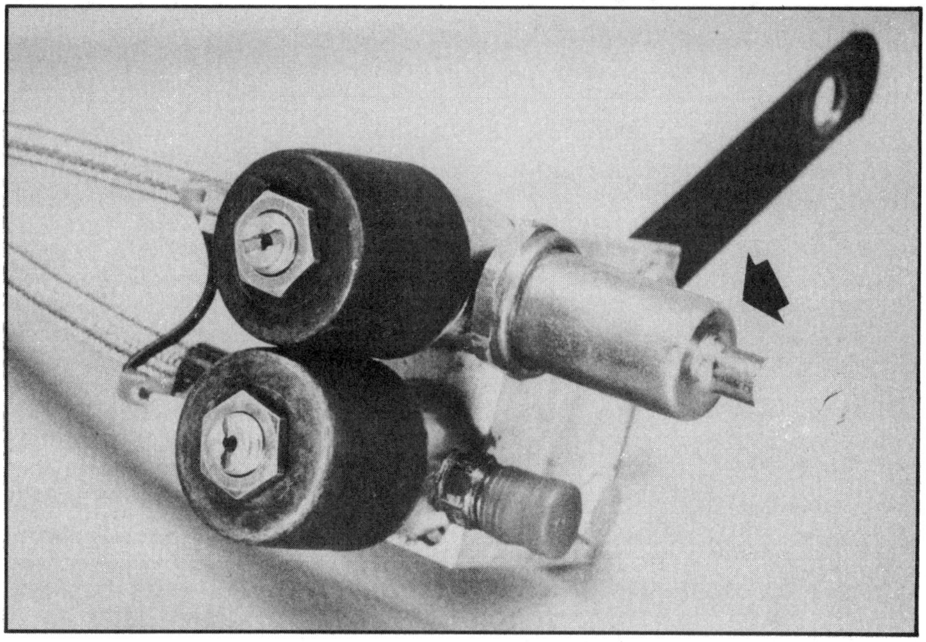

Most street kits are equipped with compact solenoid valves. The solenoid on the left activates the nitrous supply and the solenoid on the right, with an attached fuel filter, activates enrichment fuel delivery.

Solenoid-operated systems are simple in theory but they must incorporate adequate safeguards to prevent inadvertent nitrous delivery. Most systems also utilize a general "arming switch." With the arming switch off, the nitrous system cannot be operated. Turning on the switch on "arms" the system. And for safety's sake, it is important to connect an indicator light to the arming switch (that illuminates when the switch is on) so the driver knows when the system is ready for operation.

The solenoid valves used with nitrous systems must be of a type that can withstand high pressures. They must have a working pressure of at least 1000psi—some systems have a maximum working pressure as high as 1400psi—and to allow for overload circumstances, they must be able to withstand peak pressures as high as 2000psi.

The material from which the valve seat is made must be able to withstand extremes of temperature as well as pressure. The material must be suitably pliable and give a virtually 100% seal in the closed position. If it does not, nitrous can bleed into the engine and accumulate in a gaseous form. If sufficient quantities of gas are trapped inside the engine, this nitrous can cause an intake explosion—from mild to wild, depending upon leakage rate—when the engine is started. This sort of backfire can bend throttle shafts; destroy various seals; and, at worst, cause a severe underhood fire that may eventually lead to a total vehicle burndown.

Admittedly, these eventualities are unlikely, but they are possibilities. In the early days, nitrous valves were often adapted from other industrial applications and they were often less than totally reliable. Accidents did happen. Currently the valves used by reputable kit manufacturers are designed and assembled to rigid specifications and perform to very high standards.

Because the nitrous normally used for high-performance automotive applications is not 100% particle-free, it is necessary to put a particle filter in the supply line between the nitrous bottle and the nitrous valve. The most popular type is the sintered-bronze filter, which successfully screens out all particles large enough to cause problems with the nitrous valve or delivery orifices.

NITROUS DISTRIBUTION

Nitrous-oxide is normally stored in

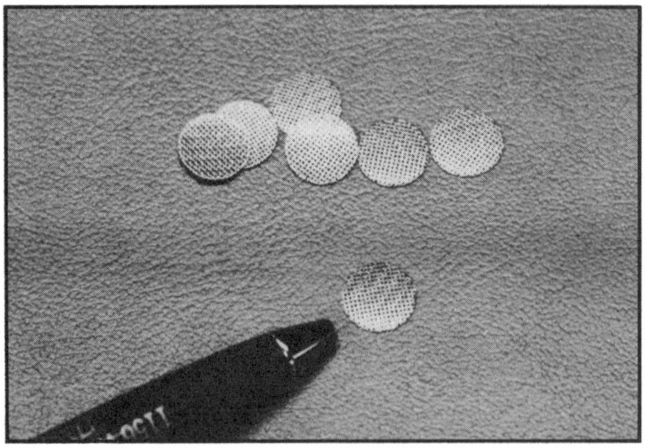

The most common filter is a simple screen located in the nitrous valve. This type of filter is not effective with a low-output system, because the open mesh can pass particles that are large enough to block the tiny calibration orifices.

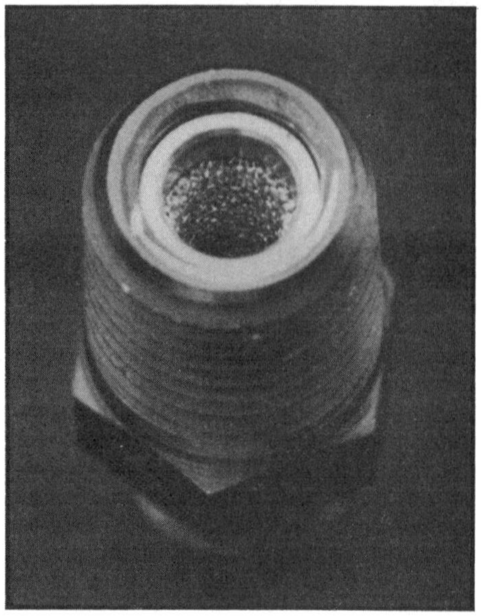

A sintered-bronze filter can be added to the nitrous supply system to remove undesirable particulates. These are excellent filters, but they are restrictive. If such a filter is used, the actual flow capability (verified) of the filter must exceed the maximum flow requirements of the system.

a pressurized bottle. These bottles must meet very rigid government specifications. When properly handled, the likelihood of a bottle failure is extremely remote. Nitrous bottles are normally painted light blue. This is a universal color code—indicating what sort of pressurized chemical is stored in the bottle—and the bottle should not be painted another color. Should your vehicle be involved in an accident, safety workers will know what the bottle contains and can take appropriate safety measures.

Conventional storage bottles are modified slightly for automotive applications. A pickup tube is added. This tube goes to the bottom of the bottle and is angled toward one corner. When correctly mounted, this ensures that all but the last drop of liquid nitrous-oxide can be drawn from the bottle. The valves used in these bottles are specially made for use with nitrous-oxide and the attendant high pressures.

Other provisions within the delivery system are also required to cope with the nitrous. The transfer lines conveying the nitrous-oxide from the storage bottle to the solenoid and from there on to the spraybar are usually steel-reinforced, high-pressure hoses capable of withstanding 5000psi. With some nitrous systems, the distribution manifold carrying the nitrous to the spraybar or nozzles is fabricated from steel tubes. These lines also are capable of withstanding very high pressures, and they can be formed into relatively sharp bends more readily than high-pressure hose.

ENRICHMENT SYSTEM

The system for supplying enrichment fuel is also controlled by a solenoid valve. This valve functions in a very similar manner to the nitrous solenoid, however, it does not need to withstand very high pressures. Most nitrous-oxide systems do not require more fuel pressure than that delivered by a typical stock fuel pump. While steel-reinforced hoses are also used on the fuel side—often for the sake of appearance—they need not be of the super high-pressure variety. Nonetheless, as a matter of convenience, many kit manufacturers use the same high-pressure hose on both

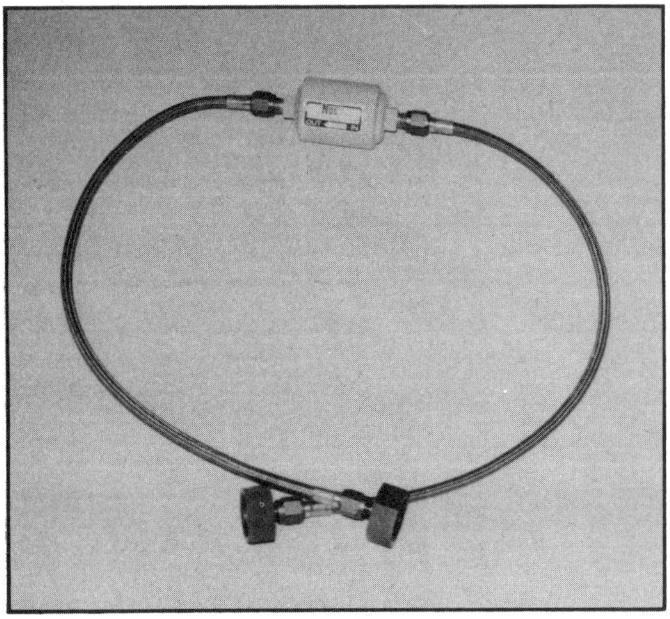

When positive filtration is required in a high-boost system, a high-capacity filter is mandatory. This excellent inline high-flow filter is available from NOS.

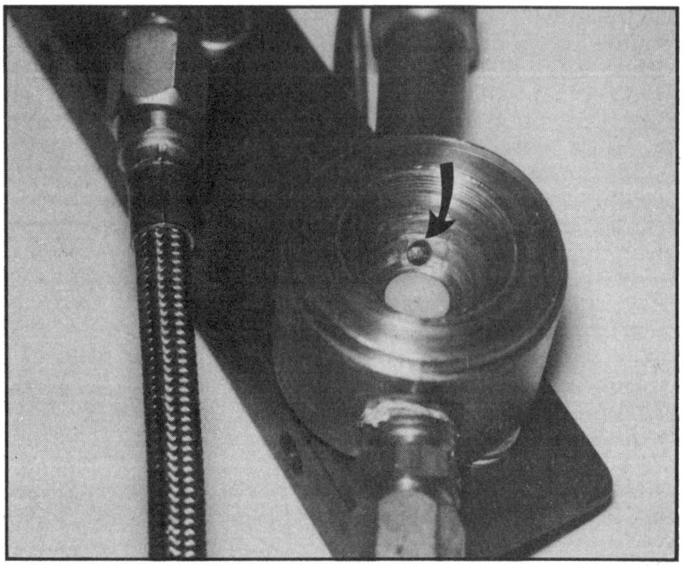

Filters won't catch everything. A large metal chip was found trapped in the orifice of this valve. This may be a rare instance; but if the system becomes unpredictable, methodically inspect the delivery paths of both the nitrous and fuel to make certain there are no unwanted restrictions.

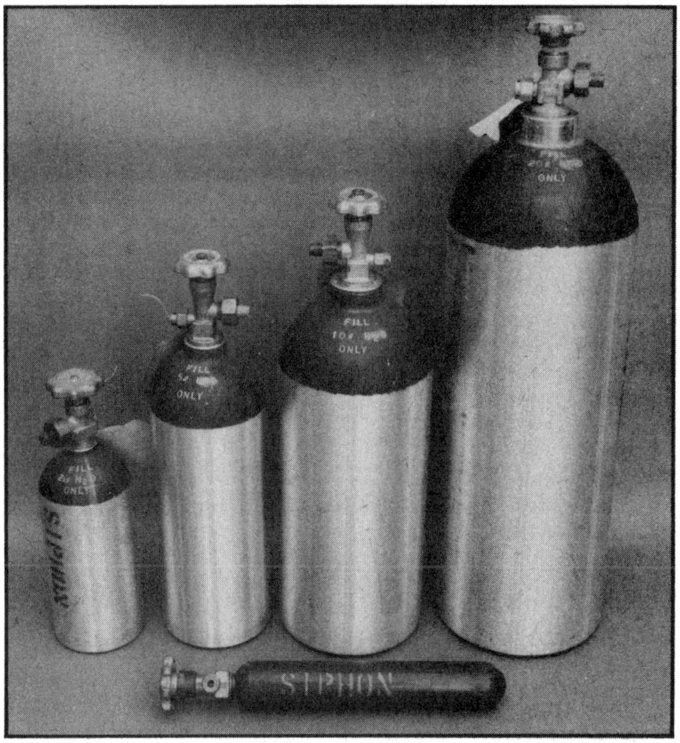

Nitrous-oxide storage bottles are available in a variety of shapes and sizes. The examples shown here are aluminum, but steel bottles are also available.

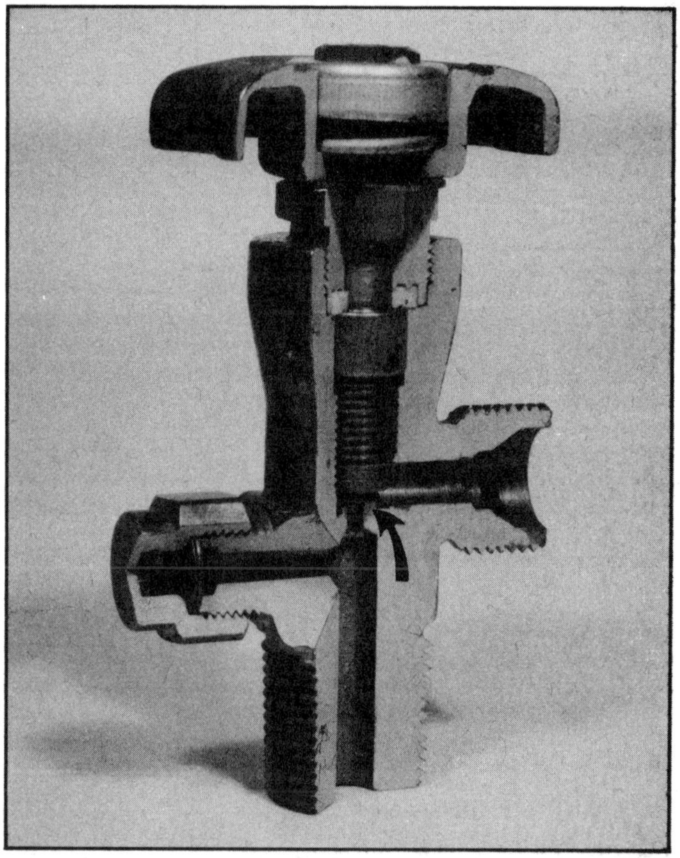

The valve in a typical nitrous bottle is more complex than it appears. The outlet on the left is the "blow-off valve," which ruptures if the pressure in the bottle exceeds a pre-determined limit. To minimize leakage past the valve stem, a heavy-duty seal is located beneath the retaining nut. Nitrous flow is shut off by a seal at the end of the valve stem that butts against the flat face of the tank orifice (arrow) deep inside the valve mechanism. When large flow rates are required for a high-boost system, this orifice may restrict the maximum amount of nitrous delivered by the system.

supply systems.

It is important to remember that *the functioning and calibration of the enrichment fuel delivery is the single biggest key to system reliability and effectiveness.* If the enrichment fuel delivery is too rich, engine power will be less than optimum, fuel will be wasted and a situation known as cylinder-bore wash may occur. This leads to increased bore wear, piston scuffing, and ultimately the possibility of piston seizure. If the fuel delivered by the system is too lean for the amount of nitrous-oxide, the combustion temperatures will become excessive and catastrophic engine meltdown is inevitable.

To avoid enrichment problems certain precautions are absolutely essential! It is very important to have an efficient fuel filter prior to the solenoid. This filter must have a large flow capacity. In the event that it collects a large amount of debris, it must still be able to flow enough fuel to satisfy the maximum flow requirements of the engine. If fuelborn debris is allowed to pass through the solenoid valve, it could block the orifices in the spraybar. If these orifices are blocked, the engine will have an excess of nitrous-oxide and experience excessively lean fuel-oxygen mixtures (along with the catastrophic consequences).

Most nitrous-oxide kits are made to function with fuel pressures of about 3.0 to 6.0psi, but some fuel

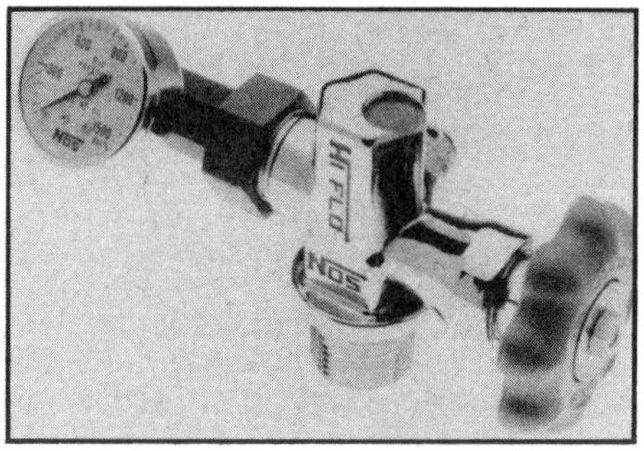

To reduce restrictions inside the bottle valve, NOS now offers an improved valve that increases maximum nitrous delivery by approximately 50%.

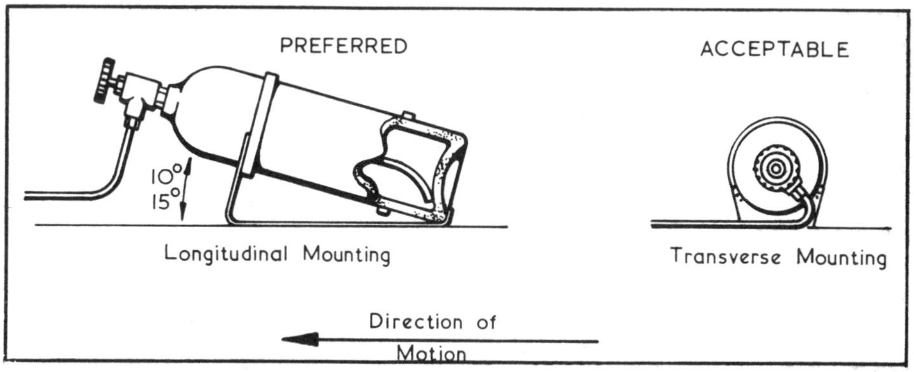

The pickup tube extends to the bottom of the nitrous bottle. The inlet of the syphon tube, as it is sometimes called, extends in the same direction as the outlet of the bottle valve. The bottle should be mounted in an inclined position, as shown above, with the syphon inlet toward the rear of the car. If space is limited, the bottle can be mounted transversely with the syphon inlet positioned slightly toward the rear. During acceleration the inlet must be immersed in liquid nitrous.

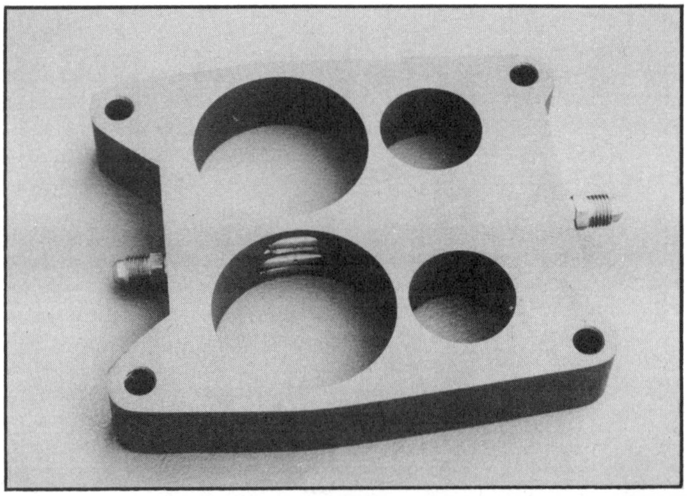

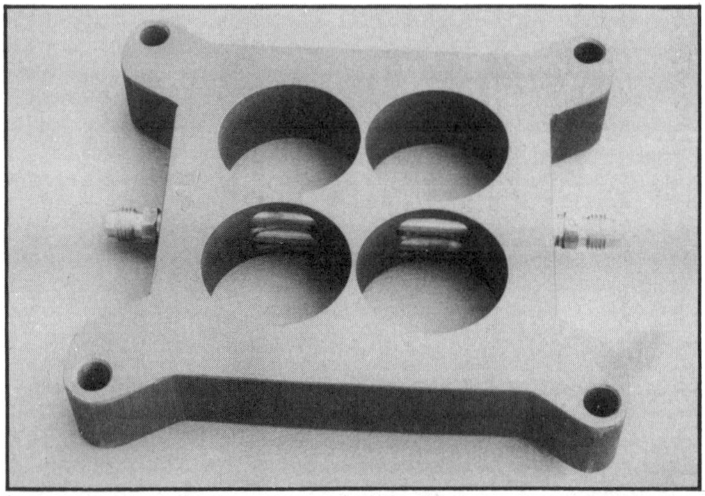

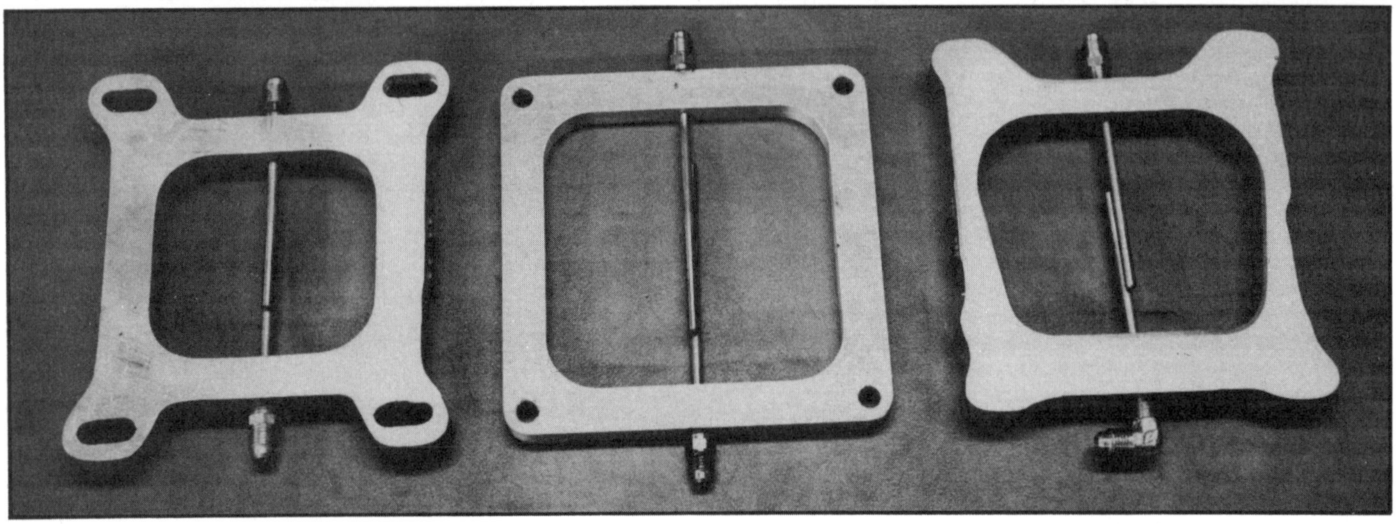

pumps can deliver well in excess of 6.0psi. The high-pressure Holley racing fuel pumps are prime examples. If a high-performance, high-pressure pump is used, it is advisable to use a pressure regulator in the system to drop the fuel pressure to that recommended by the kit manufacturer.

The schematic (Figure 3-1, page 28) illustrates a pressure regulator in the system. Although it is positioned after the fuel pump, the best physical location is to mount the regulator as close to the spraybar as possible. This provides high delivery pressure throughout the system, eliminating percolation difficulties, while the pressure is reduced to the correct level at the point of injection (the spraybar).

The spacer plate should be selected to match the carburetor. This is critical if a four-hole spacer, with bores that match the bores of the carburetor, is used. Four-hole spacers are available to match "spread-bore" (Quadrajet-type) or "square-bore" (Holley-type) carburetors. These photos also illustrate open spacers designed for (left to right) the square-bore Holley, Holley Dominator, and typical spread-bore carburetors.

SPACER-PLATE DESIGN

There are several factors to consider when choosing a particular spacer system. For instance, on many late-model cars the clearance between the air-filter case and hood is very minimal. Installing a kit that employs a 2.0-inch spacer below the carburetor will inevitably cause clearance problems. On the other hand, some companies produce kits with very thin spacers. Some thought and measuring before purchasing a kit may be worthwhile.

Incorporated into the spacer is, of course, the means for delivering the nitrous and additional fuel to the engine. Although the subject of spraybars and/or nozzles has been explored elsewhere, it will be worthwhile to reconsider the important points.

The spray-bar design and position are important. The jet of nitrous issuing from the spraybar should, in some way or other, impinge upon the jet of enrichment fuel. This promotes thorough mixing of the nitrous and fuel. In most spraybar systems this is accomplished by locating the nitrous spraybar above the fuel spraybar and positioning the orifices in the nitrous spraybar so that they are angled downward.

In a spraybar system, the number of discharge orifices seems to influence system performance. To a point, it is better to have many smaller discharge orifices, rather than a few larger orifices. Even if the total delivery area in both instances is equal, the system utilizing a greater number of smaller orifices—within reasonable limits—produces more effective mixing and distribution.

For maximum performance the spraybar and nitrous-fuel delivery must also be designed with an eye to the specific distribution eccentricities. Most V8 and V6 engines that are fitted with open-plenum manifold—with or without plenum dividers—tend to have a flow bias toward the central cylinders. As a result, the end cylinders of each bank tend to run a little lean. In this situation it may be beneficial to orient the spraybar delivery orifices to increase the flow toward the end cylinders.

If the spraybar is oriented at right angles to the crank centerline, which is normal, such biasing toward the end cylinders is difficult—indeed almost impossible—to prevent with a

FIGURE 3-2: Uniform air-fuel distribution is important, especially in high output engines. If any of the cylinders begin detonating, the damage can be swift and serious. For maximum reliable output, every cylinder must receive a uniform amount of air and fuel.

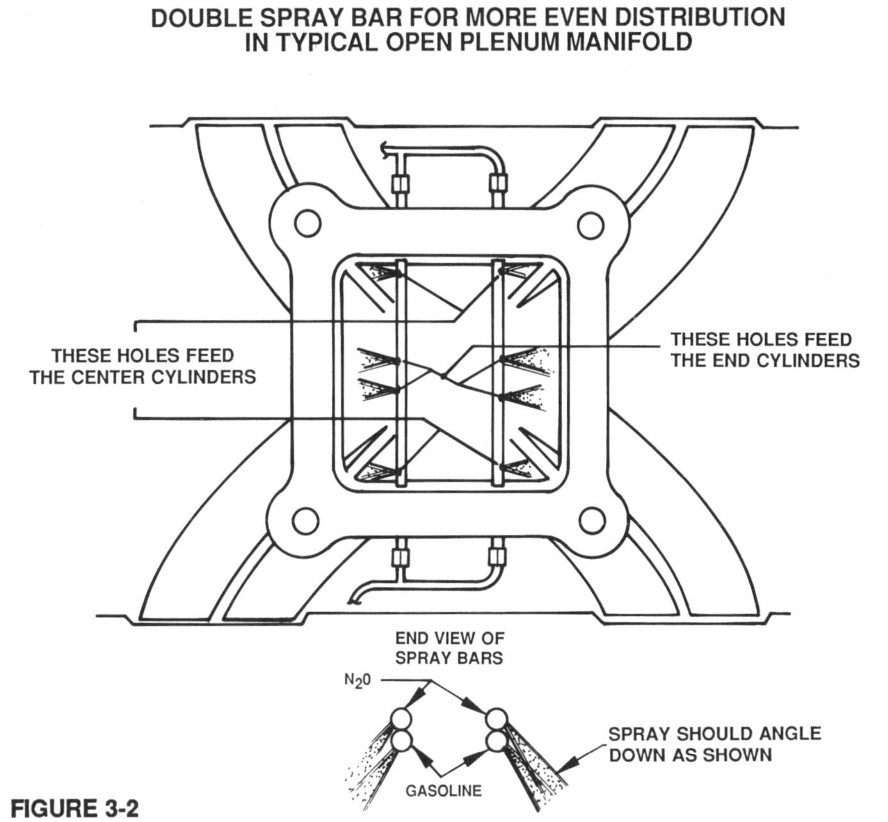

FIGURE 3-2

180-degree manifold. However, with an open-plenum manifold, the orifices can be located near the center of the tubes to increase flow (slightly) toward the end cylinders.

On the other hand, the problem can largely be alleviated by using two sets of spraybar orifices, but this will inevitably require some custom work. Figure 3-2 shows a suggested setup that tends to favor the end cylinders.

On V6 engines, irrespective of whether an open-plenum or a divided-plenum manifold is installed, the author has found that a spraybar running the length of the engine (rather than at 90 degrees to the crank axis) produces better distribution. The spraybar orifices should be situated near the edge of the manifold so that the direction of injection is toward the corner cylinders, rather than the center cylinders. Aligning the spraybar in such a manner sometimes means that installation of plate-mounted solenoids is more difficult because they may interfere with the carburetor float bowls. If this is the case, it will be necessary to use either remote-mounted solenoids or a spacer tall enough to eliminate interference difficulties. Fortunately, the widespread availability of extremely compact solenoids has gone a long way toward eliminating this problem.

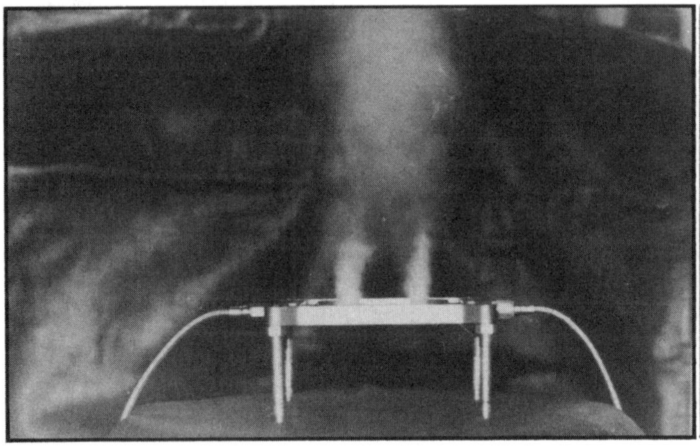

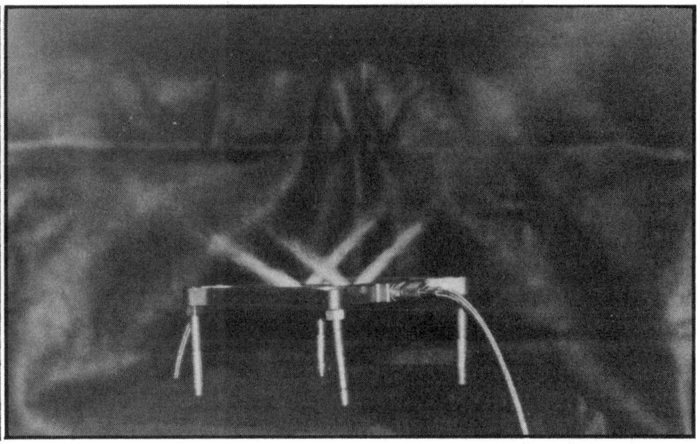

These photographs demonstrate how far the nitrous must travel from the injection orifices before it becomes a homogeneous cloud. A greater number of small orifices will more effectively disperse the nitrous inside the manifold and improve power output.

With a double-spraybar system—one spraybar for the nitrous and one for the fuel—there can be a problem with flow pulsing. This pulsing, or thermo-hydraulic resonance (discussed in Chapter 2), appears to be caused primarily by successive heating and cooling of various parts of the nitrous line and spraybar. The heat fluctuations can cause the nitrous to

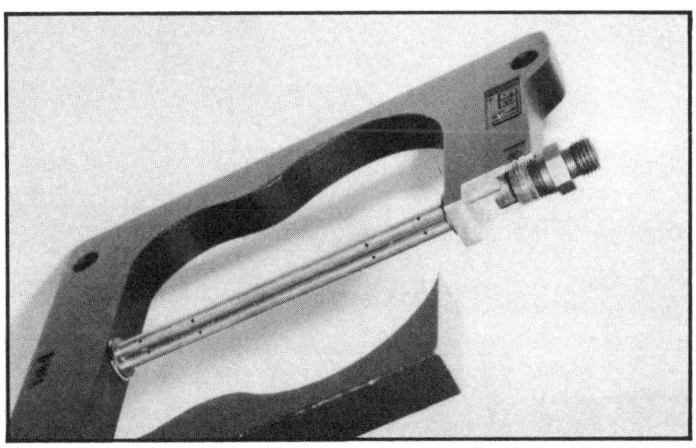

This is a cutaway of a typical NOS spacer. To achieve better nitrous distribution this unit has eight orifices in the nitrous spraybar. Experiments have indicated that further gains, although less pronounced, can be achieved with up to 16 orifices.

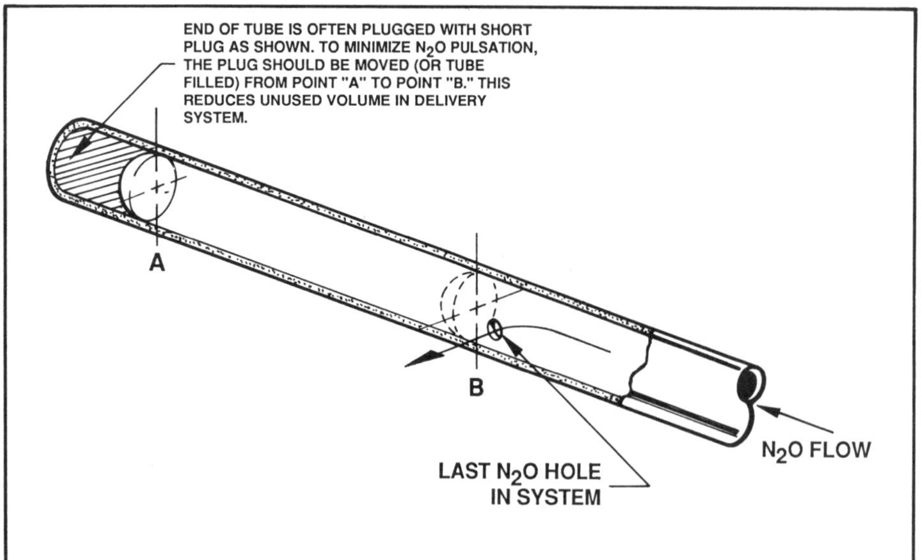

TYPICAL N_2O SPRAY BAR CONSTRUCTION FIGURE 3-3

FIGURE 3-3: Spray-Bar Construction

be injected alternately as a liquid, then as a gas. This may occur only in one or several small portions of the system, and reproducing this pulsing during bench test is often difficult because heat input to the system (from engine operation) affects the pulsing.

To reduce this tendency, it is best to block the nitrous spraybar beyond the last orifice. In other words, do not leave an empty cavity at the end of the nitrous spraybar. The modification shown in Figure 3-3 may, depending upon the particular installation, solve or reduce the severity of this problem.

Another possible source of thermo-hydraulic resonance is the delivery line between the nitrous solenoid and the point of injection. Shortening the line or simply using one of smaller diameter can reduce the resonance. Make these adjustments with caution, however, because an excessively small line may affect power output.

In this respect it is worth noting that aluminum is probably the worst material for a spacer because it conducts heat very well. Most hose and tube fittings are brass, which also conducts heat, and this aluminum-brass combination is excellent for conducting unwanted heat into the nitrous system. An effective insulator, like phenolic plastic, would be a better material for this spacer.

JET SYSTEMS

As explained in Chapter 2, jet systems do not, in general, suffer from thermo-hydraulic resonance problems to nearly the same degree as spraybar systems. A spraybar system can easily cause engine torque to fluctuate by 30 to 40 foot pounds, whereas the typical jet system may hold the torque steady to within 4.0 to 6.0 foot pounds.

If the delivery orifices in a jet system are the single type—as opposed to the combined fuel/nitrous type—the nitrous does not readily mix with the fuel to produce a homogeneous combustible mixture in the same way that spraybars (in close proximity) do. In every case tested by the author, a well-developed spraybar kit produced more horsepower for a given amount of nitrous than a well-developed jet system (provided, of course, that the point of injection was roughly equivalent). Just to make the point perfectly clear, I am referring to a jet—such as an injection nozzle—at the delivery point rather than a calibration jet or orifice in the supply line (upstream of the delivery point).

CALIBRATION

Whether they be of the spraybar variety or jet variety, *all conventional nitrous systems are calibrated by virtue of the area of the delivery orifice(s) or by restricting orifice(s) within the nitrous delivery line.* Of course, in a spraybar system there would be a number of delivery orifices. And in the case of a jet system, there would be one, two, four or more orifices, depending upon the configuration of the manifold. Except for variable-calibration systems, the flow of nitrous is governed solely by the area of the delivery orifices in the spraybar or nozzle/jet.

We must also remember, however, that the pressure in the nitrous bottle increases with temperature. Obviously, when the temperature/pressure of the bottle increases, there is greater force to drive the nitrous through the lines and out the delivery orifices. Thus it would be fair to assume that at higher temperatures, more nitrous will flow. This would, of course, have an undesirable consequence. If, in fact, more nitrous is delivered (relative to the enrichment fuel delivery), the resultant mixture will be lean.

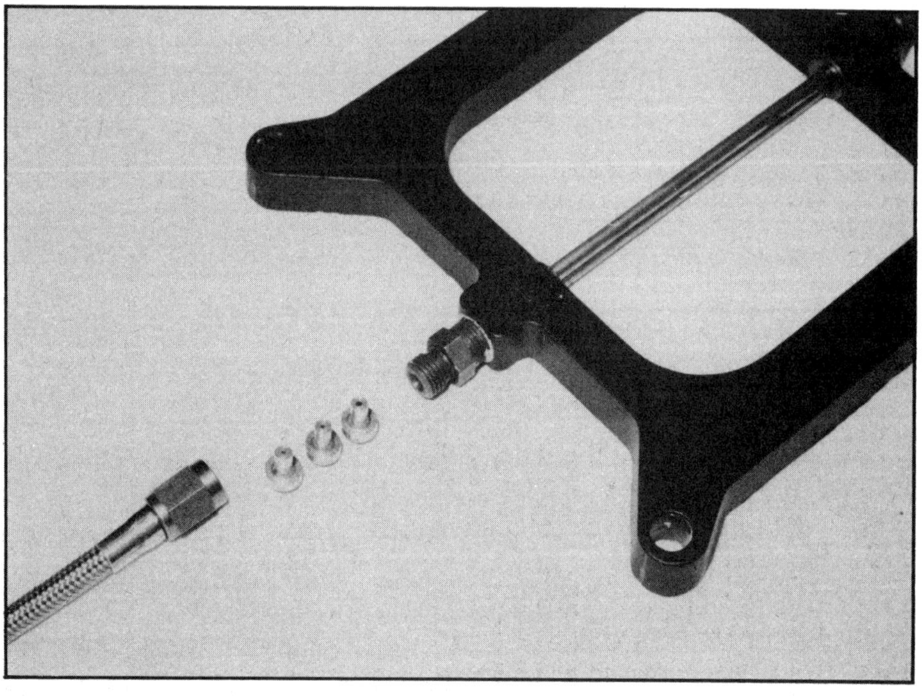

This system uses replaceable "metering jets" located inside the nitrous and fuel ports of the spacer plate. The area and shape of the jet orifice calibrates the respective delivery of nitrous and enrichment fuel; hence nitrous/fuel ratio and power boost can be readily altered.

One important aspect comes to our aid. As the nitrous temperature increases, the containment pressure increases, but conversely, the density decreases. And fortunately for us, the drop in density is such that it virtually offsets the effect of the pressure rise. The net result is that *the mass flow of nitrous through the delivery system is almost totally independent of the bottle pressure.* As pressure changes, the density changes in the opposite direction, so the mass flow (in pounds per minute) through the nozzles stays relatively constant—at least close enough for all practical purposes.

On the other hand, we must remember that operating temperature can adversely affect performance. Excessive heat at the point of injection can cause difficulties. In this instance, a relatively cool temperature in the bottle and delivery system and a sharp temperature rise at the delivery point will combine to reduce nitrous mass flow. The sudden temperature rise at the point of injection will reduce the density of the nitrous, but there will not be a complementary increase in the bottle/delivery pressure. This is a strong argument for reasonable bottle temperatures and temperatures as cool as practicable along the entire delivery system.

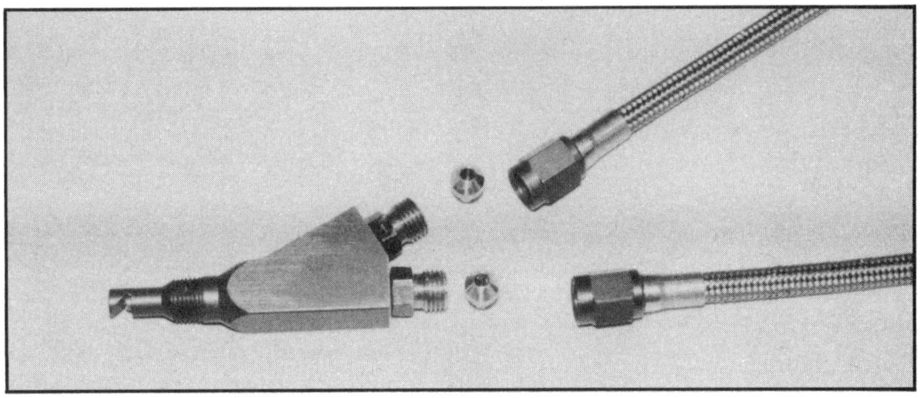

The NOS fogger nozzle is calibrated with a metering orifice retained in the supply line. The mixing of fuel and nitrous takes place at the tip of the nozzle, ensuring a homogeneous mixture is delivered to the manifold.

ADJUSTABLE SYSTEMS

Though the ideal point for metering the nitrous—and to a lesser extent the fuel—is at the point of injection, it is possible to successfully alter the point at which nitrous metering takes place. It is important to understand how this will alter system operation. If a restriction (a smaller orifice than the orifice at the delivery point) is placed in the supply line, the nitrous-oxide will expand rapidly after passing through the restriction. When the nitrous expands, a proportion of it will convert to a gas. As soon as it converts, it will cool the length of tube between the restriction and the end of the pipe (the point of delivery).

This phenomenon must be considered in the design of every system. For instance, if the solenoid passes less nitrous than the supply orifices in the spraybar, the solenoid becomes a restriction in the supply line. As a result, the solenoid valve can become supercooled and could, under extreme circumstances, freeze open.

It is much simpler, therefore, to *locate the calibration point close to the end of the nitrous delivery system.* But this does not preclude the possibility of having a calibration point that is not at the very end of the line. Some "adjustable" nitrous systems have small calibrating orifices positioned within the fitting on the spacerplate. With this type of adjustable orifice in both the nitrous and fuel lines, the user can readily adjust the power level produced by the system.

A typical adjustment range—with variable orifices—would be 75, 100, 125 horsepower. However, It is important to note that bigger is not necessarily always better. Super-impressive horsepower numbers may cause the vehicle to break traction and run slower; or they can cause melted engine parts to fall into the oil pan! So do not become dazzled by big horsepower numbers.

In addition, if the range of adjustment is too great, at lower power levels the system can become very slow-hitting, mushy, and generally inconsistent in operation. During humid ambient operating conditions the spraybar could, in fact, ice up and restrict delivery. Apart from this, it is also important to realize that there comes a time when increasing delivery volume simply does not increase power any further!

It is important to note that, when calibrating an adjustable system, the jets come in matched pairs; this means that when the nitrous jets are changed, the fuel jet must also be changed to maintain the desired nitrous-to-fuel ratio.

ELECTRICAL SYSTEM

The electrical portion of a nitrous injection system is fairly simple, but

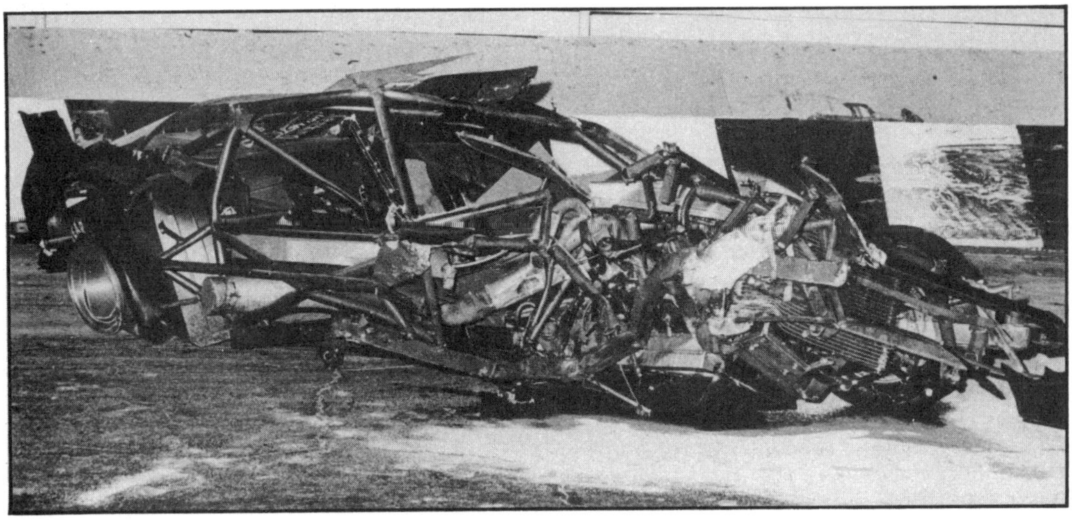

Reliable electrical operation of every component in a nitrous system is important. The nitrous and fuel solenoids of Danny Press' 370-inch Chevy failed to shut off at the end of a straightaway and the power developed by the malfunctioning nitrous system (with the throttle closed) forced the car into a wall, reducing a $25,000 race car to $25 of scrap.

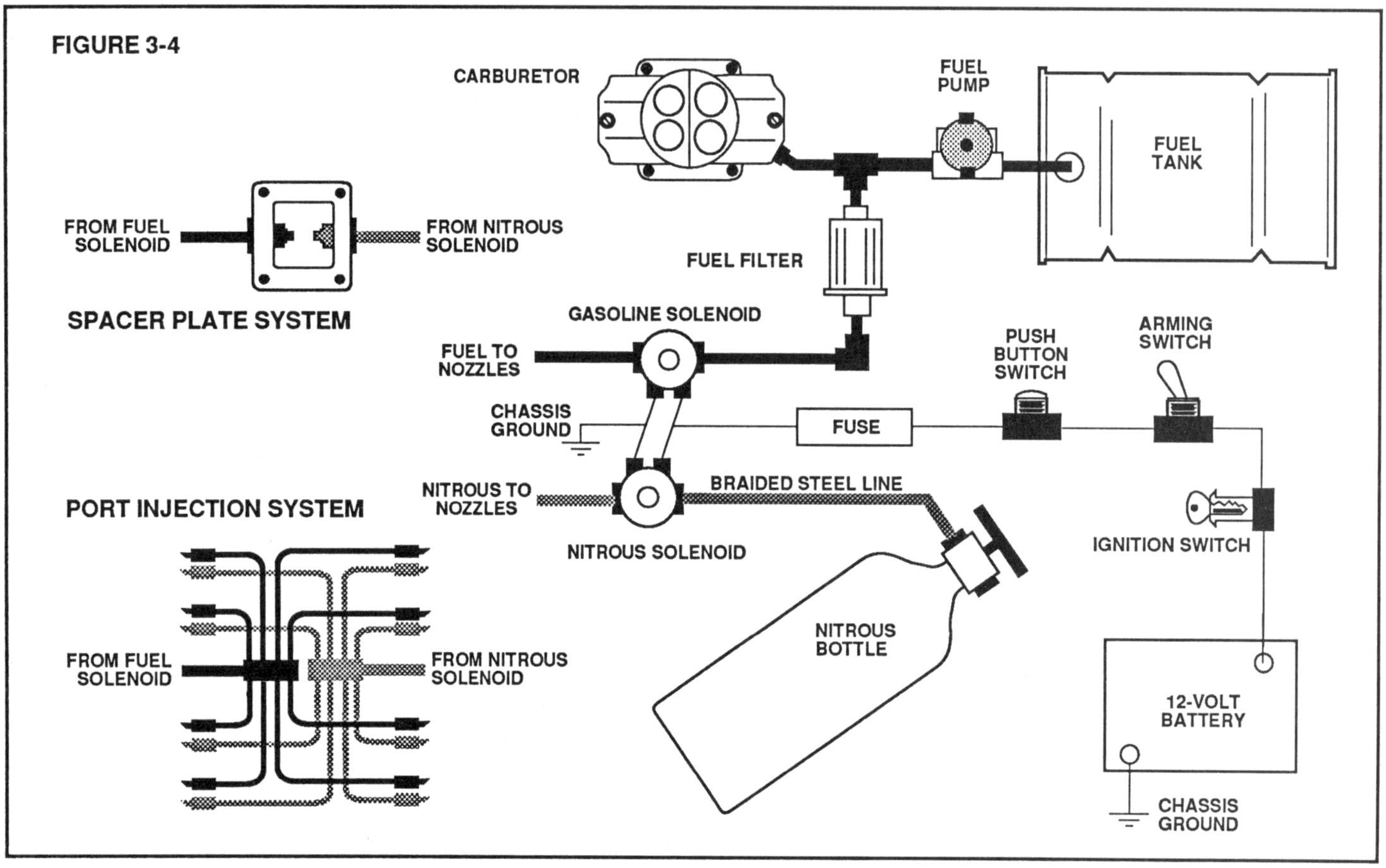

FIGURE 3-4: This is a schematic of the fuel-flow and electrical connections in a typical nitrous-oxide system. Notice that the arming switch is wired in series with the activation switch; when the arming switch is off, it prevents the system from firing even if the activation switch is accidentally contacted.

things can become somewhat complicated when the system has multiple stages or is used on a supercharged or turbocharged engine. The following information is a general discussion of the electrical system of a typical nitrous-oxide system; however, the instructions and guidelines included with a specific kit should be followed.

ARMING SWITCH

The primary circuit that activates a typical nitrous system is controlled by the arming switch. This is the switch that readies the system for activation or totally disarms the system when the driver wishes to turn it off. Figure 3-4 shows a typical example.

The arming switch is generally a single-pole, on-off switch. The switch must be able to carry all the current that the activated nitrous system will require. The manufacturer generally provides a switch that will carry enough current, plus a safety margin, but if you decide to use a non-stock switch, it is important to use one that is rated at least equal to—and possibly higher than—the stock switch.

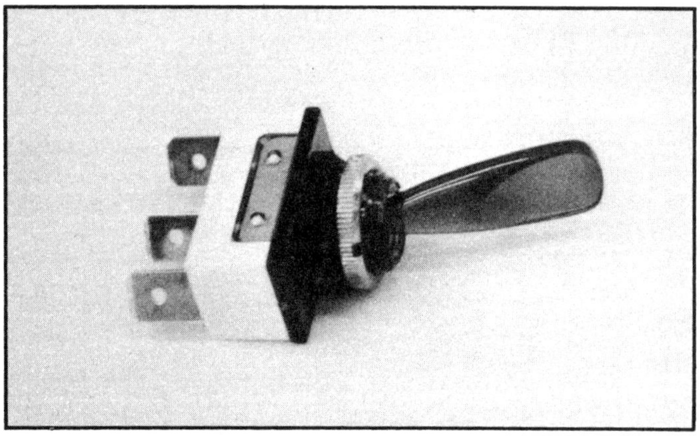

The lever of this on-off switch is made of clear, blue plastic; when the system is armed, the switch is lit by an internal lamp.

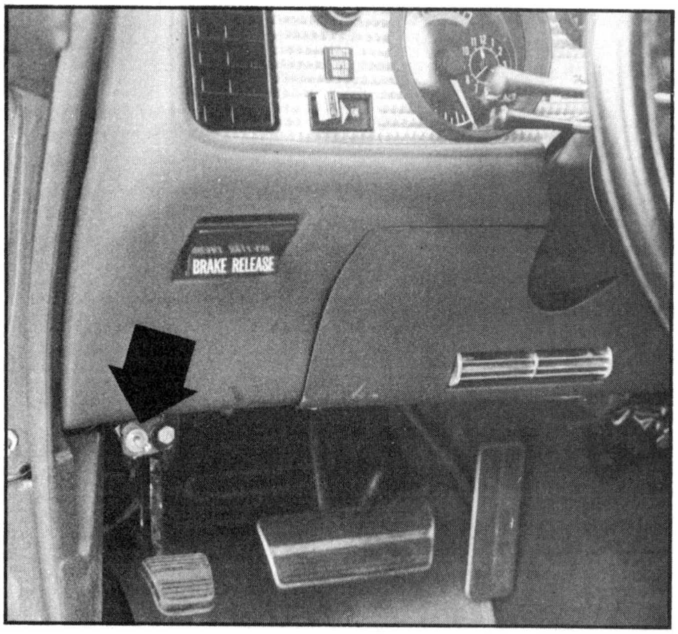

The arming switch can be mounted in almost any convenient or inconspicuous location. This innocent switch puts 150 horsepower on standby for instant use.

If you are building a custom system or are considering the possibility of combining two single-stage systems into a multi-stage setup, be certain that the arming switch is rated in excess of the total current demands of the system. With some types of solenoids—especially older models—the current demands can be quite high. This could overload the arming switch and the wiring harness.

The best way to verify the total requirement is to use an ammeter to measure the current each solenoid draws during operation. To make these measurements, connect the solenoid and ammeter to a 12-volt source as shown in Figure 3-5. Do this for all the solenoids. If an additional fuel pump is being used, check this current requirement as well. To see if the switch is within the current rating, total the current draw for all the components. If there is any doubt, buy a switch that is rated well in excess of the actual requirement.

Some arming switches have wire terminals that are located very close together—close enough for a frayed wire to short one terminal to the other. Should this happen, the system can be armed, even though the switch is off. With a powerful nitrous kit, this could be extremely hazardous. All wiring should be carefully installed with proper terminal ends and finished neatly to preclude dangerous shorts, A good way to make certain that the system is really disarmed is to use an "illuminated" switch. This type of switch has a built-in lamp that glows when the switch is on (the system is armed). Some kits do not use this type of switch; but for safety reasons, I would recommend going to an electrical supplier and buying a top-quality, heavy-duty illuminated switch, preferably with wide terminal spacing.

It is always important to think about safety when selecting and mounting the arming switch. Many kit makers supply a blue-colored arming switch. which may or may not be illuminated; but some companies supply a common-looking red switch. If there is a serious mishap, especially with a race car, a red switch can cause confusion. In the event of an accident, the safety officials, firefighters, crash marshals, etc., reach into the car and throw any switch that is red or red-illuminated. Normally, the nitrous arming switch will be off (depending, of course, on the situation at hand), but if it is red, the unaware safety workers may actually switch the nitrous system on, possibly increasing the danger. To reduce the likelihood of such a misunderstanding, I like to use a blue illuminated switch on a street-only vehicle. For a race vehicle—which by its very nature is much more likely to be involved in an accident—I prefer to use both blue and red: a blue illuminated arming switch with a large red indicator lamp placed nearby. When the system is activated, the large lamp will readily indicate the system status, even in bright sunlight.

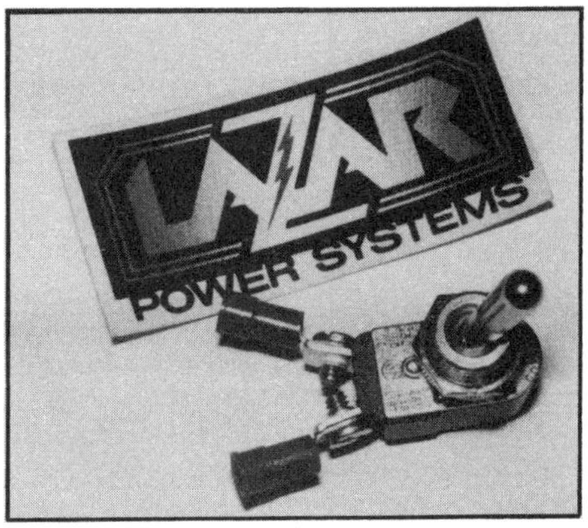

The contacts of this switch are extremely close. The screws could easily touch (from vibration), and the resulting short circuit would arm the system even though the switch is in the "off" position; a potentially dangerous situation.

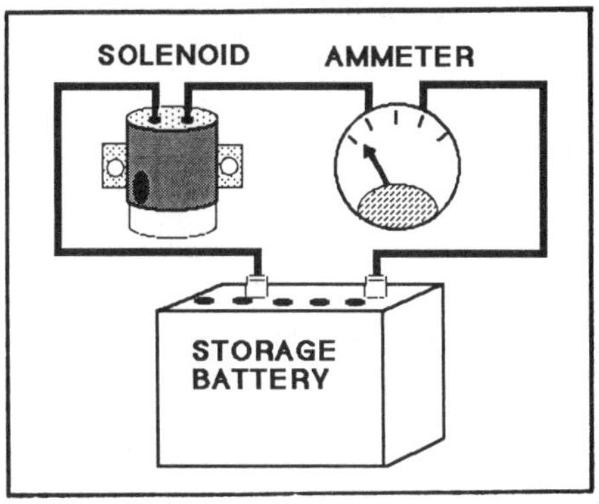

FIGURE 3-5: Current flow requirements for each solenoid in the system can be measured with a simple circuit that uses an ammeter connected in series with the solenoid and the 12-volt power source. Check each solenoid and add current flows to determine the system requirement.

SYSTEM ACTIVATION

In the early days, the nitrous system was generally activated with a simple "momentary" push switch. This type of switch makes the circuit when the button is held down and breaks the circuit as soon as the pressure on the button is released. This is the only type of switch to use if the circuit is going to be manually activated by the driver. Do not, under any circumstance, use a conventional on-off toggle switch or any type of switch that stays in the "ON" position when the driver releases pressure.

I know of at least one instance when a conventional on-off switch proved foolhardy and downright dangerous. A motorcycle enthusiast installed a 50-horsepower nitrous system on his bike with, unbelievably enough, a conventional rocker switch to fire the system. This is a lot of boost for a motorcycle engine, and

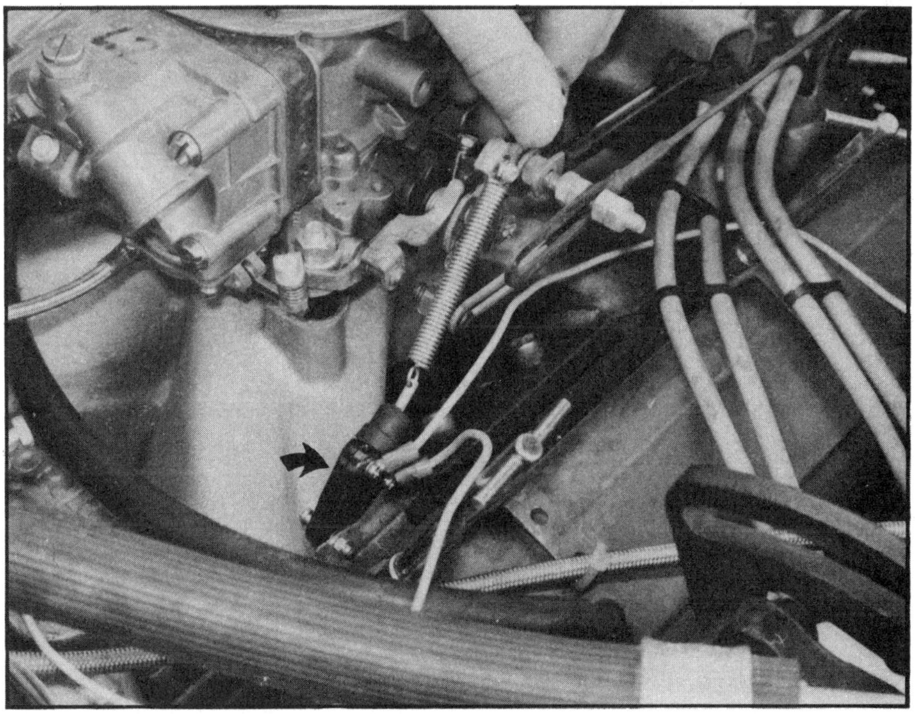

A heavy-duty spring-loaded microswitch is one of the most popular choices for throttle activation. The action can be adjusted so the switch initiates nitrous flow at the desired point in throttle travel.

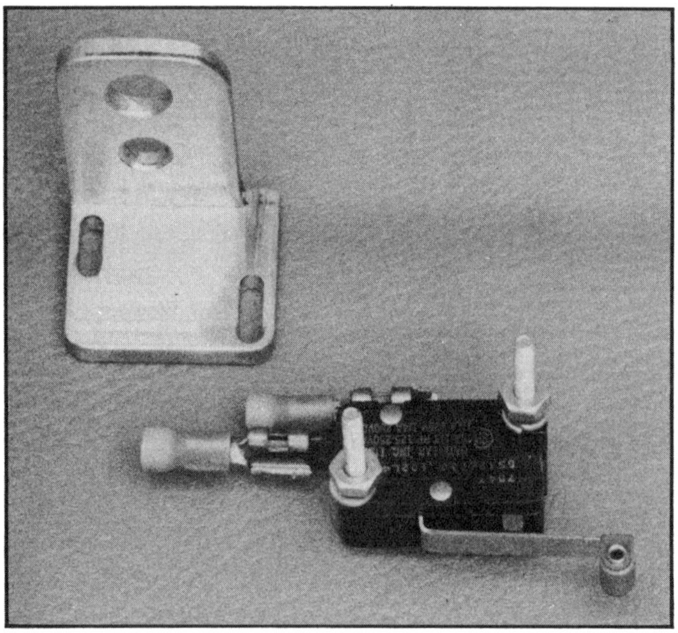

The microswitch is triggered by the throttle, but in most cases the light-duty microswitch must indirectly activate the nitrous system through a heavy-duty relay that can handle the high current needs of the solenoids.

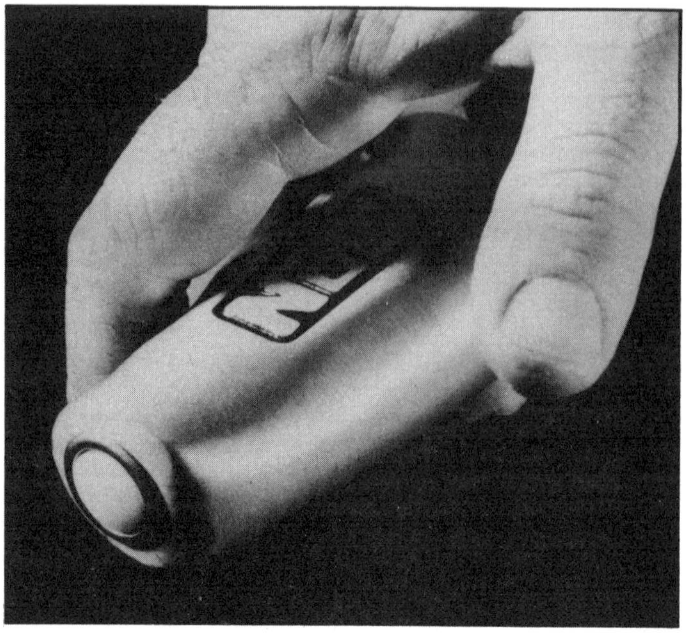

A shift knob with a built-in electrical switch is one of the most convenient and most popular firing switches for a street nitrous system.

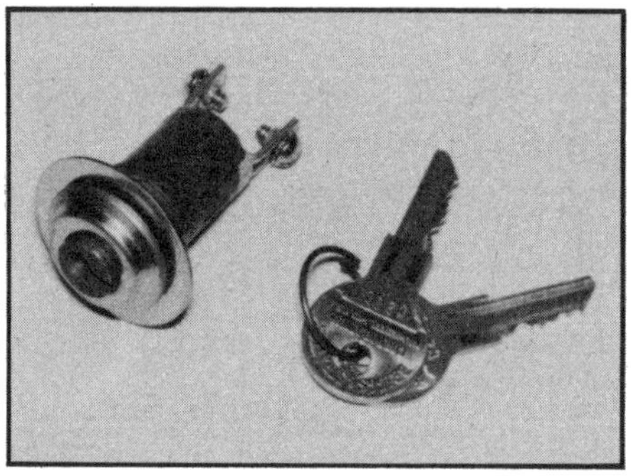

This key-operated arming switch is useful if you don't want anyone else to use the nitrous system while driving your car.

when the rider switched on the nitrous, the bike accelerated so hard that the rider lost control and could not get his thumb back on the switch to turn the nitrous off. And remember, when the nitrous system is dumping nitrous and fuel into the engine, closing the throttle does not shut down the engine. Since injection takes place downstream of the carburetor butterflies, the engine is still receiving a lot of oxygen and fuel from the nitrous system. Needless to say, the unfortunate rider had a wild ride until he bailed out.

Most basic nitrous kits are supplied with a manual momentary firing switch. This is fine for most applications: The driver simply activates the system whenever he wants boost—as long as he isn't too busy shifting gears—but while it may be functional, it lacks finesse. A more sophisticated approach is to use a throttle-operated switch. This is a simple contact switch that can be positioned to activate the system when the carburetor throttle is opened a pre-determined amount. However, it must not hinder the throttle action. In other words, even after the switch has functioned, the throttle must still be allowed to open further. (The switch shown in the photo—page 37, bottom—is perfect for this type of application and is available from NOS.)

If a two-stage system is used on a drag car, it is sometimes a good idea to activate the primary stage with a throttle switch. This is especially true if the primary stage is used for a low-power boost to launch the car without over-powering the tires and suspension. The second stage, which will provide max power boost, can then be activated at the big end by a conventional driver-controlled push switch.

Another way to achieve the same sort of thing is to use a vacuum-type firing switch to activate the primary stage. Indeed, a vacuum switch can also be used to advantage on a single-stage system. If the car has an automatic transmission, the manifold vacuum will drop off long before full throttle is reached. As a result, a vacuum switch will, in many instances, cause the engine to react a bit more quickly. Nevertheless, a vacuum switch is not without disadvantage. An override switch must be incorporated somewhere in the firing circuit to disarm the system when the engine is not running. For maximum safety under all circumstances, an override relay controlled by an oil-pressure sensor is required.

Throttle-operated firing switches are simple and reliable, but the driver must be aware of low-speed boost limitations. Many kit manufacturers do not recommend activating the nitrous system below 3000rpm. Feeding nitrous to the engine when the crank speed is below 3000rpm is not really a problem; it's just a question of how much. A single-stage system that develops 100-plus horsepower will generally deliver a lot of nitrous (and enrichment fuel) whenever it is activated, and at low engine speeds this may cause excessive combustion pressures. A sturdy big-block engine can, obviously, withstand more than a smallblock (a big engine may withstand a 100-horsepower boost at speeds as low as 2500rpm). In general, however, when the amount of nitrous (boost) is less, the *safe* low-speed activation limit will be lower.

This is where two-stage systems—especially in street applications—really shine. The initial stage of nitrous can be quite low—50 horsepower is not uncommon—and this will greatly increase the boost and power flexibility of the engine. Of course, a killer banzai system may have a primary stage that delivers 100-horsepower, and the high initial boost level with this type of system will greatly reduce low-speed flexibility. Nonetheless, these systems are normally used on engines with long-duration camshafts, which reduce low-speed combustion pressure. When used with low gears and an automatic transmission with a "loose" torque converter—a combination that will reduce low-speed engine loading—this type of system will often work surprisingly well in the lower speed ranges.

The biggest problem centers around the amount of control the driver has over the system. The situation is especially difficult when a vacuum switch is used on an engine that is coupled to a stock torque converter. Under some conditions, the system may be activated when the engine speed is below the safe minimum limit. To avoid this circumstance—most common with street engines—a mechanical firing switch should be used.

Vacuum switches are unpredictable at low engine speeds because a slight change in the throttle position can cause the manifold vacuum to drop below the activation point (determined, of course, by the preset threshold of the vacuum switch). On the other hand, a mechanical switch operated by the throttle arm will only activate the nitrous when the throttle reaches a specific position. It is easy, normally, for the driver to feel the throttle respond as it touches the contact switch, and by "feathering" the throttle he can delay the exact moment when the nitrous activates until the engine speed reaches the optimum level.

It is up to the driver to determine, under actual operating conditions, which system he prefers. Often, it is a good idea to test the system response at reduced boost levels before finalizing the type and adjustment of the firing switch. However, if there is some possibility that the system may activate when the engine speed is too low, a throttle-operated switch would be the safest and most reliable selection.

A more sophisticated solution is to use an rpm-sensitive switch (see photo, page 69). This type of switch—available from NOS—delays system activation until the engine speed reaches a preset level, irrespective of whether full throttle has been reached. With this switch, a system can be dialed in to very specific conditions.

Obviously, an rpm-sensing switch can be a big help on a drag-racing machine. For instance, if the system delivers too much nitrous at low engine speed, the tires may lose traction leaving the line on a slick track. With an adjustable rpm-sensing switch, the activation threshold can be "fine tuned" to allow the engine to gain more speed, allowing more time for weight transfer to assist traction before the nitrous hits.

Greater flexibility to adjust the activation point should be helpful, but under some circumstances, setting the nitrous to come in a few hundred rpm higher may not cure the problem. The car may simply leave very lazily and suddenly explode to life—again losing traction—a few yards down the track. An rpm-control switch is not going to fix this; the problem, as discussed earlier, is that too much nitrous is being fed to the engine at relatively low engine speeds. Here, once again, the ultimate solution is a two-stage system: a relatively low-power first stage activated by a throttle switch and a high-power second stage activated by an adjustable rpm-sensing switch.

There are, apart from these three basic systems, other "unconventional" ways of firing the nitrous. The specific effect can differ slightly and will vary with the situation. For instance, by using a relay, almost any switch on the vehicle can be made to fire the nitrous. This can be useful if it is important to camouflage the firing switch. One novel approach is to use the horn button as a firing switch. When the system is armed, a relay can bypass the horn circuit and activate the solenoids of the nitrous system. Thus, when the horn button is pressed, the nitrous system will fire!

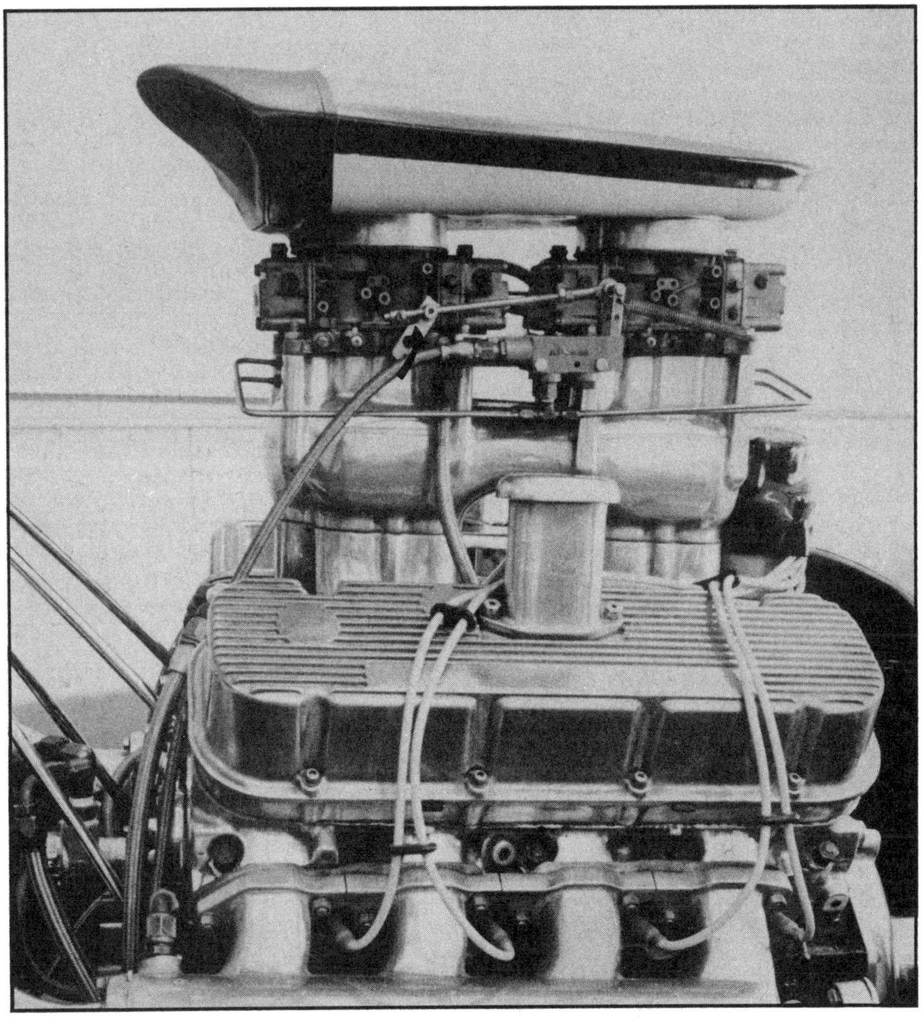

It is also possible to use an entirely mechanical activation system. This setup from 10,000 RPM employs a mechanical valve; the throttle lever incorporates an adjustment to vary the activation point relative to throttle position.

SOLENOID FUNCTIONING

The primary operating mechanisms in a nitrous injection system are the solenoid valves that control the flow of the nitrous and enrichment fuel. These valves are relatively simple; however, *the single most important consideration is that the valves must seal reliably time after time.* As mentioned earlier, many kit manufacturers have spent a lot of time and effort perfecting control valves that are not just reliable, but VERY reliable. Since the valves are the heart of the system, they must be selected and properly installed strictly according to the manufacturers' recommendations.

An important, but often overlooked, aspect of valve design is the electrical requirements of the solenoids. When current is applied to the coil inside the solenoid, heat is produced as a natural byproduct of the resistance in the coil. Obviously, the

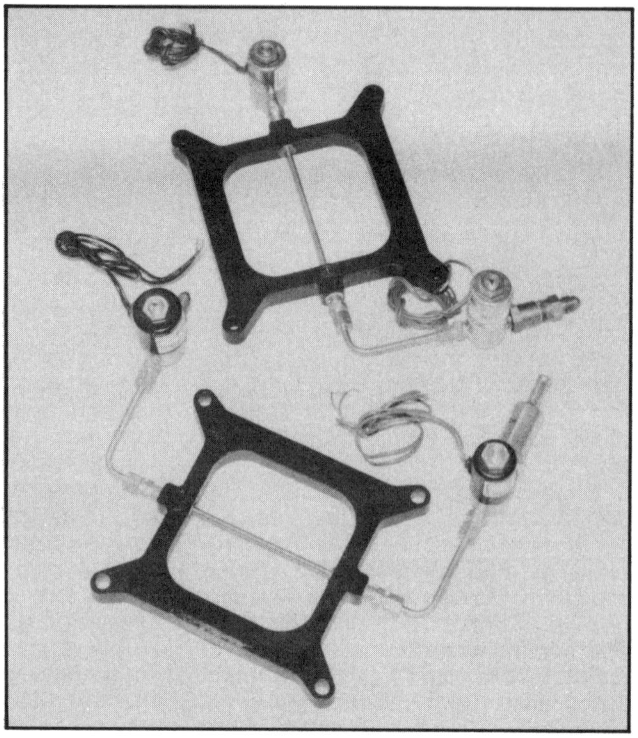

Modern high-flow solenoid valves are compact and reliable. The small size eases installation in tight quarters, yet these valves will flow enough nitrous or enrichment fuel to develop 200 horsepower.

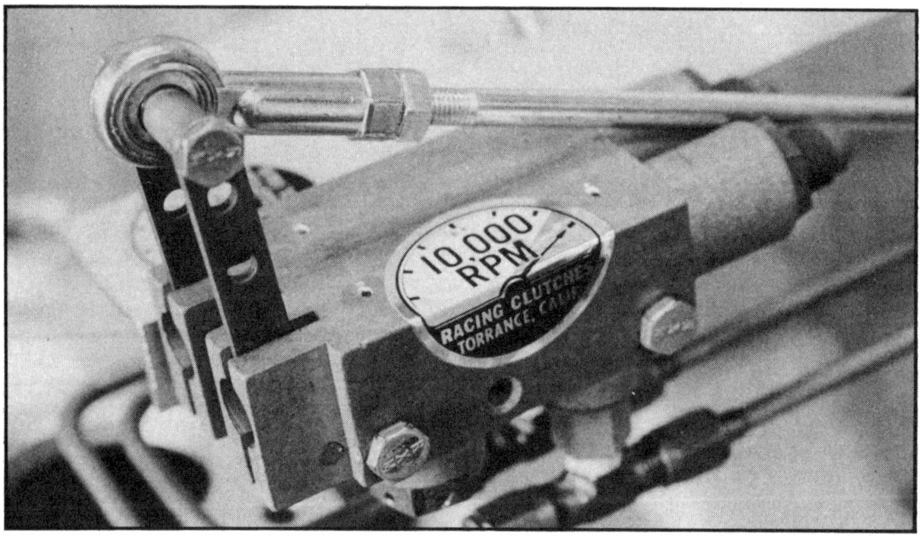

The nitrous and fuel valves do not have to be actuated by electricity. The mechanical valves used on this 10,000 RPM system serve the same function as solenoid-controlled valves.

coil has to be designed so that the relationship between the electrical current, the magnetic field, and the magnetic energy requirements of the solenoid do not produce an excessive amount of heat. If excessive current is applied to the solenoid or if the design of the coil is not properly matched for the amount of applied voltage, the windings in the coil may overheat. Portions of the coil may then burn and semi-weld together. When this occurs, the valve may still function, but the electrical short created across portions of the coil windings may cause sporadic operation (particularly on a hot day when system pressure is high) and eventual failure.

On the other hand, the solenoids in a nitrous system are operated for relatively short periods; and they are, to an extent, cooled by the liquid going through them. As a result, it is possible to select the number of windings and diameter of wire so that the coil can, in effect, be temporarily overloaded, thus producing a greater magnetism from a smaller coil. This allows the use of a compact solenoid, because the bulk of any solenoid is primarily in the electrical coil and the armature—or plunger—that the coil must move when it is energized.

For most street applications, the amount of current drawn by the solenoids is rarely a problem, simply because most street applications will use fairly small solenoids due to the limited amount of nitrous involved. Such limitations are dictated largely by the stock or near-stock nature of a street-worthy engine and chassis. Also, with a street vehicle, the alternator usually has sufficient output to keep pace with the current required by the solenoids.

On a race car, there may be only a battery as a source of power. Plus, the amount of nitrous and fuel needed for a race engine is generally greater. This, in turn, means bigger solenoids. Ultimately, the current draw of the solenoid becomes an important factor on a race car because other electrical equipment will also require current from the battery (which is not being replenished if, as is fairly common, the race car does not have a recharging system).

Assuming that reliability is always a primary priority, the other major factors that need to be considered are the size of the valve and the amount of nitrous that it will flow. *A point of considerable importance to note here is that the nitrous valve must always be capable of flowing a substantially greater amount of nitrous than the flow requirements of the metering orifice.* A 2:1 valve-to-orifice flow ratio should be considered minimum. In other words, if the metering orifice flows a maximum of 6.0 pounds a minute, the nitrous valve should be capable of flowing at least 12.0 pounds a minute.

In some instances, kit manufacturers have modified the seat area of the valves in an effort to increase flow. The intent is to provide more mass flow through a valve that occupies less space and draws less current (relative to the nitrous flow requirements). It appears to be simply a matter of drilling the orifice in the center of the valve to a larger size. On the face of it, the maximum size that does not interfere with the seat radius should give the best results; but a larger orifice requires some additional considerations. These valves are designed to have the pressure inside the system act against the backside of the plunger and hold it on the seat. This system pressure is in addition to the pressure applied by the plunger spring; however, the system pressure is probably the major force holding the plunger in place. So, when the flow orifice is enlarged from 0.050-inch to 0.060-inch, the operating pressure of the valve may be reduced as much as 40%. A modification such as this could mean that a valve that would open at 1200psi will now open against a pressure of 860psi. The result is that some day the nitrous valve will refuse to function.

Early in the development of nitrous systems it was common for designers to drill valves oversize, but unfortunately, they did not actually test the flow capabilities of the modified valves. Often the expected flow increase did not materialize; or if extra flow was achieved, it was usually very

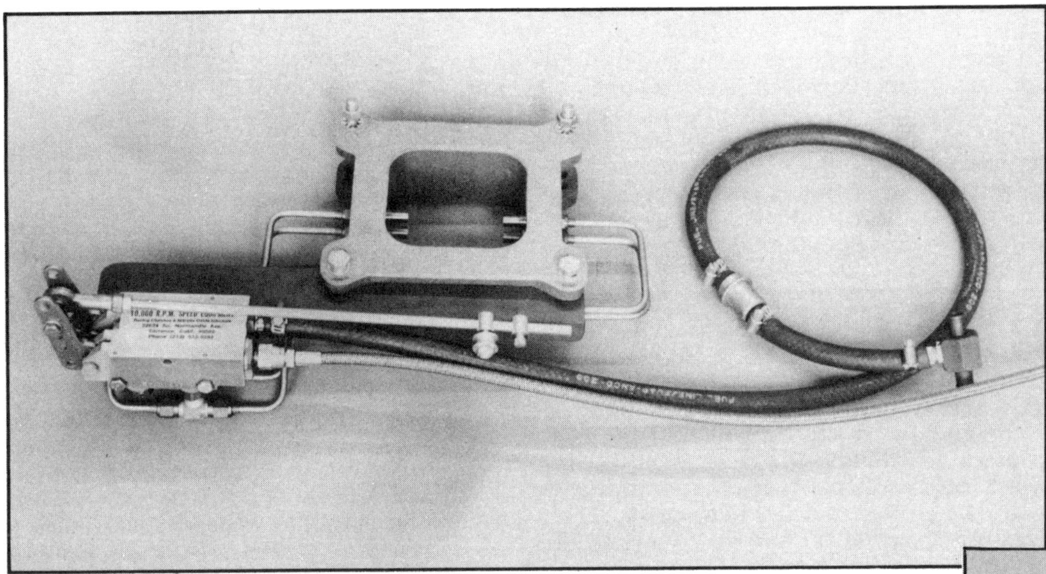

When electrical power is not available (e.g., a dragster), or if electric solenoid valves prove unreliable (e.g., in adverse conditions, long-distance off-road racing, etc.), a completely mechanical system may be the only answer. The 10,000 RPM system pictured above uses a pair of "spool" valves ganged together. The valve controlling enrichment fuel is closest to the spacer plate, while the nitrous valve can easily be identified by the high-pressure line leading to it. Throttle linkage determines how the valves will open: incrementally for nitrous assist at part throttle, or staged for boost only at near full throttle.

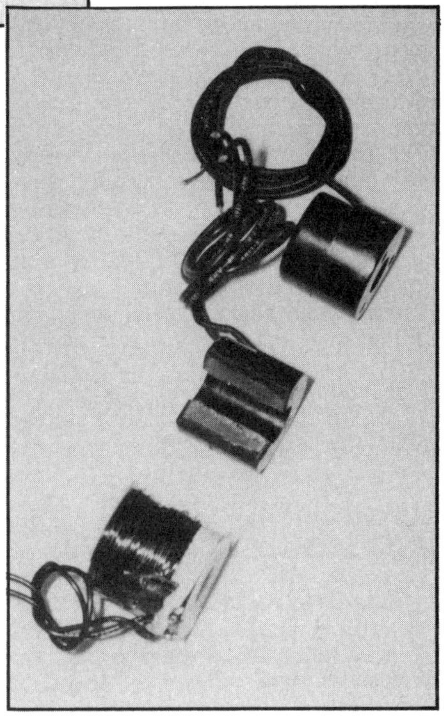

The magnetic field developed by the coil operates the valve, but the strength of the magnetism depends on the electrical current fed to the coil and the number of turns in the winding. The center coil has thousands of turns of very fine wire. The coil on the right has heavier gauge wire but fewer turns. To obtain optimum performance and reliability, it is necessary to strike the proper balance between the number of windings and the current draw.

minimal. The principal reason for this is that many solenoid valves previously used in the nitrous industry (and in some instances, are still used) have a very low *armature lift.*

The armature can be likened to an intake valve and seat arrangement. When the solenoid is operated, the valve is lifted away from the seat a prescribed amount. When the armature—or piston or valve, whichever you choose to call it—is positioned at full lift, it may impede flow unless it is raised high enough from the seat to provide sufficient area between the valve head and the seat surface. In fact, to allow unimpeded flow *it is necessary to lift the valve from the orifice seat a distance that equals at least 0.40 times the diameter of the orifice.*

For instance, if the valve has a 0.100-inch diameter flow orifice, the solenoid armature must be lifted at least 0.040-inch to provide full flow through the orifice. Nonetheless, it is not uncommon to find solenoids supplied with some nitrous kits that have 0.100-inch, or larger, flow orifices and only 0.020-inch of armature lift. Depending upon the requirements of the application, this may not provide enough flow area for reliable system functioning.

If a compact solenoid valve is going to flow well in relation to its size and electrical requirement, it must have a relatively high armature lift. Figure 3-6A (in the sidebar) demonstrates how armature lift, relative to the diameter of the flow orifice, affects gross flow. To gather this data a number of nitrous valves were tested in stock form and with some port enlargement. As demonstrated in these tests, the principal factor affecting flow is adequate armature lift in relation to the flow orifice diameter.

The bottom line of all the foregoing is simple: there is more to solenoid design than meets the eye. If solenoid size and current requirement are not important, it is better to use a large valve. If you err on the high side, i.e., a solenoid that is far too big for the job, performance and reliability will not be adversely affected. On the other hand, if space requirements and current draw are important considerations, smaller valves are the only answer. In this situation, *it is important to make absolutely certain that the flow capabilities of the valves will meet the system requirements.*

Kit manufacturers are always concerned about ease-of-installation and reliability. Consequently, most reputable kit manufacturers have spent considerable time and money to research valve and solenoid design so that they can, as nearly as possible, optimize their systems. Even if you consider buying solenoid valves and building your own nitrous installation from scratch, *it is a good idea to buy solenoid valves from a company that has experience with the unique and specific requirements of nitrous-oxide injection.*

SUPPLY LINES

Supplying the enrichment fuel for a nitrous system is relatively simple. The fuel must be delivered at the correct pressure and it must be filtered to ensure against blockage of the metering orifices. In almost all cases these requirements can be met with standard, off-the-shelf fuel-delivery components.

The same cannot be said for the nitrous supply. On the nitrous side of the system it is important to achieve as little pressure drop as possible from the bottle to the point of injection. Most installations use a bottle mounted in the rear of the vehicle with long supply lines to carry the nitrous to the engine. These lines tend to be relatively small in diameter. Tube sizes of 3/32- to 1/8-inch are not uncommon, but larger diameters are often used on all-out competition kits.

First, let's consider the smaller lines. It appears that nitrous-oxide flowing through a small line would experience a considerable pressure loss between the storage bottle and the solenoid valve. Experiments by Don Laughlan, of Alden Automotive in England, showed that a pressure drop of 100psi is not uncommon during normal operation. This is a surprisingly high pressure drop, bearing in mind that even a 3/32-inch line has a far greater cross-section area than the combined area of the orifices in the spraybar on a typical street system. The moral here is that a larger line is better. If the line is not sufficiently large, the ultimate limiting factor to flow may not necessarily be the metering orifices. It is very likely that a major portion of the pressure loss is created by wall friction. In other words, even though the restricting orifice (jet) may be the smallest area in the system, *wall friction in the*

SOLENOID SCIENCE

The nitrous solenoid must be able to flow more nitrous than the minimum system restriction (calibration jet or orifices) at maximum boost. If it cannot, the solenoid will restrict nitrous delivery and become an unintended calibration orifice. In addition, the restricted nitrous flow may super-cool the solenoid and cause the valve to freeze in the open position.

Current state-of-the-art nitrous solenoids are substantially better than earlier models. In the "good old days" make-shift systems often used solenoid valves that had been adapted from other applications. This is no longer necessary, fortunately, but there may still be some kits available with solenoid valves that limit the boost potential.

The author tested several valves—in both stock and modified form—with a simple fixture and a rotometer to measure the flow. In general, "modified" valves flowed less nitrous than stock valves; and if the flow did increase, the change was very marginal. It is interesting to look at a typical example. A stock NOS valve was altered to duplicate the most common type of modifications. The entry and exit to the central port were drilled oversize and the central port was enlarged from 0.110- to 0.125-inch. The stock solenoid valve (test #3) flowed 220 units; the highly modified valve (test #4) flowed 217. This is an impressive performance loss, and a lot of work!

The disadvantage of a modified valve doesn't stop here. The original valve would operate with nitrous pressure up to 1025psi; the modified valve would not operate at pressures above 900psi. Obviously, the increased area of the central port made it more difficult for the magnetic field to pull the plunger off the seat.

When the central port is enlarged it is also essential to re-machine the plunger seat that surrounds the port. The drilling operation inevitably distorts the seat, and if the seat is not reformed, the plunger will not seal properly.

At this point it looks like modifications are in vain and the best alternative is to use a larger valve. However, something else enters the picture. Most solenoid-actuated valves have armature lifts in the region of 0.015- to 0.025-inch. This is not enough lift for most nitrous applications!

Unless the armature rises away from the seat by a distance that equals 0.4 times the diameter of the flow orifice, the armature itself will restrict flow. In other words, if the armature is not lifted high enough, the open area between the armature and the seat will not be large enough to flow the same amount of nitrous as the main flow port in the valve body. However, most nitrous solenoids have a central flow port that is about 0.060 to 0.125-inch in diameter. With this much flow area in the body, the

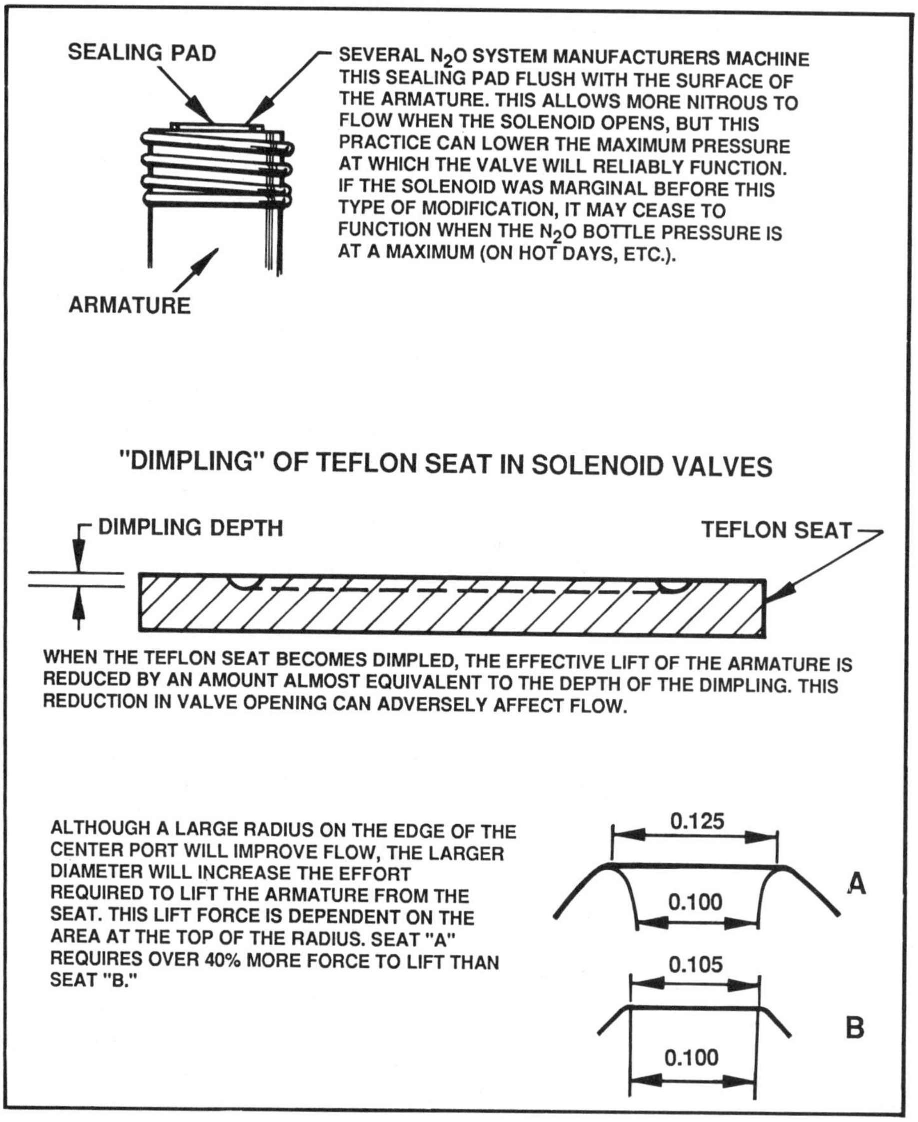

FIGURE 3-6A: Effects of Seat Dimpling on Armature Lift

supply pipe will dictate using as large a line as is practical between the bottle and the solenoid.

If the conditions under which the vehicle is operated are constant, a supply line with a relatively small internal diameter may not be of great importance as far as consistent performance is concerned; but if the vehicle is operated under a wide variety of conditions—temperature is the most likely factor to vary—the pressure in the supply bottle will rise or fall considerably. Under certain conditions, pressure decline in the system and pressure loss due to wall friction in the supply line may adversely affect engine performance. This ultimately can affect car performance and consistency, which may be important in certain types of racing cars (particularly bracket drag-race cars).

LINE COOLING

The greatest cause of inconsistent nitrous performance is temperature variation in the supply line between the solenoid valve and the spraybar or jets. If the solenoid is located in a

SOLENOID NUMBER	ORIFICE DIA	LIFT	FLOW UNITS	FLOW/THOUSANTHS OF SQ-IN DIA.
1–N.O.S. CHEATER	0.076	0.040	132	29.1
2–N.O.S. POWER SHOT +	0.072	0.025	85	20.9
3–N.O.S. PRO SHOT	0.110	0.040	220	23.2
4–N.O.S. PRO SHOT DRILLED OUT	0.125	0.040	217	17.7
5–UNNAMED BRAND SOLENOID WITH DIMPLED SEAL	0.095	0.036	*	*
6–AS ABOVE WITH NEW SEAL GROUND FLUSH	0.085	0.036	165	23.3
7–N.O.S. MODIFIED PRO SHOT	0.110	0.050	237	25.0

* DID NOT REGISTER ON GAUGE THAT MEASURED A MINIMUM OF 70 UNITS OF FLOW

\+ A VERY COMPACT SOLENOID FOR PLATE MOUNTING (FOR KITS IN THE 110–130 HP RANGE)

FIGURE 3-6B: These are the results of flow tests performed on various nitrous solenoids. In general, flow efficiencies improve when the armature lifts higher in relation to orifice size. Although flow efficiency is important, high-boost systems must deliver large quantities of nitrous, therefore, gross flow becomes the most important factor. Test #5 demonstrates how much flow can be lost by a "dimpled" seat.

armature lift should be at least .030 to 0.050-inch.

A few numbers will give you an idea of how much flow can vary. An NOS "Cheater" solenoid with a 0.076-inch central port and a 0.040-inch lift flows 132 units; restricting the lift to 0.025-inch drops the flow to 85 units. Many older valves had an 0.072-inch port and an armature lift of only 0.020-inch. This type of valve flows less than 80 units.

Of course, if the valve flows enough nitrous to satisfy the delivery requirements, the foregoing is of no real consequence. The problem arises only when the flow capability of the nitrous valve is inadequate for the boost levels desired.

Another point to remember: don't use outdated valves with Teflon seats (newer valves use a neoprene-type material). Teflon provides a good initial seal, but eventually the pounding of the plunger distorts the Teflon; and if the plunger doesn't land on exactly the same spot, the valve will leak. In fact, Teflon seals may leak so badly that prolonged seepage (overnight) into the intake manifold can cause a severe backfire or a substantial engine explosion upon start-up.

The flow capability of the valve will also be reduced if the Teflon seat "dimples" (see accompanying drawing). Test #5 indicates that a valve with a dimpled seat is so restrictive that the gauge did not even register (the lowest measurable reading is 70 units). On the other hand, when a new seat was installed, the valve registered a flow of 165 units. The lesson is simple: don't use valves with Teflon seats. Over a period of time the seat will inevitably dimple and the restricted nitrous flow will cause the system to produce less boost.

Certain kit manufacturers supply solenoid valves that have a "specially formulated material" on the seat. This material is supposedly pliable enough to return to the preformed shape—even at very low temperatures and over an extended period of time. I was not able to test one of these valves, but if this material lives up to the manufacturers' claims, it should improve the reliability of the valve.

Based on the foregoing it would seem wise to leave the solenoid valves alone (unless you have equipment to accurately test the result of any modification). If there is clear evidence that the valves are causing a restriction, buy new valves that are rated for the intended application.

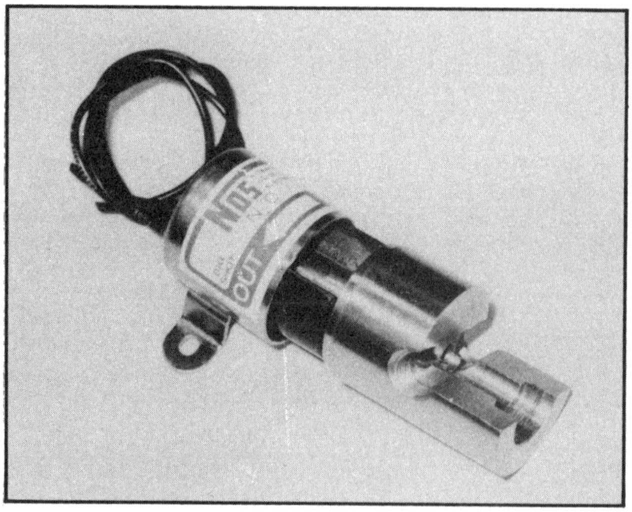

This cutaway illustrates the basic simplicity of a solenoid-operated valve. These valves are reliable but must be matched to the flow requirements of the system.

high-temperature area, the operating temperature of the solenoid valve will rise considerably, and this will undoubtedly contribute to inconsistent performance.

Here's what happens. Ambient heat (from the surrounding environment) will be absorbed by the solenoid and the supply line(s) leading from the solenoid to the spraybar or jets. When nitrous flow is first initiated, the high temperature in the solenoid and supply lines causes the nitrous to boil and turn to gas. This boiling action absorbs heat and within a short time—one to two seconds—the line cools sufficiently for the nitrous to remain in a liquid state right up to the point of injection. In those first few seconds, however, the operation of the nitrous can be very inconsistent because the nitrous is being injected as a low-density vapor. If a relatively large dose of nitrous is being used and line temperatures are high, the mass of nitrous injected into the engine will be unusually low; nonetheless, the engine will still receive a full dose of enrichment fuel. This causes the fuel/air ratio to momentarily go very rich, and the engine bogs.

Fortunately, there are several ways to circumvent this problem. The simplest is to "prepare" the system for action just prior to making a pass by depressing the control button very briefly while the engine is running. This purges the line of the gaseous nitrous and cools the supply lines sufficiently so that the system is primed with liquid nitrous. In racing vernacular this maneuver is sometimes known as "burping" the system.

It is possible to achieve the same results with a nitrous bleed valve. In essence, this is an additional solenoid valve—a small one is sufficient—that bleeds nitrous from the supply line. In effect, this primes the supply line with liquid nitrous-oxide. When it's time to punch the system for real, all of the supply lines are sufficiently cool to feed dense liquid nitrous-oxide into the engine.

Taking this one step further, some Pro Stock racers (and I believe the late Lee Sheppard tried this on one of his Pro Stock cars) have developed a system that bleeds nitrous into a sleeve-like tube surrounding the nitrous supply line. The end of this sleeve is open to atmosphere. As the nitrous converts to a gaseous state, heat is absorbed, and the nitrous supply line is, in effect, super cooled. When the system is activated during a race, the cold line instantly feeds liquid nitrous into the engine.

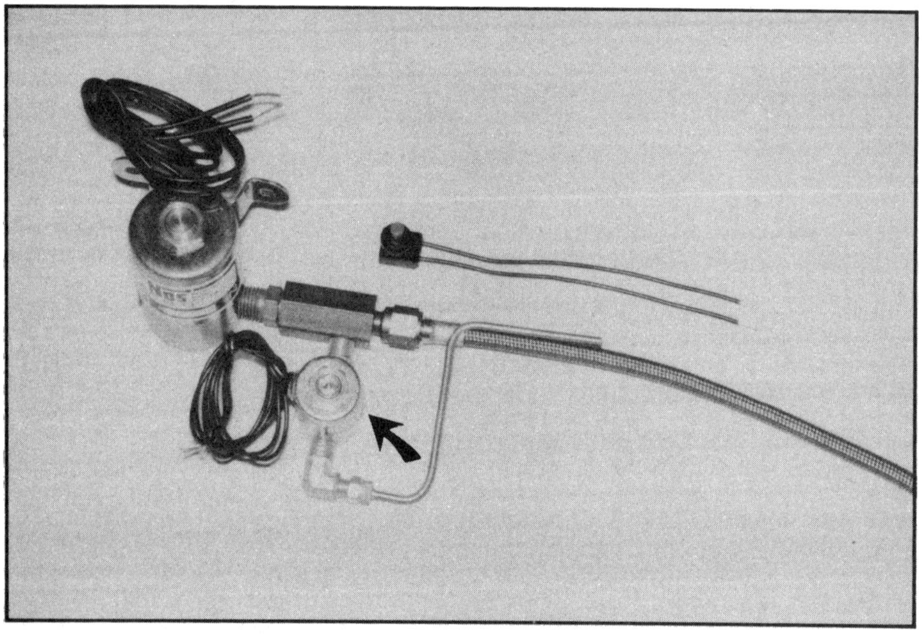

The initial response will improve if a bleed solenoid (bottom) is used to prime the supply line with super-cold liquid nitrous. The blast from the bleed line should be diverted toward the nitrous supply line to cool it even more. This effect can be increased if a shroud is used to direct the nitrous along the length of the supply line. The distribution line(s) leading from the solenoid to the point of injection should also be cooled; but considering the number of lines involved, this could be difficult with a port-injection system.

FUEL PUMP

Though fuel pumps are rarely included in kits, they are one of the most important factors contributing to reliable engine operation and performance. If the fuel pump capacity is inadequate during system operation, the fuel supply will drop off and the mixture will become extremely lean. Naturally, this leads to detonation and/or melted pistons.

The fuel pump must have sufficient capability for the job at hand. This means that the fuel pump must deliver not only adequate pressure but also adequate volume. It is important not to confuse these two factors. The fuel pressure produced by a "stalled" pump—one that is pumping against a blockage or restriction on the pressure side—can be considerably higher than the fuel pressure delivered when the pump is operating without a downstream restriction. In the second case the actual *volume* delivered by the pump will be a lot higher, even though the pressure may be lower.

For proper functioning, most nitrous kits require a fuel pressure of about 4.0 to 6.0psi. Although for some European vehicles 3.0psi is an acceptable pressure, simply because on many European vehicles the fuel pumps deliver a lower pressure. There is a basic reason for this difference. Most domestic engines are fitted with pumps that develop higher delivery pressures because the engines are usually larger in displacement—requiring greater delivery volumes—and some of the performance models, especially those from the muscle-car era, are capable of exceptional acceleration performance. And, as the car accelerates forward, the mass of gasoline in the fuel line is pushed toward the rear. This means the pressure and delivery volume measured at the carburetor will be relatively lower during hard acceleration. To compensate, most performance fuel pumps are preset to deliver around 9.0psi (whereas most European vehicles deliver 3.0 to 4.0psi). This higher pressure ensures adequate pressure and volume at the carburetor float bowl during all normal (non-nitrous) operating conditions.

Assuming the vehicle is capable of rapid acceleration—as would be typical of a performance or racing car—when a nitrous system is added, it is necessary to keep the fuel pressure as high as is practicable, all the way to the point of injection. Just prior to the point of injection, a pressure-regulating valve should be installed in the system to reduce the fuel pressure to that specified by the kit manufacturer.

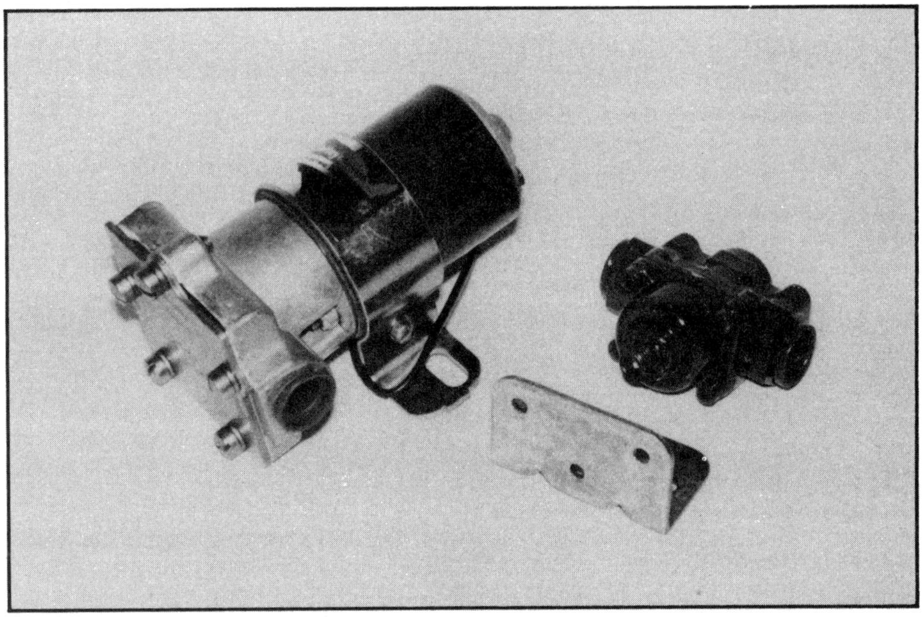

Enrichment fuel delivery to the nitrous system must be adequate in pressure and volume. If there is any doubt that the existing fuel system can deliver adequate fuel, a heavy-duty electric pump and a pressure regulator (mounted near the fuel solenoid) should be added.

On some vehicles, the fuel pressure delivered by the stock fuel pump may meet the pressure requirements specified by the kit manufacturer. However, delivery pressure is critical to ensure proper fuel enrichment when the nitrous system is activated, therefore, the pressure must be checked and verified accurately. Bear in mind that when the vehicle accelerates, the fuel pressure measured at the front of the vehicle will drop, so there is not much room for error. Too much is generally better—within reason—and too little can easily be disastrous.

If the car hooks well and leaves hard it is possible to lose between 4.0 and 6.0psi of delivery pressure at the carburetor due to the acceleration force. Here, I am talking about a car that is capable of producing forward acceleration of about 1.0g (i.e., 32.2 feet per second per second of acceleration). This is a relatively high acceleration rate for a car. Most street vehicles are not likely to hook this hard (due to tire and chassis practicalities for street use) and the initial acceleration for this type of vehicle will probably not exceed 0.5g (16 feet per second per second). Under these conditions, about 2.0psi of fuel pressure will be lost.

Based on these general performance levels, it is essential for a street car to have at least 2.0psi higher fuel pressure at the carburetor—just prior to the pressure-regulating valve—than is specified by the nitrous kit manufacturer. On a drag-race car with good suspension, *the delivery pressure to the regulator must be at least 4.0psi and sometimes as much as 6.0psi in* <u>*excess*</u> *of the minimum delivery pressure specified by the kit manufacturer.* The pressure regulating valve should be adjusted to produce the delivery pressure specified by the manufacturer. If the valve is mounted near the point of injection there will be very little pressure loss on the delivery side of the regulator.

Most domestic vehicles utilize an engine-driven mechanical fuel pump (usually a lever-operated diaphragm-type pump) to deliver fuel to the carburetor. This type of pump must draw fuel through the long supply line leading forward from the rear-mounted (in most cases) fuel tank. In general, these pumps are susceptible to "stalling" problems because they are designed for late model (low-power) engines and can draw only a limited amount of fuel through the supply line. To ensure adequate fuel delivery for a nitrous system, it is often necessary to install an auxiliary electric pump near the tank to work in conjunction with (or in place of) the stock mechanical pump.

This is not always necessary. If the vehicle is stock or near-stock in every other respect and the nitrous kit is not excessively powerful (i.e., it produces less than about 125 horsepower), the stock mechanical pump may be adequate or there may be a high-performance model that will produce sufficient fuel delivery. If you think this may be the case, it is a good idea to check with the kit manufacturer to determine if they have had experience with the specific mechanical fuel pump and delivery system you are considering. They may be able to tell you if the pump and kit are compatible.

The high-output mechanical pump fitted to some Chevrolet performance engines has changed very little in the past 15 years. This is a pretty good mechanical pump, and if the vehicle is to be used for street applications with street tires, this pump will probably handle gross power outputs up to about 300 horsepower. If the projected power output will exceed 300 horsepower, it is necessary to test the pump to ensure that it will meet the delivery requirements specified by the manufacturer of the nitrous kit. Motors producing over 350 horsepower will almost certainly require an auxiliary electric pump at the tank. If the car is to be used for drag racing and is on slicks, a mechanical pump simply will not be adequate (if the car is really capable of hooking) and a high-pressure, high-volume electric pump or multiple pumps will be mandatory.

If there is any doubt about the ability of the existing pump, be it mechanical or electrical, to supply the required amount of fuel for additional power given by the nitrous kit, then *it will be necessary to test the flow under working conditions.*

The most common high-performance electrical unit is the competition Holley pump. This is a good

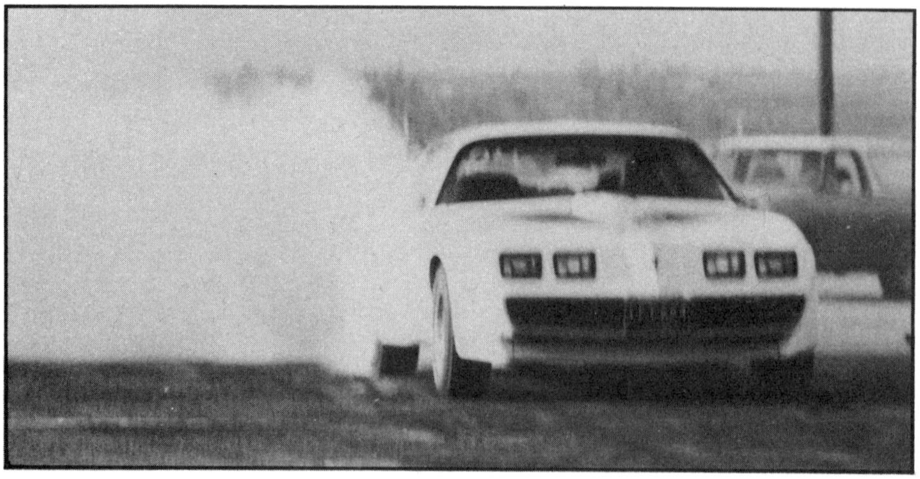

The author warms the tires of his 350cid Chevy-powered Firebird during drag testing. This engine develops 550 horsepower and 570 lbs/ft of torque. Needless to say, this requires a lot of fuel; an electric pump was mounted close to the tank.

pump, however, it is not always necessary to opt for a competition pump. Most production fuel pumps will deliver pressure and volume in excess of that needed by the carburetor. As long as the pump delivers a pressure adequate to supply flow requirements for the nitrous system, it will work just fine. Most pumps designed for V8 engines will meet this requirement. This is mentioned primarily because high-pressure and/or high-volume competition fuel pumps are expensive. One of these pumps would be a good choice for a street or racing nitrous system but not always essential.

Another good fuel pump to consider is the Walbro pump. This pump has a very high stall pressure, so precautions must be taken to prevent difficulties. But before discussing this, let's consider how an electric pump is hooked into the system. Figure 3-7 shows the recommended method of wiring an electric fuel pump in a typical nitrous system. The point to note here is that the additional "boost" pump is wired to activate when the *arming switch* is turned on, not when the firing switch is actuated. This is important. If the pump is turned on by the firing switch, there will be a delay in fuel delivery when the system is fired. It will take a few seconds for the pump to fill the fuel lines that carry the enrichment fuel—especially if this line is relatively long—before flow is actually initiated at the injection nozzle. When this happens, the nitrous-oxide—which is delivered immediately due to the pressure in the nitrous cylinder—will reach the combustion chambers before the enrichment fuel. This results in a momentary lean condition that will lead to overheating and almost certainly to detonation.

If a Walbro pump is used in the system, the line pressure will be very high—in fact, up to 125psi (under "stall" conditions). In some situations this may be too much fuel pressure. It will be necessary, in this instance, to install a *return line* to the tank. This line must be fitted with a suitably-sized restriction or bleed jet so that the Walbro pump develops a maximum delivery pressure of about 50psi.

The Walbro pump is ideally suited for a dual-fuel engine that uses gasoline for the main system and alcohol for the nitrous enrichment. Under these circumstances, a nitrous system originally designed for a gasoline engine can be used; but to achieve sufficient fuel flow for the alcohol enrichment, the *minimum* delivery pressures must be in the 35 to 45psi range. This is higher than the max pressure a Holley competition pump can develop, but quite within the capability of the Walbro. However, though it develops high pressure, the Walbro does not deliver as much volume as the Holley pump. As a result, depending upon the horsepower boost produced by the system, the fuel requirement must be checked to ensure that it does not exceed the capability of the Walbro pump. (Remember, when alcohol is used, the fuel requirement will be 2.5 times the comparable gasoline volume.)

Another thing to remember is that most automotive fuel pumps do not cope well with alcohol for extended periods. The synthetic rubber used in virtually all diaphragm-type automotive pumps will inevitably swell when exposed to alcohol. However, the Walbro pump—which has steel internal components—can cope with alcohol for extended periods of time.

If the engine is equipped with a Hilborn fuel-injection system, the Hilborn mechanical pump has enough capacity to supply the enrichment fuel (alcohol) for the nitrous system. This can be accomplished easily by teeing into the high-pressure line (at the appropriate location), routing the fuel through a pressure regulator and then to the enrichment-fuel distribution lines. The pressure regulator must be able to handle an input line pressure of 100 to 120psi and regulate the output pressure down to about 40 to 50psi. (A standard Holley pressure regulator is not built for these very high pressures.)

An interesting alternative on an alcohol engine is to use gasoline as an enrichment fuel. If there is enough room in the chassis to carry a small additional fuel tank and a battery, this type of system may be worth considering. Less enrichment fuel— less volume relative to alcohol—is required with this system. In addition, a conventional electric fuel pump will deliver the required pressure and volume.

A point worth noting here is that many of the basic kits for street use

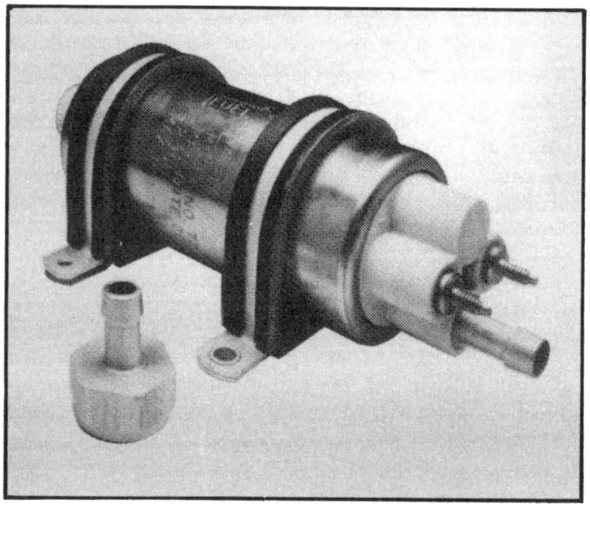

This high-performance fuel pump is manufactured by Walbro Automotive Products. A powerhouse of a pump, it can deliver over 100psi from its rotary vane design. The Walbro (OEM on some Bosch injection systems) is readily available from Toyota, Nisson and Cadillac dealers, and directly from Walbro (see buyers guide, pgs. 126-127).

do not include a pressure-regulating valve. In fact, very few nitrous kits—street or racing—include a pressure regulator. Almost all kit manufacturers sell fuel regulators as an extra "option." It would be wise to purchase a suitable pressure regulator along with the kit. One of the most convenient pressure regulators is the one that has an extra port to accommodate a pressure gauge. With a gauge installed at the regulator it is very simple to adjust the delivery pressure accurately and the driver can monitor the gauge to ensure that the system and regulator are functioning properly.

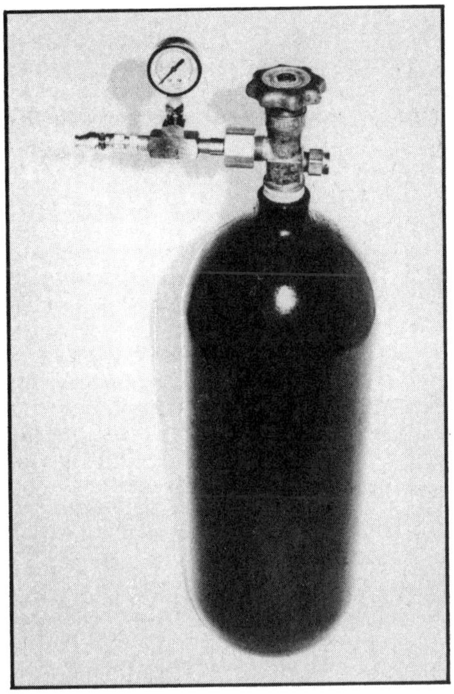

A bottle that holds 15 pounds of nitrous is supplied with most kits. Larger bottles substantially reduce the storage space in a small trunk. Smaller bottles restrict the total available activation time of the system.

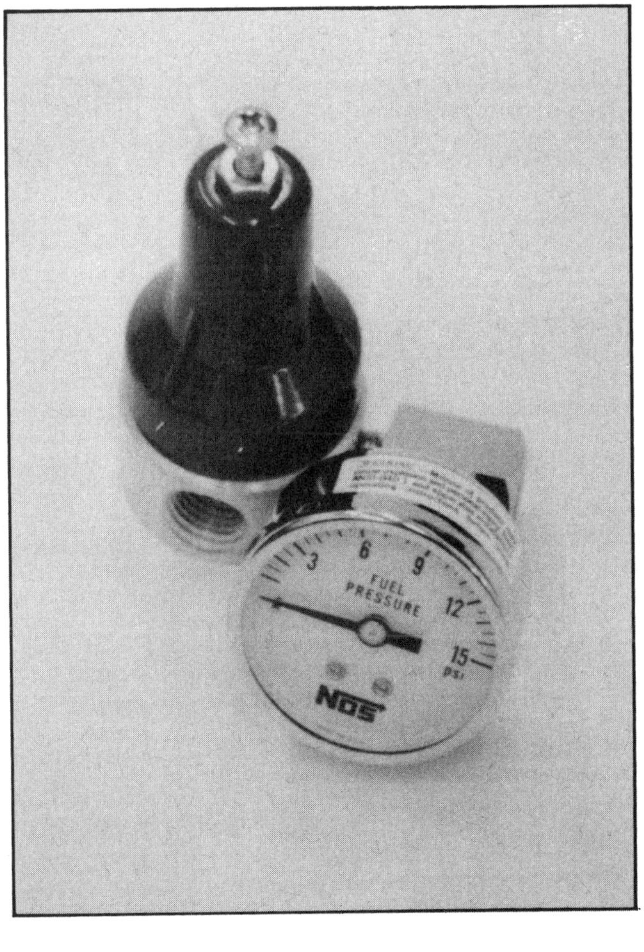

An adjustable pressure regulator and a fuel pressure gauge are essential tools for tuning the nitrous system to track conditions.

BOTTLE PRESSURIZATION

Apart from the ability to contain high pressure, it is easy to believe that a nitrous-oxide storage bottle is a relatively insignificant component. This is not the case. Apart from mounting the bottle in an appropriate and, as near as the installation situation will allow, optimum position, there are certain factors about the bottle that greatly affect the consistency of the power output.

The most obvious factor is bottle temperature. If the bottle temperature is elevated and nears the critical temperature of 98 degrees (F), when the nitrous-oxide is injected, it can, in certain areas downstream of a minimal point, convert to a gas and further restrict the flow. Conversely, if the bottle temperature is too low, the internal pressure drops. In combination with engine heat input at the injection point, this may cause the system to react slowly when first activated. A good compromise is achieved when the bottle temperature is about 65 to 80 degree (F). These temperatures will produce an internal bottle pressure of about 700 to 850psi.

If a nitrous system is operated under extremely high ambient temperatures—such as on a hot summer day—the bottle temperature rises to substantial levels, even if the bottle is not in direct sunlight. Under these conditions (and if time will allow) it is a good idea to cool the bottle. This can be accomplished by placing a wet cloth(s) on the bottle and using a fan to cool the surface (via evaporation). If possible, a better solution is to put the bottle in a bucket of ice.

A measure of cooling can also be achieved by releasing some of the nitrous-oxide. This causes the nitrous to boil off and absorb some of the heat, reducing the bottle temperature. There are certain obvious drawbacks to this method. The vented nitrous-oxide is wasted and when the bottle contains less nitrous, the system may lose some efficiency. Many racers feel that nitrous systems produce more power when the bottle is over half full. This is not an illusion. This is substantiated by several reliable sources, but knowledgeable experts seem at a loss to explain this phenomenon with total assurance.

The most probable reason for the initial part of a nitrous-oxide bottle giving more power than the remnants of a near-empty bottle stems from a situation arising from the ratio of liquid to gaseous content of the bottle. The best way to envisage this situation is to imagine a bottle that is totally full of liquid nitrous-oxide. In other words, no gaseous nitrous-oxide exists in the bottle. Let us also assume that the bottle is sitting under pressure of 750psi. Now imagine that we can instantly remove a certain amount of nitrous-oxide from the bottle, say 5.0 cubic inches. This would, of course, go as a liquid; and for an infinitesimally instant in time, there would exist a vacuum above the liquid nitrous-oxide. Under these circumstances, the nitrous-oxide would boil violently to give off gas so as to re-establish the 750 pounds pressure, known as the vapor pressure, in the bottle.

Let's now assume that we instantly remove another 5.0 cubic inches of nitrous-oxide from the bottle. This time, we have 750psi of gas pressure above the liquid nitrous-oxide. Removing 5.0 more cubic inches and creating 10.0 cubic inches of space above the liquid nitrous will cause the gas to momentarily drop to 375psi. The liquid nitrous-oxide will now boil but not as violently as it did in the first instance to rebuild that 375psi back up to 750psi. As you can see, if this chain of events is followed on down the line until the bottle is almost empty, we find that at the far end of the scale, when only a few cubic inches of nitrous remains in the bottle, taking some more out of the bottle will only cause the nitrous to boil at a relatively low rate. In other words, what happens is that as the nitrous is used, the rate at which it reestablishes the vapor pressure becomes slower. So the rate of flow of nitrous toward the end of the bottle will be reduced compared to flow rates from a full bottle.

This situation was appreciated by early experimenters (during World War II) and, more recently, by unlimited hydroplane engine builders, who currently use generous quantities of nitrous in war-surplus V12 engines. These developers found that it was necessary to stabilize the flow of nitrous-oxide to the engine, no matter how much nitrous was contained in the bottle. One of the workable solutions is to pressurize the nitrous-oxide bottle with nitrogen gas (see Figure 3-7).

When the nitrous-oxide container is pressurized to 3000psi and the container temperature is held below 98 degrees, the nitrous-oxide in the container remains in liquid form. If a pressure-regulator valve is used downstream to regulate the nitrous-oxide back to some pre-determined pressure—usually about 1000psi—totally consistent results can be achieved, no matter if the bottle is 90% full or 10% full.

With this type of system the engine performance will be very consistent, but if the bottle is totally exhausted of nitrous, the engine will suddenly cease to function. Instead of injecting the oxygen-rich nitrous-oxide, the system will deliver pure nitrogen to the engine. Nitrogen very effectively *dampens combustion.* This dampening effect, combined with the super-rich fuel delivery (caused by the added enrichment fuel from the nitrous system), will cause the engine to cease running just as surely as if the ignition system were turned off.

It is also essential to use a *nitrogen bottle*—as opposed to a nitrous-oxide bottle—to store the nitrous-oxide in this system. The very high pressures created by the nitrogen can put an ordinary nitrous-oxide bottle dangerously near the maximum pressure limit. In fact, if you wish to use a system like this, it will be necessary to have it engineered by an experienced professional, because modified nitrous-oxide bottles will no longer conform to government specifications and they will be considered illegal.

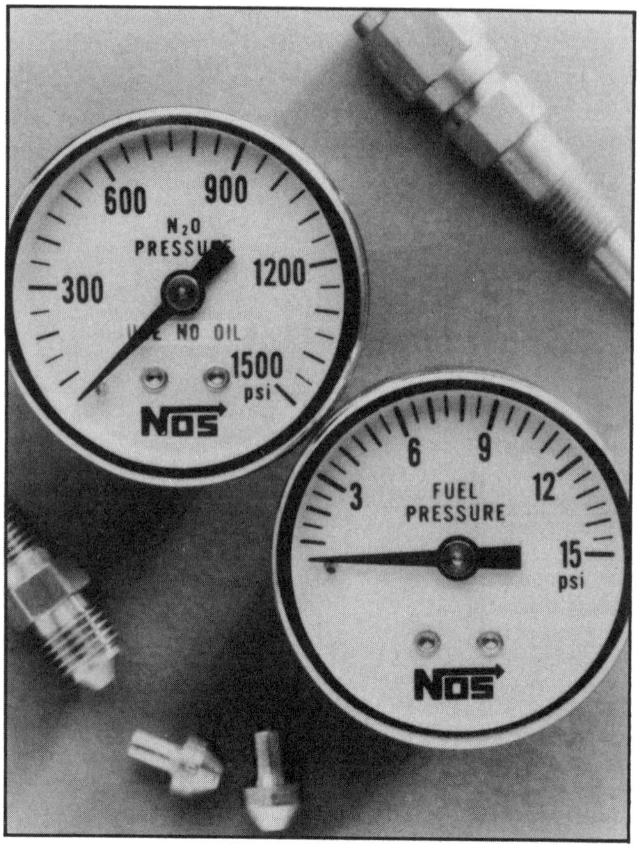

A nitrous pressure gauge is a useful accessory. It does not indicate the amount of nitrous remaining in the bottle; it reads the internal pressure (in pounds per square), which, in turn, reveals the temperature of the contents.

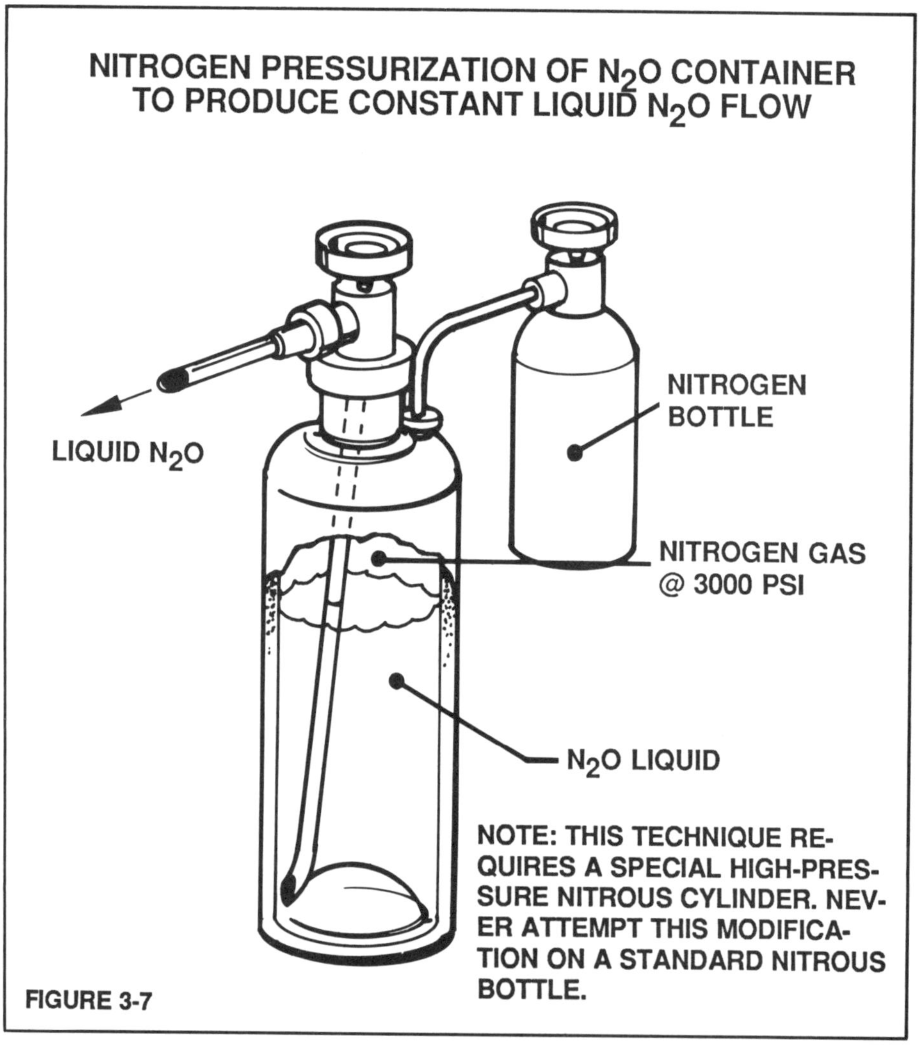

FIGURE 3-7

FIGURE 3-7: Regulated nitrogen pressure applied to the airspace inside a nitrous bottle will facilitate constant flow throughout the entire bottle life. (This is a general representation, not a detailed schematic of how to accomplish the job.)

ACCESSORIES

Some of the most useful nitrous accessories are part of the system "plumbing." This includes many of the components required to easily and safely install the nitrous bottle and supply lines: T-fittings, bulkhead fittings, distribution blocks, and various hose adapters. And remember, if you are installing a port-injection system and plan to bend the distribution tubes yourself, you are undertaking a relatively difficult job. A careful survey of the available components to aid such a plumbing job will almost certainly make this task easier.

VALVES AND FILTERS

Sooner or later, there is the possibility that the nitrous solenoid will leak—especially if it is an older solenoid with a Teflon seat. If the solenoid allows nitrous to collect inside the intake manifold, a backfire during start-up will cause an intake explosion. If the car has been sitting for a long time with even a slight leak, a lot of nitrous will collect in the manifold. And make no mistake about it, if a highly volatile mixture of nitrous and fuel lights off inside the confines of a manifold, it is going to do a lot of damage. The carburetor throttle shafts will almost certainly be severely bent, and the manifold may even be fractured. In almost every case, this unhappy event is going to result in a heavy-duty repair bill.

It is, therefore, wise to take precautions against nitrous leaks. When the vehicle is parked or left overnight, it is always a worthwhile precaution to turn off the valve on the nitrous bottle. However, this can be a hassle: the driver has to get out of the car, go around to the back of the vehicle, open the trunk—the most usual place to install the bottle—and turn off the valve. Easy enough, but nonetheless a hassle. And next morning, of course, if the driver is distracted, he forgets to reverse the procedure, and just when he wants to use the nitrous, he remembers that he forgot to open the bottle valve. A good accessory to bypass this difficulty is a remote valve. This valve is placed in the nitrous supply line and allows the driver to turn the nitrous supply off from inside the vehicle. The bottle valve need only be turned on or off when the bottle is installed or removed from the car.

It is important to prevent dirt and particles from entering the supply lines. This unwanted debris can damage the sealing surfaces of the all-important valves and solenoids. Some nitrous-oxide kits have filters in the supply line. Some of these filters will only catch large particles, while others will trap even the very tiniest bits of jetsam. Obviously, a fine filter is better, but whatever filter is used, *it must be capable of flowing more volume than the nitrous restriction that controls the delivery volume.* If not, the filter will reduce the volume of nitrous flowing through the system, and the system will not react properly when the jet or primary flow restriction is altered.

Some manufacturers use a small piece of steel wire mesh to filter the nitrous as it flows through the bottle valve. This is only barely adequate. This screen no doubt catches most of the troublesome debris; but in some cases, the orifices in the spray bar have a greater total area than the combined area of the holes in the wire screen. As a result, the screen ends up "jetting" the system. Sometimes the reverse applies, and the holes in the screen are individually larger than the spray-bar orifices. The result is that particles can go through the screen but not through the orifices. This will eventually allow the spray orifices to become blocked by debris.

When buying a kit, it is important to determine if the manufacturer has included a filter somewhere in the system, and to check that the flow

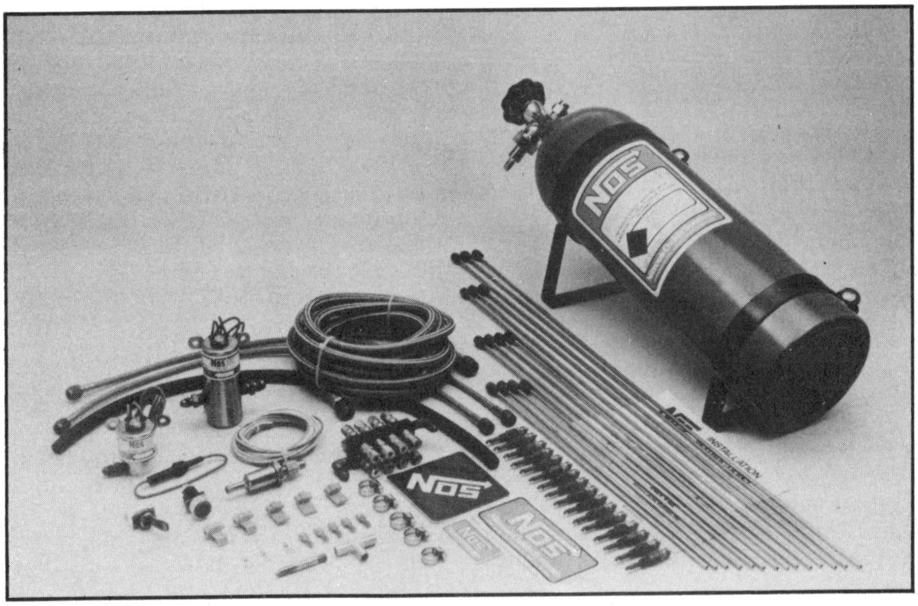

All of the accessories shown in this photo are available from NOS. High-quality accessories add considerably to the convenience and reliability of a nitrous system.

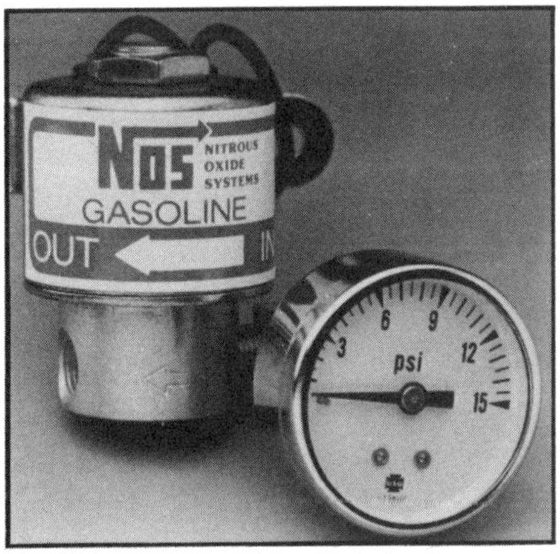

A fuel pressure gauge should be considered more of a system necessity than an accessory. This high-quality gauge combined with an accurate fuel-pressure regulator can help prevent expensive engine damage from insufficient enrichment fuel pressure.

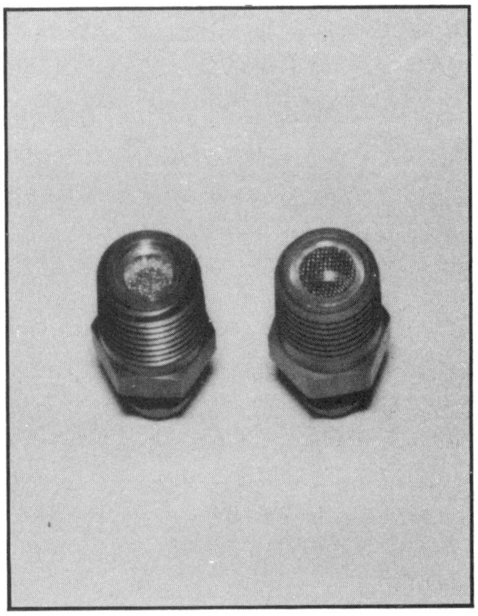

The screens or filtering elements of the nitrous and fuel filters should be inspected and replaced regularly.

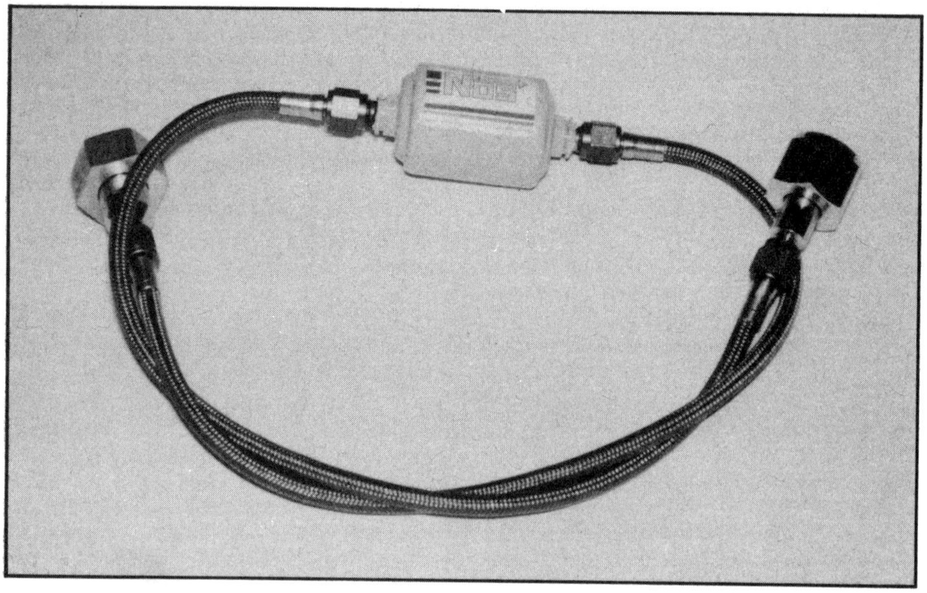

A large-capacity nitrous filter is an essential component of any high-output system. The flow capability of the filter must exceed the maximum flow requirements of the system (determined by the nitrous restriction orifice).

capacity and filtering capability are suitable. If the system does not have a filter, it is important to buy and install a proper one.

From my experience, the best type of filter to use is the so-called "sintered-bronze" filter. These filters are made of tiny bronze spheres (balls) pressed together and heated to a high temperature to bond them together. These filters look like they would be very restrictive, but they flow amazingly well. Of course, flow capability is still important; so the filter must be big enough for the job. You should be able to determine the flow requirements of the system and check this against the flow rating of the filter. However, if this is not possible, just make certain to use a very large filter! Problems can generally be avoided in a street application by using a large filter—about 1.25-inch in diameter—from a competition-type kit. Sometimes an adapter, like the 0.25-inch NPT adapter shown in the nearby photo, may be required. However, if you use this type of filter, remember this: because these filters do such a good job, they are prone to clogging and must be cleaned regularly. A good bet is to remove and clean the filter after each 10 to 12 bottle refills.

The primary consequence of blockage in the nitrous supply is a loss of horsepower, however, *if a fuel line, metering orifice or jet has become blocked, the engine air-fuel ratio will become lean when the system is activated and engine damage will almost certainly occur.* It is, therefore, extremely important to use a filter in the enrichment fuel system. Several different makes and models of fuel filters are available. Most of them do a good job, but once again, a large-capacity sintered-bronze filter will be an excellent choice. And of course, capacity is again important. The filter must be able to flow more fuel capacity than the total flow volume required from the fuel-enrichment system at wide-open throttle (max power). Remember, if the fuel system becomes blocked, the engine *will* melt down.

BOTTLE CONTENTS AND FLOW MEASUREMENT

The onboard storage bottle usually contains pressurized liquid nitrous-oxide until just a few moments before it is empty. However, the question of the *state* of the nitrous-oxide is important to performance. This is dependent, as we have already discussed, on the temperature and pressure of the bottle. It is useful to know these conditions, along with the amount of nitrous remaining in the bottle. Let's first deal with bottle temperature.

The temperature and pressure within a nitrous bottle vary in direct relationship with each other. (This is discussed in Chapter 1.) Therefore, if the nitrous bottle is fitted with a pressure gauge, the temperature can be determined by using the chart in Figure 1-4.

If the pressure gauge and chart prove too cumbersome, a temperature gauge can be fitted to the bottle. But be aware: A temperature gauge will react relatively slowly (compared with a pressure gauge). If the pressure gauge is used to monitor temperature, it reacts virtually instantaneously. A temperature gauge will not record a significant change until the temperature variation has spread throughout the contents. The amount of delay will depend on the volume of the contents and whether the bottle is made of steel or aluminum. However, if pressure is used as a means of determining temperature, the response time for the pressure gauge is a matter of

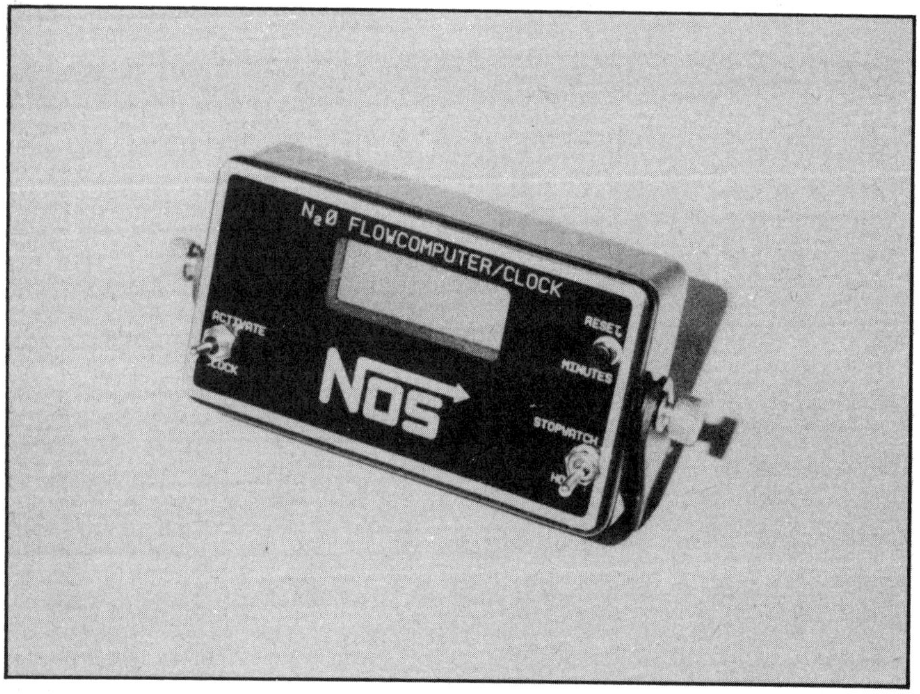

If the user knows the amount of nitrous in a full bottle and the rate of nitrous consumption, the total available operating time can be calculated. A system timer allows the user to accurately determine the remaining operating time (in seconds).

seconds, at the most.

Nitrous flow "counters" are also available. In effect, these are more accurately described as flow timers. They are nothing more than a simple stopwatch that starts when the nitrous system is fired and stops when it is released. This provides a reasonable estimate of the number of seconds (of usage) remaining before the bottle is empty. For instance, if the driver knows that a full bottle will last 20 seconds and the timer shows the system has been used for a total of 12 seconds, approximately 8 seconds remain before the nitrous is expended.

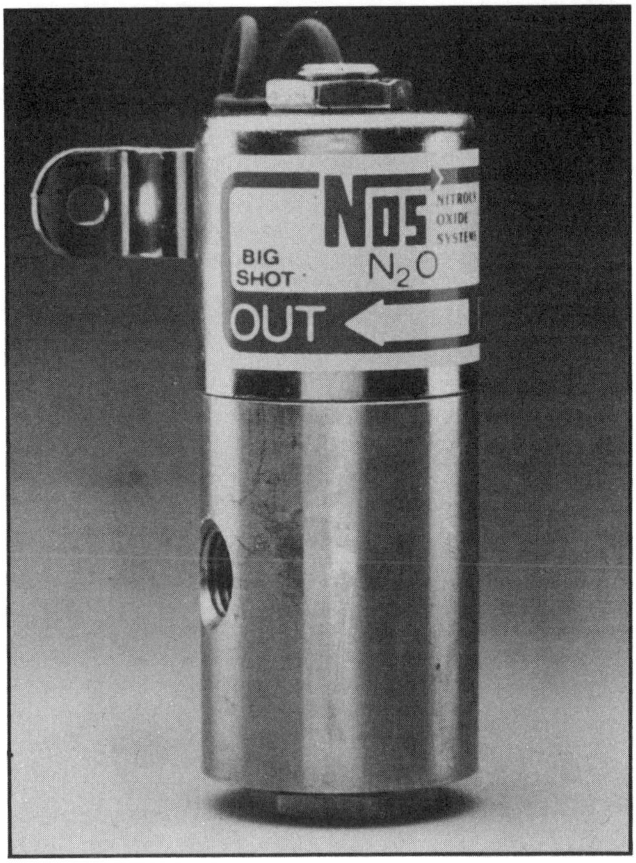

The major flow restrictions in most systems are the solenoids. This "Big-Shot" solenoid from NOS is typical of the high-flow solenoids used in nitrous systems on all-out racing engines.

A timer will give useful information if the user knows how much nitrous the system uses *in a given period of time* and the amount—the weight—of nitrous in the bottle. A bottle is usually "rated" for a nominal capacity. For instance, the most common nitrous bottle is usually rated at 10 pounds. This means it will hold a maximum of 10 pounds, but in actual fact, the bottle usually holds a little less than the rated weight when it is refilled.

To calculate the *actual weight* of the nitrous in a bottle, weigh the bottle after it has been refilled with nitrous and subtract the *tare weight* ("empty weight," which is normally stamped somewhere on the bottle). For instance, if the tare weight of the bottle is 10 pounds, 8 ounces and the bottle weighs 20 pounds, 2 ounces when filled with nitrous, the *actual contents* of the bottle weigh 9 pounds, 10 ounces (remember, there are 16 ounces in a pound). If the bottle is rated at 10 pounds, the user knows that it is not quite filled to maximum capacity.

The *rate of nitrous expenditure* can be determined by calculating the weight of nitrous in the bottle (using the method above), operating the system for a set number of seconds—say, 5 seconds—and again, determining the weight of the nitrous remaining in the bottle. When the remainder weight is subtracted from the starting weight, the result is the total amount of nitrous-oxide—in pounds—expended during the 5 seconds. Then, the total expenditure is divided by 5 (the total amount of time) to determine the rate of nitrous expenditure: *the amount of nitrous used by the system during each second of operation.*

For example, if we weigh the bottle at the beginning of the test and calculate that the bottle contains 9 pounds, 10 ounces of nitrous, and after the test firing we again weigh the bottle and calculate that it now contains exactly 7 pounds, 2 ounces—we would subtract the remainder from the beginning weight and determine that the system used 2 pounds, 8 ounces of nitrous during the 5 seconds of operation. Then, dividing the amount of nitrous expended by 5 (total seconds of operation), we determine that the system used exactly one-half pound of nitrous during each second of operation (2lb-8oz divided by 5.0 seconds equals 8oz/sec, which in decimal equivalent is 0.5 pounds per second).

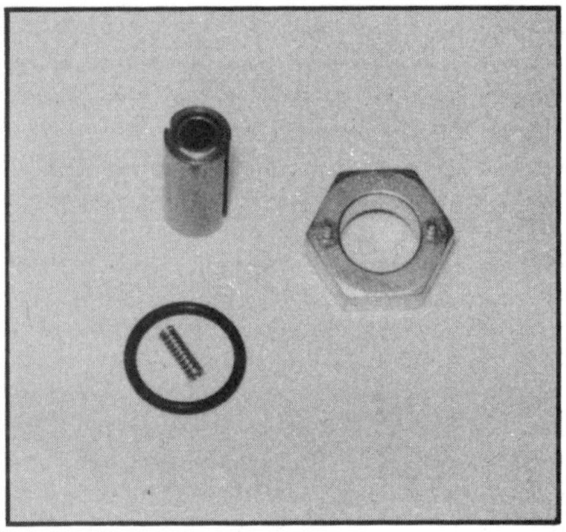

The components of the system must be inspected and serviced regularly to prevent malfunction or engine damage. Overhaul kits are available for solenoids supplied with most systems.

Once the rate of expenditure—the amount of nitrous used for each second of operation—is known for a specific system, we can calculate the *total available operating time* by dividing the rate of expenditure into the total weight of available nitrous. For example, let's suppose that we have a 10-pound nitrous bottle full of nitrous. We weigh the bottle (and contents) and calculate that, for the sake of this example, it contains a full 10 pounds of nitrous. In the example above, we determined that the rate of expenditure would be 0.5 pounds of nitrous for each second of operation. We divide the rate (0.5 pounds per second) into total nitrous weight in the bottle (10 pounds) and determine that the bottle contains enough nitrous for 20 seconds of total available operating time.

Once the total available operating time of the system is known, a flow indicator or system timer can be used, with a reasonable degree of accuracy, *to determine how long the system will operate before engine power drops off* and a bottle refill is required. However, there is, as the saying goes, a fly in the ointment. In actual practice the first pound of nitrous will be expended more quickly than the final pound. If, using our previous example, the first 5 pounds of nitrous lasts for 10 seconds of system operation, the last 5 pounds may last as long as 12 seconds before the bottle is totally empty. In actual practice this provides a comfortable margin for error, but performance will drop off as the bottle nears the "empty" condition. If you are in a serious racing situation, remember that *it is not wise to deplete the bottle even close to the empty weight because the engine horsepower will drop off.*

CHAPTER 4

NITROUS STREET SYSTEMS

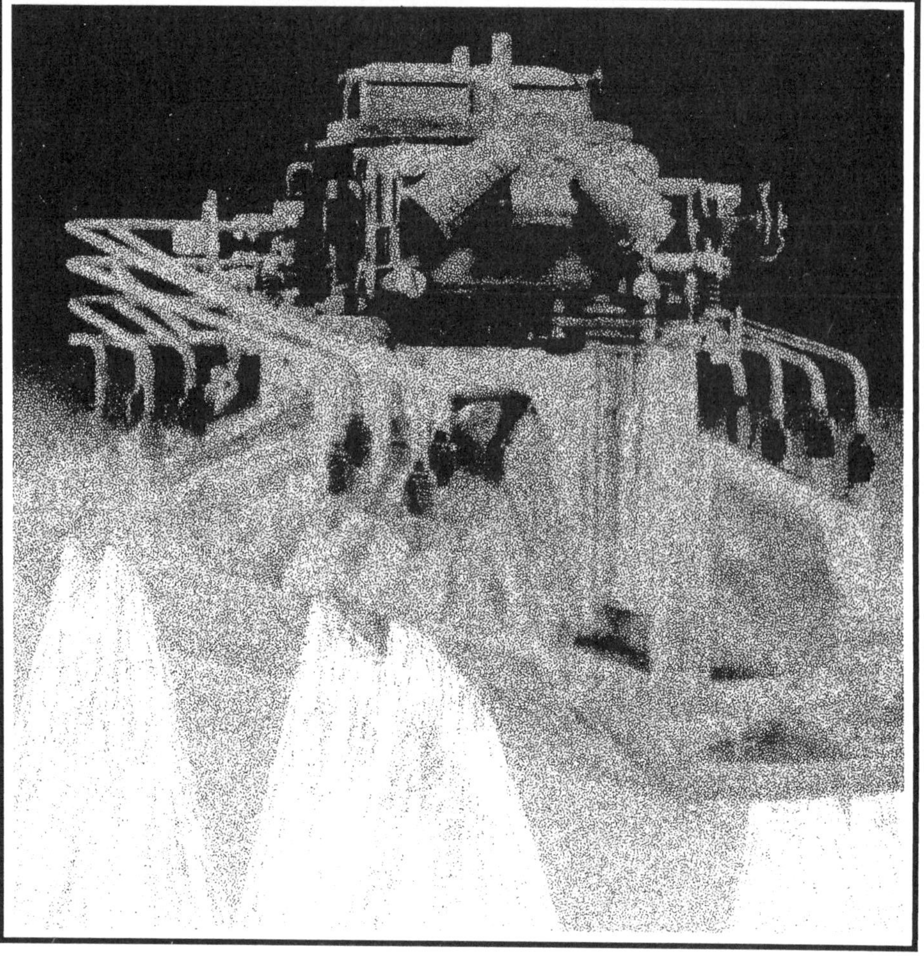

It's one thing to talk about the potential power of a nitrous kit, but it is quite another to actually demonstrate the power on the dynamometer or at the race track. In a previous chapter we discussed the power potential of some currently available kits. However, these were special race kits that had been extensively "tuned" to provide maximum effect. Although this is useful and valid research for a racing-type nitrous system, the results are not representative of those a typical user might expect. Therefore, in this chapter I will show the results that can be achieved with stock, off-the-shelf kits. Initially the kits were installed straight from the box and tested in totally stock form. In addition, though most users will install a kit and leave the calibration untouched, I think it will be worthwhile and interesting to see what improvements can be expected from a little fine tuning.

First, a word of caution. Virtually all of the tests results shown throughout this book were developed with my own fully instrumented dynamometer, which is highly sophisticated compared to some dyno installations. Also, in the interest of this research, I was quite prepared to "scrap" an engine or two. (Fortunately, despite all the measurements that were taken, very few serious engine problems occurred.) But most performance enthusiasts cannot afford a lot of dyno time to fine-tune a nitrous system, so it is important to note the following caution: *If any reader attempts the modifications or alterations described herein, it would be wise to do so in very small increments and to monitor the results very carefully. Often an engine will produce the very best results when it is on the verge of self-destruction!*

And always remember: If you desire more power, it is better to increase the flow of both nitrous-oxide and enrichment fuel delivered to the engine, rather than trying to "optimize" the effects of the current mixture flow. For the average user this boils down to a simple axiom: It is relatively safe to get 170 horsepower from a 200-horsepower kit, but it is very dangerous to modify or "tune" a 150-horsepower kit to produce 170 horsepower. In this instance, the 150-horsepower kit—operating beyond the design level—will almost certainly create excessive temperatures. However, the 200-horsepower kit—operating below the maximum design limit—will, in all likelihood, not cause any thermal problems. The author hopes that all readers will understand and remember this important axiom; and with this firmly in mind, let's look at some typically available street and competition kits.

At this point, it may be helpful to explain just how the dyno tests were conducted. To measure the power increase, the engine speed (rpm) was raised to the desired level and the computer-controlled load was set to hold the engine at that level. The nitrous was then activated. Of course, the power would increase dramatically, but the dyno load was readjusted to hold the rpm at the desired level. The nitrous system would remain activated for a period ranging from two to as much as ten seconds to allow the engine to stabilize and the load to be readjusted. The power reading was determined by simply pushing a button, which automatically recorded the instantaneous power level., This was done three times, at about one second intervals, and the three readings were averaged. In most of the tests shown here, power figures were taken at intervals between 3000 and 5500rpm.

If the system displayed any unusual tendencies, the nitrous was activated for longer than ten seconds in hopes that the level would eventually stabilize. In these instances the primary problem was usually power "surge." If the level did not stabilize after a reasonable period, the average of the minimum and maximum levels was recorded.

NOS STREET KITS

The first results that we'll explore are the tests of the Stage-1 street kit from Nitrous Oxide Systems. This kit was developed by NOS several years ago. It is quite popular, and while it is still available (at the time of writing), it has been superseded by the Power Shot system, which is simpler, cheaper, and apparently as effective—according to subsequent tests—as the Stage-1 kit.

Because both kits are similar, the Power Shot system was not tested to the same degree as the Stage-1 kit, and the accompanying chart contains only one set of power readings for the Power Shot kit. Prior to the first NOS system test, the author contacted Nitrous Oxide Systems to determine the power boost to be expected from the Stage-1 kit. They speculated that—on the particular engine used for this series of tests—the system should produce 115 to 125 horsepower.

As can be see from the data in Figure 4-1, the NOS Stage-1 kit produced 115 horsepower (rounded off to the nearest whole number). This is a substantial increase, but a secondary point that is worth noting here is that this company made an accurate estimate of the power produced by the kit. This is significant in view of the fact that some kit manufacturers have, at least in the past, sometimes been given to exaggerations.

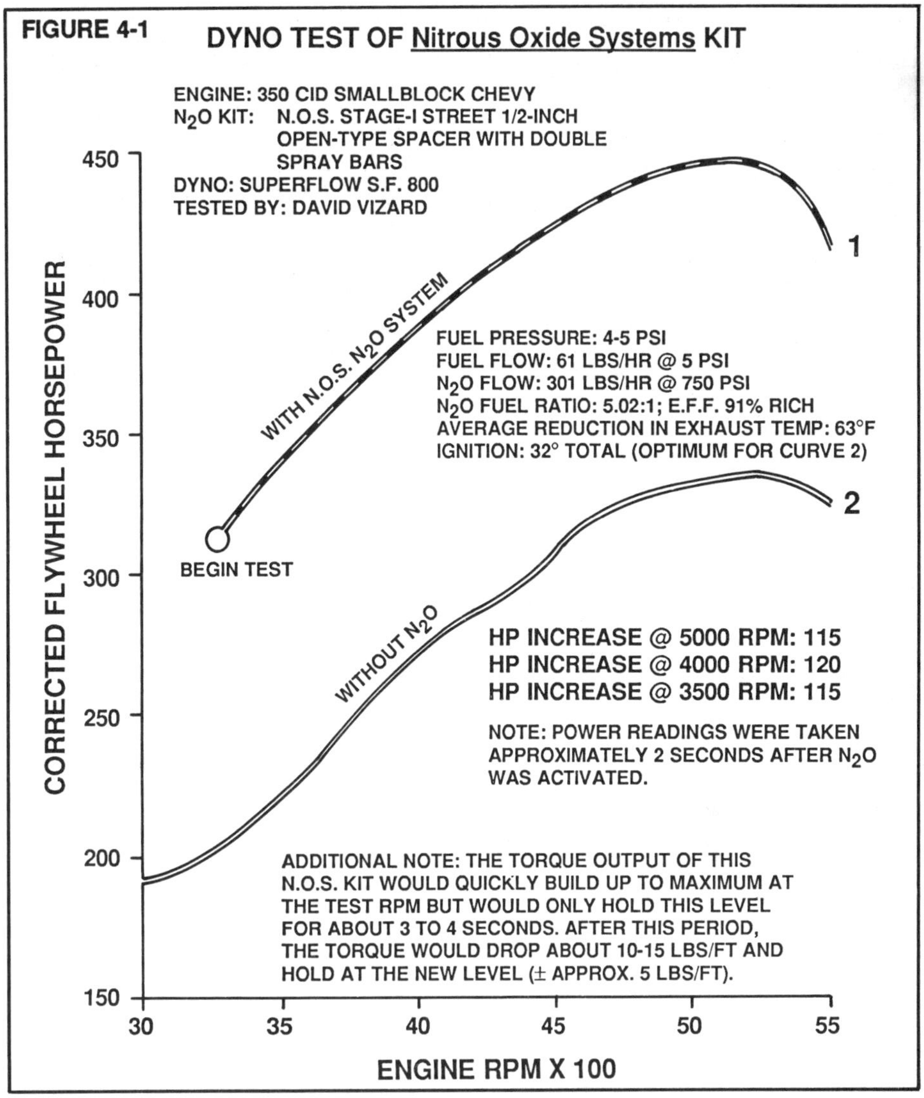

FIGURE 4-1: Dyno test of a NOS double-spraybar kit on 350cid smallblock Chevy

During testing, the NOS Stage-1 kit demonstrated a tendency to surge. Figure 4-2 shows the torque variation over a period of about ten seconds. You will note that there are two curves on this graph. It was discovered during testing that a shorter supply tube between the bottle and the solenoid would reduce the surging, so a second series of tests was performed with the shorter tube.

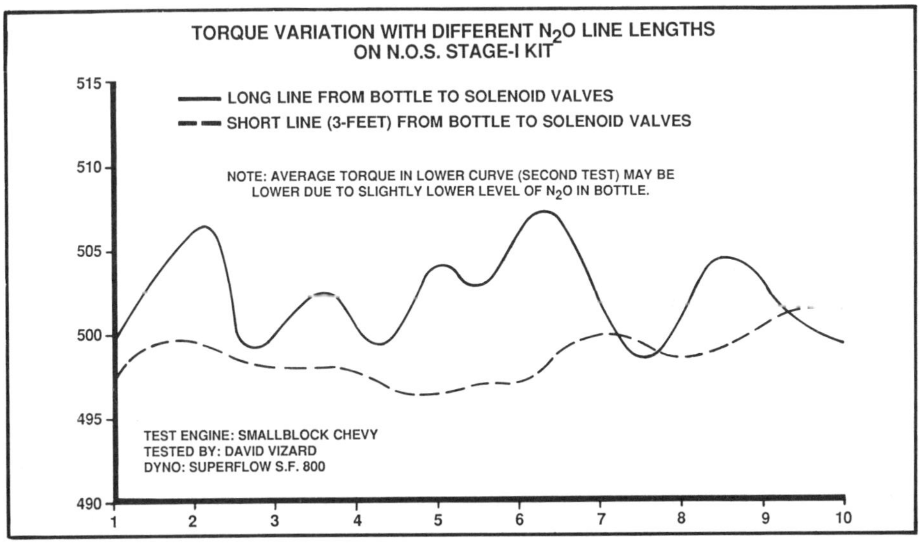

FIGURE 4-2: Torque changes with various nitrous line lengths

At first, this suggests that the reduced friction between the nitrous and the inner wall of the shorter delivery tube has a bearing on thermo-hydraulic resonance. However, it might be expected that friction in the tube would dampen the tendency for surge to develop and a longer tube would be better. But this proved not to be the case. It is possible, however, that pressure reduction at various points (restrictions) may have caused a certain amount of the liquid nitrous to convert momentarily to a gas, reducing the flow of liquid nitrous. A possible cure might be to use a larger line between the bottle and the solenoid valve.

The NOS system caused the torque to rise quickly—the torque increase at 3000rpm was about 160 pounds-feet—however, as noted earlier, surge was a problem. In a typical test the torque held steady for the first two or three seconds; then the level dropped by about 10 to 15 pounds-feet. When the system was activated for a period of 20 seconds or more, the torque

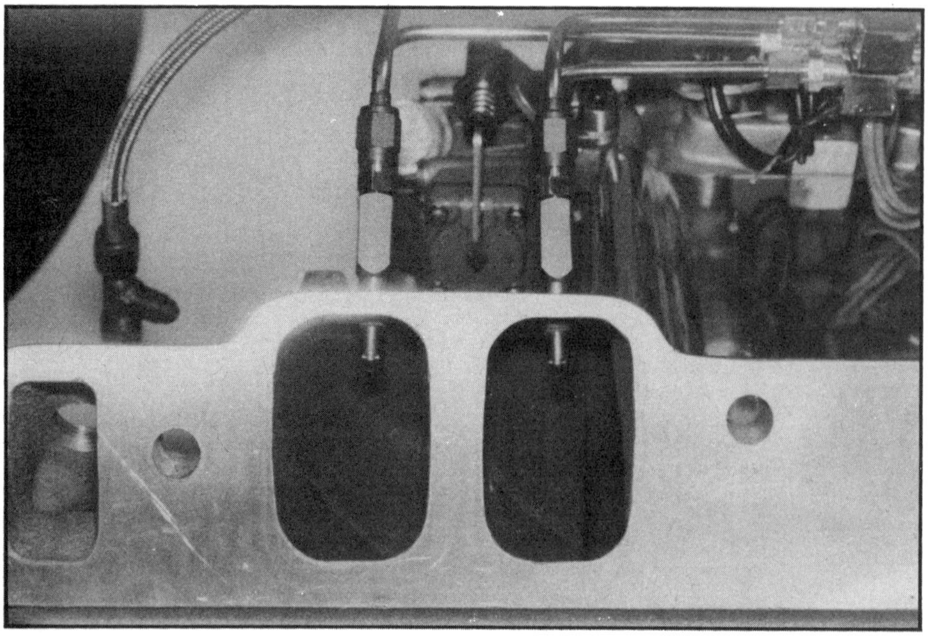

When NOS "fogger" nozzles are used, the fuel and nitrous are mixed right at the point of injection.

dropped even further, usually another six to ten pounds-feet. During system operation the torque fluctuated—over a relatively short time—by as much as four or five pounds-feet, sometimes as high as eight pounds-feet.

As indicated in Figure 4-1, the kit was calibrated sufficiently rich that the average exhaust temperatures dropped 63 degrees when the nitrous was activated. This is a good reason to suspect that the gradual drop-off in power when the system was activated for periods of 20 or 30 seconds was not due to excessive combustion-chamber temperature. Rather, the drop-off in power may be related to vaporization peculiarities in the nitrous-oxide bottle (as discussed in Chapter Three).

Another interesting feature of the NOS kit was the relatively economical use of nitrous-oxide. Within the scope of the author's experience, only one or two kits proved to be marginally more economical—in relation to the power they produced—than the NOS systems.

Testing of the Power Shot system showed that it did not produce a notable surge effect; but by the same token—in a "non-adjustable" mode—it also developed a lower power increase. This consequence appears to be more by design than pure happenstance, and is probably an effort to provide a margin of safety for the sake of reliability. The system tested here could not be re-calibrated to give more horsepower, but recently all of the NOS kits have been altered to make them re-calibratable. This would probably affect the ultimate performance of the kits.

Before the Power Shot kit was installed, the baseline engine produced about 250 horsepower and 360 pounds-feet of torque. As you can see from Figure 4-3, the power boost at 5000rpm amounted to 105 horsepower and at 3000rpm the torque jumped 140 pounds-feet. This same system on a smallblock producing 440 horsepower (unboosted) pushed peak power to 563 horsepower. The additional power boost on the high-power engine was probably due to the better exhaust flow characteristics of the racing heads—the heads were ported to all-out drag-racing specs.

If we look more closely at Figure 4-3, we can see that, with the addition of nitrous-oxide injection, the 250-horse smallblock produced almost as

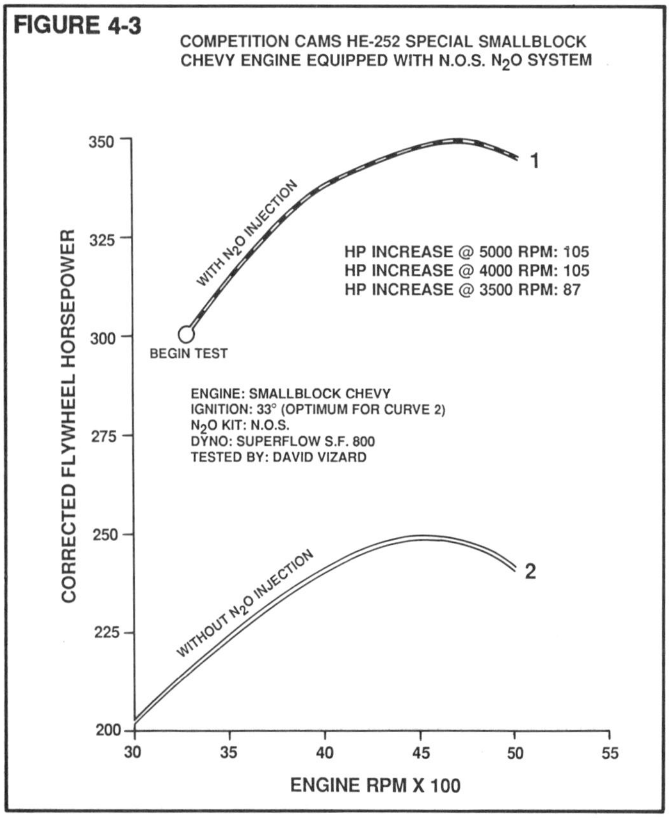

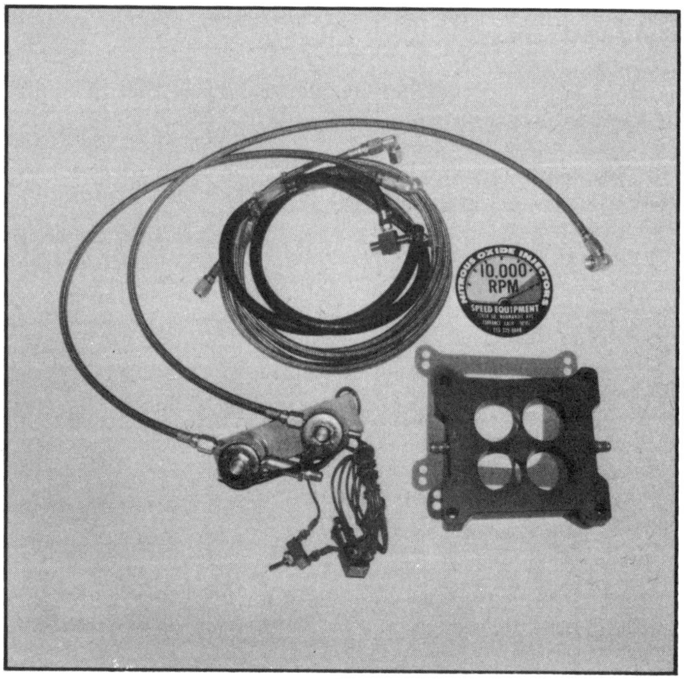

The 10,000 RPM Stage-1 nitrous kit features a 4-hole spacer. To a large degree, this system is pre-wired.

FIGURE 4-3: Power output with NOS Power Shot system.

much torque as a strong big-block. In any reasonable street machine the 500 pounds-feet of torque developed by this combination will almost inevitably cause a severe traction problem (unless the chassis has been suitably modified to withstand the extraordinary load).

As of this writing, the engineers at NOS feel that the Power Shot kit provides an excellent balance between cost, power boost, ease-of-installation, and reliability. For a kit of relatively modest cost, it performed very well—better, in fact, than some kits costing much more.

10,000 RPM STREET KITS

Ron Hamell of 10,000 RPM Speed Equipment is a veteran proponent of nitrous-oxide injection. Ron has over two decades of experience in nitrous-injection design. Perhaps as a result of the countless hours he has spent testing nitrous systems on the dynamometer, his products are very effective.

Although 10,000 RPM offers open-spacer kits, both kits used in this test employed 4-hole spacers that match the bore spacing of the Holley throttle body (model 4150 and 4160). One of the kits was a Stage-One kit and employed two spraybars in a more or less conventional manner. The Stage-two kit employed three spraybars situated one above the other. With this arrangement, the top two spraybars distribute nitrous-oxide and the bottom sprays gasoline.

The Stage-One kit has two spraybars mounted in a conventional manner in a one-inch tall aluminum spacer that is anodized blue. What was especially novel about this kit is that it came with all the wires attached to the relevant switches. This would, in most instances, make the installation simple and fast. Although this is a nice feature, it is of relatively minor importance compared with another feature of this kit—and indeed all kits from 10,000 RPM.

It has been Ron Hamell's practice, for most of the time that he has been building nitrous-oxide kits, *to dyno-test and calibrate the kits on his dynamometer.* Rather than attempt to calculate the flow requirements and then see if it works in practice, Ron tackles the situation from the other end.

First of all, the fuel calibration will have a direct bearing on engine reliability. If too little fuel is used (in relation to the nitrous), the engine will overheat. If the right amount or a little too much is used (within reason), the engine temperature will remain within limits. Ron uses these precepts and measures the effect the nitrous has on engine temperature. This is fairly simple. He runs the test engine on a dyno and measures the exhaust temperatures both with and without the nitrous injection. These temperatures indicate, with reasonable accuracy, the corresponding operating temperatures of the piston crown and combustion chamber surfaces. If the exhaust temperatures are lowered somewhat when the nitrous is activated, there is every likelihood that the peak temperatures in the combustion chamber are also lower. And the reverse is true. If the temperatures rise when the nitrous is activated, the combustion temperatures are probably higher because the fuel ratio is too lean (not enough enrichment fuel is being added).

Ron prefers to establish the fuel-to-nitrous ratio to give an appreciable drop in exhaust temperature. He feels this ensures that the piston-crown temperatures are no higher and possibly even lower than those achieved when the nitrous is not functioning. By calibrating the systems in this manner, 10,000 RPM achieves good power output consistent with the most economical fuel consumption (during system operation). In addition, this provides an added measure of reliability to prevent engine damage.

When tested, the 10,000 RPM Stage-One kit ran with only a 41% rich mixture. This dropped the average exhaust temperature from 1476 degrees (F) to 1440 degrees. Like most kits that utilize relatively long lines

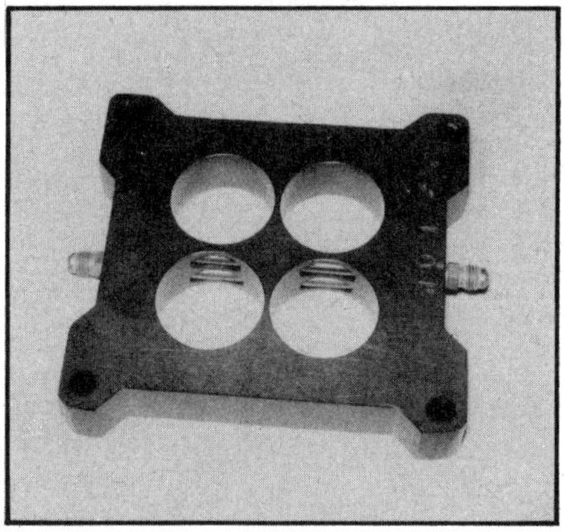

This closeup of the 10,000 RPM spacer shows the relationship between the spraybars and the throttle bores of the carburetor. This spacer system is conventional in all other respects.

between the solenoid valve and the spacer, the torque increase was progressive. In the case of the Stage-One kit, torque increased about 90-94 pounds-feet in the first two or three seconds, and then climbed slowly to the peak torque increase of 127 pounds-feet. Once the torque stabilized, the 10,000 RPM kit demonstrated less of a tendency to surge than most spraybar kits tested. Torque fluctuations were typically under 6.0-8.0 pounds-feet. Because of generally good spacer design and fuel-calibration characteristics, 10,000 RPM kit produced good nitrous brake-specific consumption figures (amount of ni-

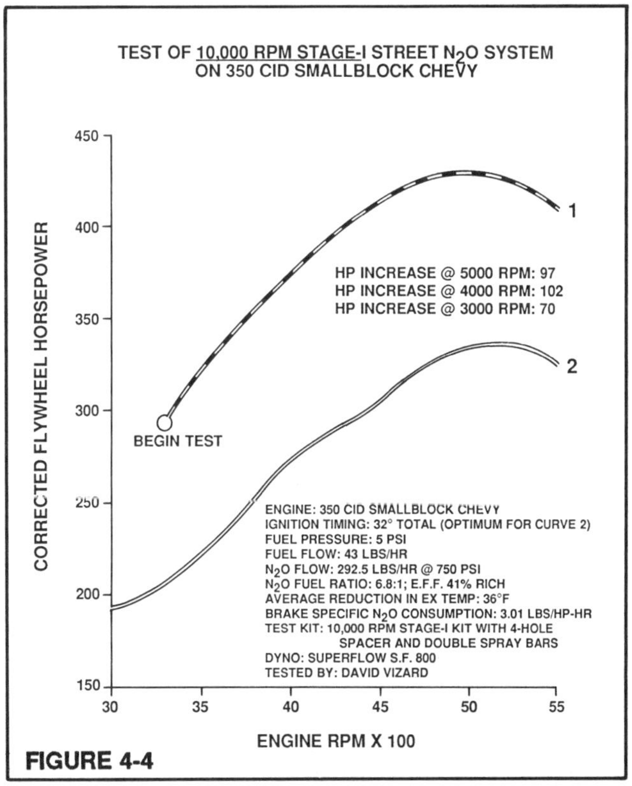

FIGURE 4-4: Note that torque boost comes in two "steps." About 75 percent of the total torque boost appeared immediately, the rest comes on two or three seconds later. From this point on, torque output held quite steady.

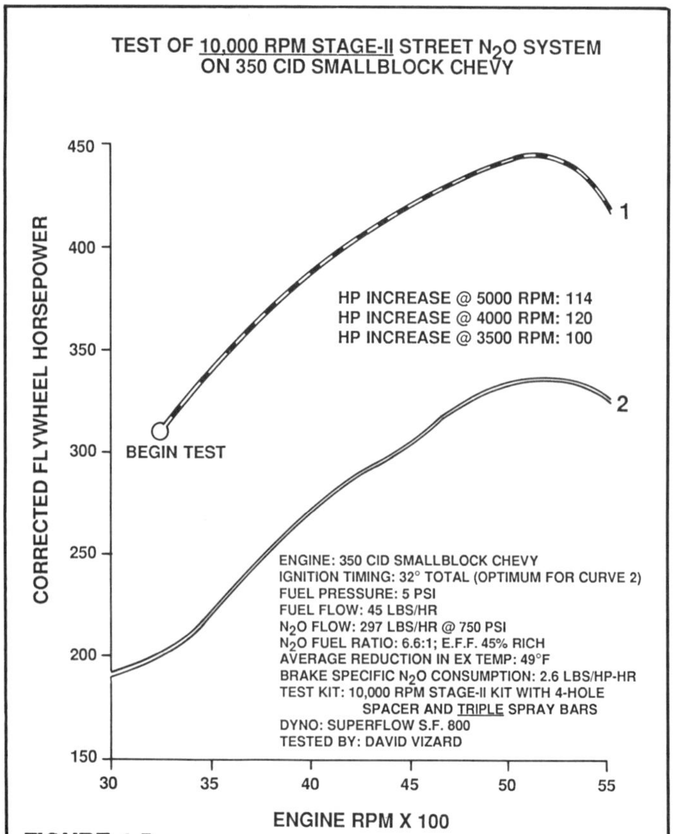

FIGURE 4-5

FIGURE 4-5: This system hit relatively softly and progressively, with about 70 percent of torque boost in the first second and the rest coming in over the next two seconds. After about 20 seconds, however, a surge developed. The 4-hole spacer has a venturi shape with triple spraybars.

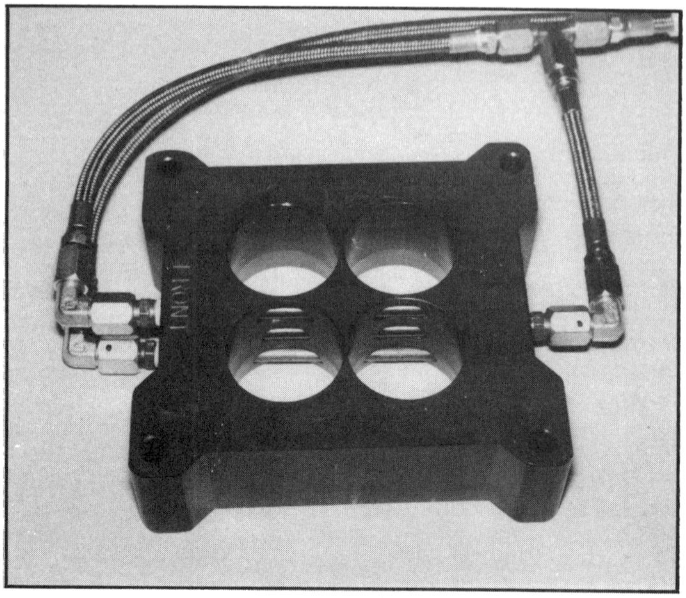

trous consumed in relation to the measured power increase), especially when it was used on a dual-plane manifold. Figure 4-4 shows the power curve produced by this kit.

The Stage-Two 10,000 RPM kit was tested on an engine similar to that used for the Stage-One test. The results are shown in Figure 4-5. The spacer used in this kit is 1.34 inches tall, and according to Ron, this spacer improves performance throughout the power band. The kit is designed for engines that will operate at engine speeds up to 6500rpm. However, the test engine was fitted with a relatively short cam (short valve-open duration), so the system was not tested to its fullest potential.

In very much the same manner as the NOS system, the Stage-Two 10,000 RPM kit tended to surge. It would load relatively quickly to a maximum torque increase of 158 pounds-feet. After a second or two at this torque level, the output would begin to fluctuate by as many as 20 pounds-feet. This caused the torque boost to vary between 138 and 158 pounds-feet.

This system also made very efficient use of nitrous. It used only 2.6 pounds of nitrous per horsepower-hour; Thus making it, as of this writing, one of the most efficient box-stock spraybar systems that the author has ever tested. This may be attributed to the triple spraybar arrangement—though I am not exactly certain of this. Some of the conventional double spraybar systems have nearly equaled this level of nitrous efficiency, and some nozzle systems that utilize deliberate mixing of the fuel and nitrous-oxide at the delivery point can better this efficiency. However, the fact remains, the 10,000 RPM system, in out-of-the box form, ranks as the most efficient system among all those tested during research for this book.

The 10,000 RPM Stage-2 kit employs a triple spraybar system: the top and middle one are for nitrous and the lower one is for enrichment fuel.

NELSON PRO SYSTEM

In the recent past, an interesting street/strip nitrous system was available from Nelson Fuel Systems and

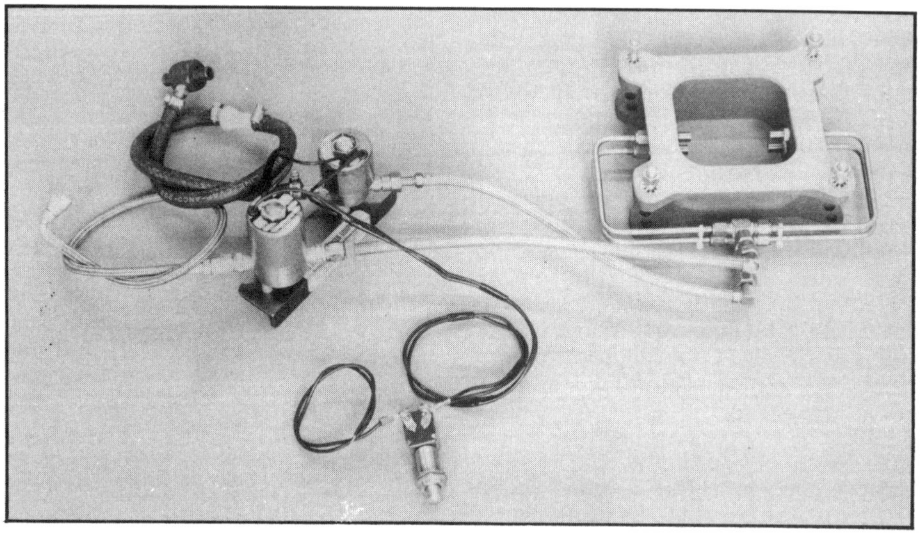

The 10,000 RPM "pseudo-jet" system is unique. Since the delivery orifices for the nitrous are located at the end of tubes projecting into the spacer, it reacts in much the same manner as a true jet system. Nitrous emitted from the upper nitrous nozzle impinges on the fuel exiting the lower nozzle.

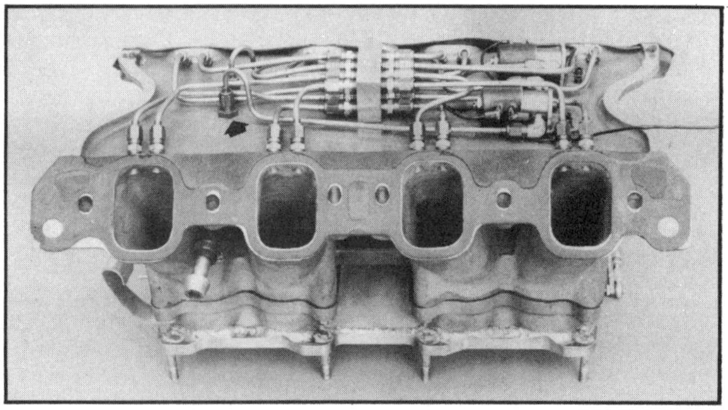

This system is not designed to encourage mixing of fuel and nitrous. Each component is simply injected into the port, the mixing taking place randomly.

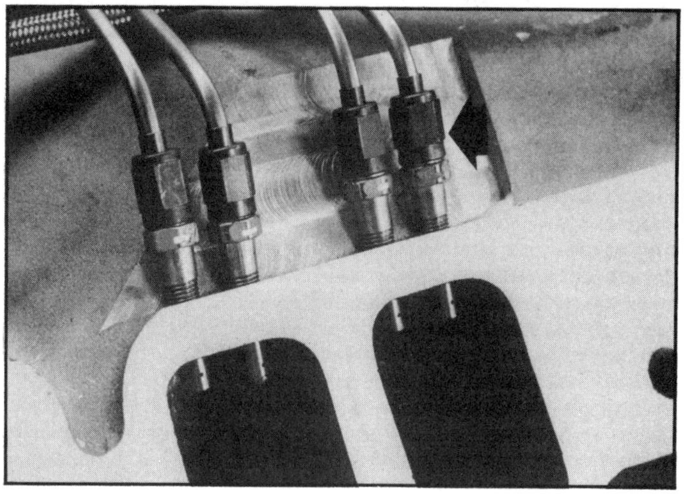

In this system the orifices in the nitrous nozzles are pointed roughly in line with the flow of incoming air. This is helpful, but unfortunately, the nitrous and fuel nozzles are directed away from each other, reducing the degree of mixing at the point of injection.

Equipment. As of this writing, the company is supposedly no longer in business, however, in the opinion of the author, among all the nitrous kits tested for this book, the Nelson kit ranked as the best engineered system. The results are included here because they provide an interesting comparison.

Unlike the other kits, the N_2O Pro employed axial-flow solenoids; i.e., the nitrous or fuel enters one end, passes through the length of the solenoid and exits the other end. These solenoids are very compact, and though they were not tested by the author, Nelson claimed these valves have a very high flow rate, especially in relation to their size. This means that they can be installed in confined spaces where a conventional solenoid may not fit. Apart from this, there doesn't seem to be any intrinsic advantage to the axial-flow solenoid. The author noted, however, that these solenoids require less electrical current, and this may be an important feature when limited electrical power is available.

The system was supplied with three gasoline jets. The instructions advise starting with the richest jet and doing spark-plug checks to determine whether the mixture needs to be leaned. Of course, in an effort to improve reliability, all reputable nitrous kit manufacturers calibrate kits a bit (sometimes a lot) rich. As would be expected, Dyno testing established that the N_2O Pro was very rich, too rich, in fact, to produce best power even on the leanest jets supplied. The

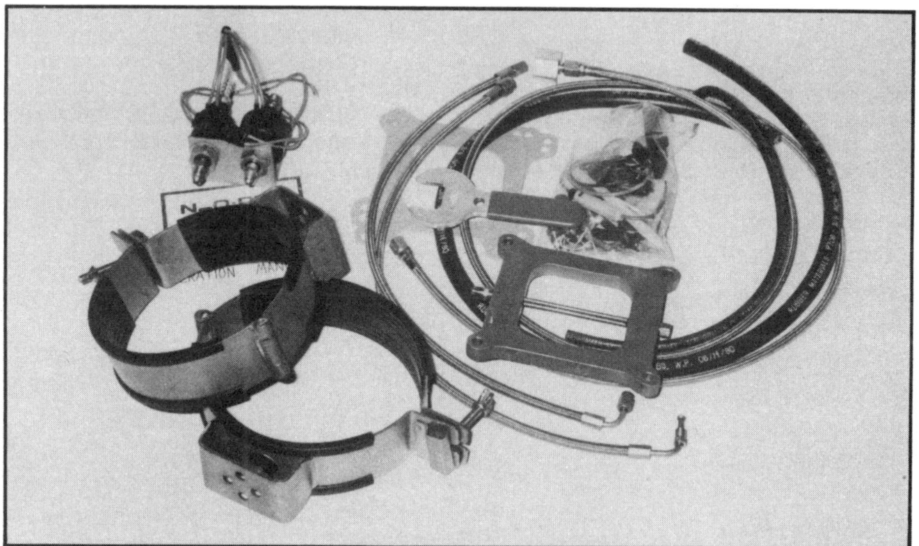

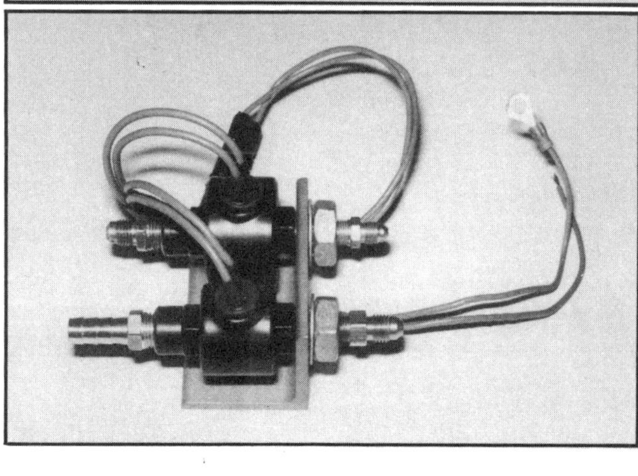

The Nelson N_2O Pro proved to be a well manufactured kit. It had an adjustable fuel system and unique axial-flow solenoids manufactured expressly for this company.

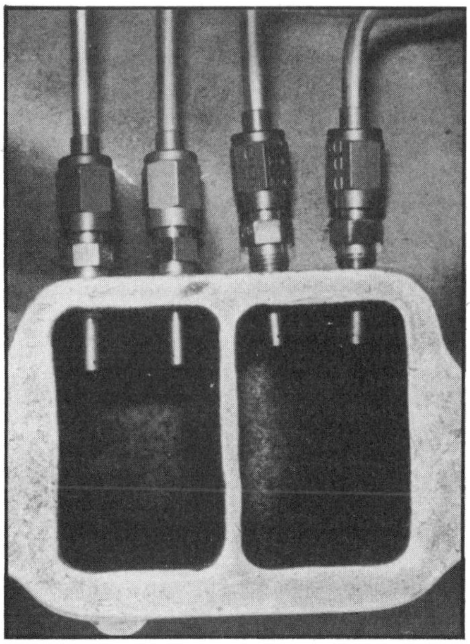

This view shows how the discharge orifices can be angled toward each other so the streams of nitrous and fuel will mix about one inch from the point of injection.

kit produced a power increase of 97 horsepower at 5000rpm on an engine producing 350 horsepower, unboosted, at 5000 rpm.

These are out-of-the-box figures with the system set up totally stock. However, the fuel system used during dyno testing has an adjustable pressure regulator, and it was discovered that when the fuel pressure was reduced to give an excess fuel factor around 45%-rich, the power increase jumped to 119 horsepower at 5000 rpm and the torque output was notably improved at 3000rpm.

The plots in Figure 4-4 shows both the out-of-the-box results and the "dialed-in" results. Bear in mind, though, that the other kits tested here may or may not have produced more power if similar efforts had been made to maximize efficiency. This would be difficult to predict. However, the author must point out that attempts were *not* made to dial-in all of the systems.

It is also interesting to note that the Nelson system could be recalibrated to power levels as high as 175 horsepower. Even if the other systems had been re-calibrated during the testing, it is doubtful that any of them could reach this level without substituting solenoids that have greater flow capacity. This would increase the cost of these systems and would probably put them into the all-out competition category.

FIGURE 4-6: This is a calibratable system. Initial fuel delivery was rich, but the #2 curve was recorded with fuel pressure reduced to 2.8psi. Exhaust temperatures indicated that the system was still "reasonably safe" at this setting. According to the manufacturer the nitrous side of this kit can be recalibrated to produce boost of up to 175 horses.

INTERNAL COMBUSTION ENGINEERING JET SYSTEM

In the following sections we will look at the general functioning and design of jet-type (adjustable) and port-injection nitrous systems that are suitable for street performance use. These systems are somewhat more complex than plate-type systems and are, therefore, generally more expensive and less common.

The first kit that we'll examine is the street kit from Internal Combustion Engineering (ICE). This particular kit is a cross-breed, because it uses nozzles for the nitrous-oxide injection and a spraybar for the gasoline. This configuration has both good and bad points. The primary advantage is that the nitrous flow is much steadier, and tests on the dyno show that the system "hits" harder when activated and is much less prone to surging than a conventional spraybar system.

On the other side of the coin, the nitrous and enrichment fuel are distributed into the plenum/manifold at different locations, therefore the nitrous and gasoline do not mix as thoroughly as with a conventional dual or triple spraybar system. Just how important this is, in the total overall scheme of things, is not totally clear. Certainly, injecting the nitrous at a substantially different location, remote from the fuel delivery point, produces comparatively less horsepower per pound of nitrous consumed.

The degree of effective fuel and nitrous mixing that occurs inside the manifold and the proportions of nitrous or fuel that are distributed into each intake runner seems to depend, to some extent, on the type and design of the intake manifold. I have not encountered problems when testing this type of system on an open-plenum, single-plane manifold. Such manifolds include the Edelbrock Tarantula, Victor and Victor Jr; the Weiand Team "G" StreetRam; and the Offenhauser Port-A-Sonic. All of these manifolds, incidentally, were tested on a 350cid smallblock Chevrolet engine; and I have no direct experience with these manifolds and this type of system on any other make or model of engine.

Nonetheless, I have heard reports of instances wherein the engine has detonated in just one or two cylinders—with the nitrous operating—while other cylinders appeared to be running very rich. These symptoms are generally indicated in the following manner: the spark plugs color uniformly when the engine is operated without nitrous, but a plug check after the nitrous is activated (upon immediate shut-down) will show definite indications that some cylinders are lean, others rich. In extreme cases, the spark plug electrodes have

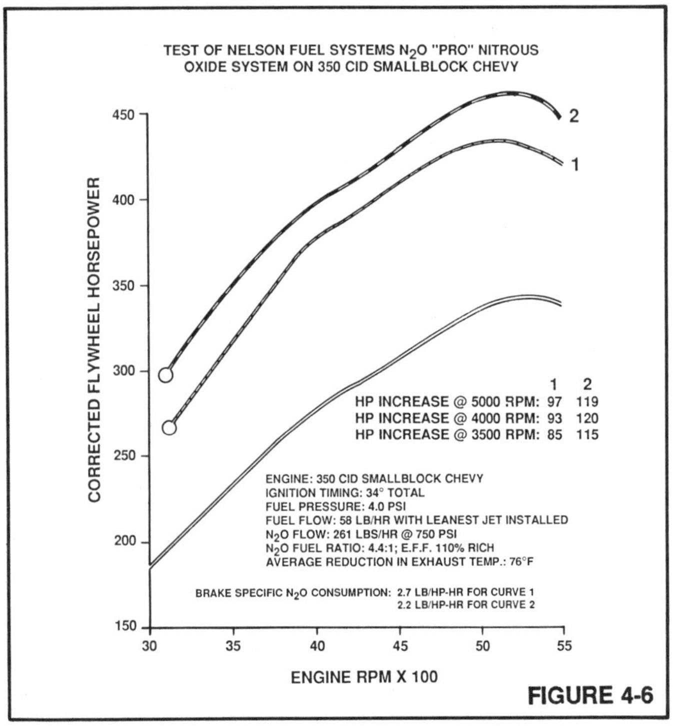

FIGURE 4-6

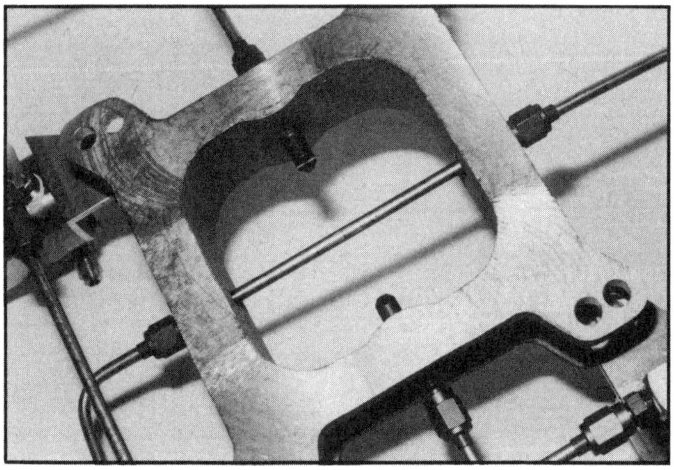

The ICE jet system is a combination system: enrichment fuel is delivered through the spraybar running across the width of the spacer and nitrous is injected through the nozzles on either side of the spacer.

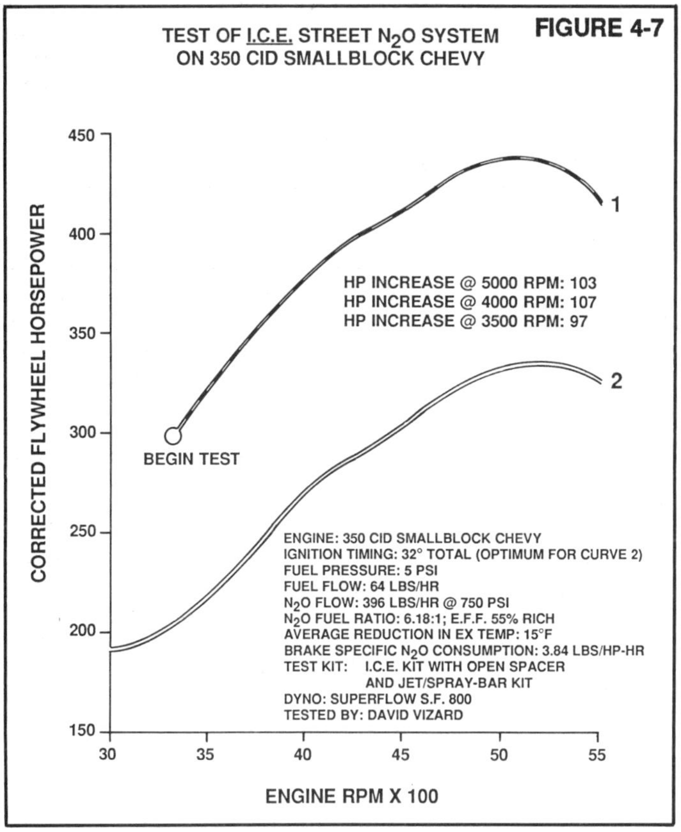

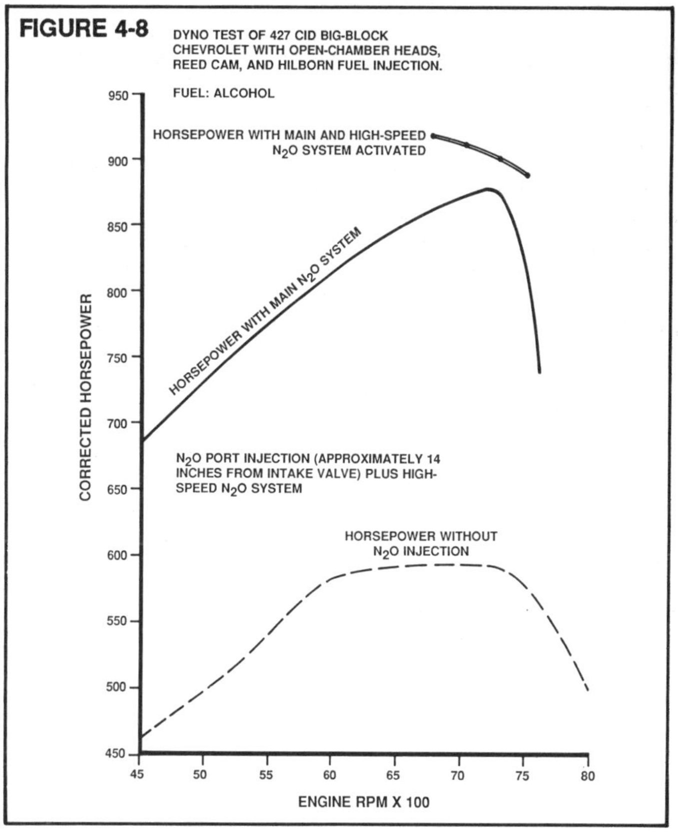

FIGURE 4-7: When this system was activated the torque jumped quickly to the boost level and held steady for prolonged periods. Easy calibration--matched pairs of fuel and nitrous jets allow various boost levels up to a peak of 150 horsepower--is a boon to the tuner. The measured power output was considered a safe level by the manufacturer for most street applications.

FIGURE 4-8: This engine, built by Ron Hammel, features a simple 2-stage nitrous system. Jets positioned near the top of the stacks inject second-stage nitrous and the fuel injection was designed to deliver a rich mixture at high rpm (thus supplying enrichment fuel). Horsepower output was a respectable 585hp without the nitrous system activated. When the engine was boosted by the main N_2O system, horsepower jumped to 845hp and when the second stage (high-speed) system was added, the final horsepower level exceeded 925hp. Only two power levels were recorded near peak engine speed. This potent engine was a 427cid big-block Chevy running on alcohol.

melted in the lean cylinders (during the nitrous operation). Obviously, during actual operation, this type of severe imbalance can cause engine damage.

Nonetheless, a setup like the ICE system tested here, which has acceptable distribution—and, providing it is functioning correctly—is a useful system for the bracket racer. It produces very consistent results! Figure 4-7 shows the power curve produced by the ICE system. It demonstrates a smooth and consistent power output.

In addition, there is yet another important advantage to this type of system. The ICE system, unlike any of the systems mentioned so far—with the exception of the Nelson N20 Pro and the latest NOS systems—can be calibrated with jets. It can be calibrated on both the nitrous side and the fuel side. Jets are supplied in flow-tested, matched pairs—in a variety of power levels—thus the user can dial-in the power to suit specific track and vehicle circumstances. The kit is supplied for typical street use with 100-horsepower jets installed; however, alternative jetting can be obtained to give up to 150 horsepower (claimed).

PORT-INJECTION

Over the years there has been a lot of controversy about whether port-injection is better than plate/spacer injection. In this section we will examine the pros and cons of port-injection systems.

Port-injection eliminates some of the primary problems arising with plate-injection systems. Most plate-injection difficulties are due to irregular fuel/nitrous distribution through the manifold. With a properly calibrated port-injection system, flow distribution in the manifold will not affect the mixture quality delivered to each cylinder. When the system is properly tuned, all cylinders will receive very nearly the correct amount of fuel and nitrous (in relation to the required power increase). This eliminates the spread between "rich" and "lean" cylinders; and the excess enrichment fuel that is required for cooling purposes (in "lean" cylinders) can be reduced to a minimum—just enough to keep the pistons and exhaust valves at safe temperatures. The amount of enrichment fuel can, in fact, be adjusted for each cylinder—provided of course, that temperature-sensing equipment is available. However, even without expensive test equipment, the fuel-to-nitrous ratio can be very nearly optimized by carefully observing spark plug readings.

In most cases, the excess fuel factor can be held to about 35% to 40% rich. This will generally produce a greater power increase in relation to the amount of nitrous used. In fact, port-injection systems that are designed to thoroughly mix the fuel and nitrous consistently show brake-specific nitrous consumption figures as good as the very best plate-injec-

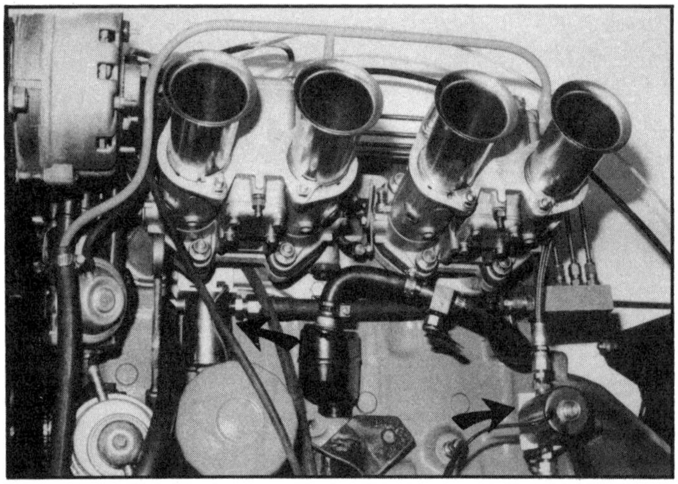

This view of the port-injection system used for the tests in Figure 4-9 shows the position of the nitrous and fuel solenoids. The plumbing of a port system is straightforward up to the distribution blocks, but from there on things get complicated.

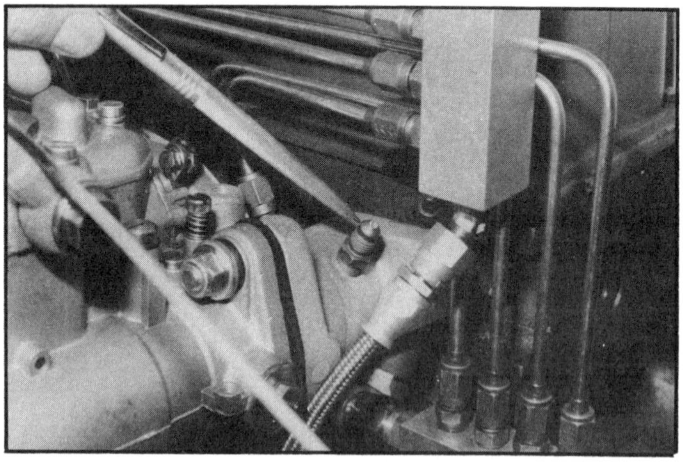

The pointer indicates one of the jets for the calibratable port-injection system designed by the author. Note that the delivery orifices are angled toward each other so that the pressurized streams of fuel and nitrous will impinge upon each other. This improves mixing and promotes uniform distribution.

tion system—and in most instances, better.

Without a doubt, there is also a disadvantage to port-injection. This type of system is more complex to build—because of the extensive plumbing required—and as a result, is more expensive. But if expense is not an overriding limitation, a port-injection system will generally offer superior performance.

Port-injection systems can be subdivided into two general groups. First, there are those that inject the fuel and the nitrous at distinctly separate locations. In these systems mixing of the nitrous and fuel is produced more or less by the natural turbulence inside the port. In these systems there is no overt effort to mix the nitrous and fuel at the point of injection. In the second type of system there is a specific attempt to mix the nitrous and fuel at the immediate point of injection. Generally, the discharge of nitrous is in close proximity to the fuel discharge and the spray of nitrous is directed toward the fuel spray. In this instance the mixing of nitrous and fuel may begin within 0.05-inch of the injection point. This produces a very homogeneous mixture of nitrous and enrichment fuel.

My original experience with a port-injection system was with a Pinto engine. The system was well designed (at least for 1978) and had replaceable jets that could be calibrated to produce an estimated 50, 100, or 150 horsepower increase. As shown in the accompanying photographs, the amount of plumbing in this home-brew system made the engine look somewhat "elaborate." However, it was worth the effort because the system worked well, despite some problems. The power curve in Figure 4-9 show the results achieved with the 50-horsepower jets. The system produced nearly 50 additional horsepower throughout the tested engine speed range.

There were some difficulties encountered during the testing of the 100-horsepower boost system. These tests were performed on a Go-Power dynamometer, and the torque increase with the greater nitrous/fuel flow was so dramatic that the engine speed would climb faster than the dyno operator (myself) could apply the load and safely prevent the engine from overspeeding. Because of the similar torque boost, it was nearly impossible to accurately test the 150 horsepower configuration.

The point here is that the power levels—in relation to the total power output of the engine—were very high. The base engine produced 140 horsepower. The 50-horsepower boost represented a power increase of about 35%. This percentage of increase is achieved fairly easily with modern nitrous systems, even with big V8's. However, the 100-horsepower system represented a 71% increase. This is a large relative power boost. It is equal, on a percentage basis, to 230 extra horsepower out of a V8 that produces 340-350 horsepower without nitrous. A 150 horsepower increase represents a 107% boost over the original output. Ultimately, this equals almost 2.2 horsepower per cubic inch! If a 350cid smallblock Chevyrolet engine was successfully built along the same lines, it would produce approximately 833 horsepower. These horsepower levels are *not* impossible, by any means.

Because of the difficulty involved in making each test, only spot readings were taken; however, some interesting indications were revealed in this initial testing. Some of these characteristics were only suspicions at the time, but were verified during later tests when more sophisticated equipment was available. However, these early tests indicated that a port-injection nitrous system has several advantages when compared to an under-the-carburetor injection system.

One factor that was observed, at least on systems that inject into a relatively cool manifold, is that surging was minimal—and in some instances, nonexistent. Though somewhat affected by the length of the nitrous supply lines, in general, the system would hit fairly hard, reach peak power quickly, and hold at the peak for a considerable period of time. At least this was the tendency on the lower power levels. At higher power levels the Pinto test engine was held at max engine speed only briefly—about seven to ten seconds—to take a stabilized power reading. Long-term operational tendencies were not observed.

Testing on 4-cylinder engines is useful, but how would this port-injection system apply to a V8? To see how effective a port-injection system can be, look at Figure 4-8. This data was developed with a 427-inch big-block Chevy engine designed for a dragster and fitted with a relatively sophisticated port-injection nitrous system. The engine is not in an exceptionally high state of tune. It has a racing camshaft, open-chamber iron heads, and Hilborn fuel injection.

The nozzles for the nitrous injection are situated in the port runner about 14 inches from the intake valve.

In addition, there is an additional nozzle situated in each port runner. At the top end of the dragstrip this nozzle injects "additional" nitrous. A complementary portion of "additional" fuel enrichment is achieved by virtue of a very rich top-end fuel delivery from the Hilborn fuel-injection system. This "top-end-only" power boost raised peak power from 875 horsepower to 920 horsepower.

It is important to point out that it is not necessary to use fuel injection to produce the power levels achieved with this engine. With modern nitrous systems, the choice between fuel injection and carburetors is largely a matter of convenience, personal preference or racing regulations. The test engine could have been carbureted, and though it may have produced less horsepower on carburetion and without the nitrous-oxide, the power could have been bumped up to a comparable level with an effective multi-stage, port-injection system!

It is also important to note again that this is not a highly developed engine. As my own tests with a 4-cylinder engine indicate, it is possible to achieve power levels as high as 2.2 horsepower per cubic inch. This means that the 427 shown in Figure 4-8 still has some margin for additional development. If it produced 2.5 horses per cubic inch, it would be well over 1000 horsepower. Indeed, even a modestly prepared 350cid smallblock engine fitted with an effective nitrous port-injection system can produce power levels in the region of 700 to 800 horsepower, with drag-race reliably. In fact, such engines are becoming common, and modern smallblocks readily power dragsters to elapsed times in the high sevens and speeds over 175mph. The point is, though, that this type of engine is not necessarily an expensive, high-strung powerplant.

Essentially, we can summarize the comparison in a few words. If the same amount of nitrous-oxide is used in a port-injection system—as compared to a plate-injection system—and the fuel is set to give about a 40%-rich mixture, the horsepower levels achieved generally will be as good as the best plate systems or, optimally, 10% to 15% higher.

POINT OF INJECTION

According to theory, if a constant flow of nitrous-oxide and enrichment fuel is injected into an engine, the power increase should be uniform throughout the engine-speed range. However, in actual fact we must look at a few other factors, but first, let's consider why the power increase should be uniform.

The power output of an engine is roughly proportional to the amount of oxygen consumed per minute. Under normal circumstances, as engine speed (rpm) increases, it consumes more oxygen (more induction strokes means more oxygen) and produces more horsepower. With a nitrous engine, we find that at low engine speeds, a cylinder will take in a lot of nitrous because there is relatively more time per cycle. On the other hand, at high speeds the engine will take in only a small amount of nitrous because the available time per cycle is relatively shorter. In other words, it is like feeding a piece of string into a chopping machine. The string represents the stream of nitrous-oxide; the chopping action represents the individual engine intake strokes. At low engine speed a large piece of string is chopped off; at high engine speed a small piece of string is chopped off.

In actual practice, *if the nitrous and enrichment fuel is mixed effectively*, things work out pretty much along the lines indicated by this logic. And, as might be expected from the aforementioned theoretical considerations, the torque curve generally drops off more quickly on a nitrous-injected engine.

This makes several assumptions: First, it assumes that the nozzles are not installed in the manifold in such a way that they interfere with the airflow into the engine. Second, it assumes that the nozzles are positioned so the fuel and nitrous can gain at least "adequate" mixing before reaching the cylinder. When the fuel and nitrous nozzles are close to the intake valve, there is less time for them to mix. In this respect, plate systems have a slight edge. If the plate and spraybars are properly designed and matched to a suitable manifold, the nitrous/fuel mix will be fairly homogeneous by the time it reaches the cylinders.

When considering the point of injection we have to remember that airflow in an intake port is not uniform. All intake ports have, to a greater or lesser extent, an *airflow gradient*. In other words, the flow in one part of the port may be moving at very high speed, whereas in another part, the flow may be very lazy. This is generally the result of numerous compromises forced on the designer by manufacturing limitations or other restrictions. As a result, selecting the point of injection for nitrous-oxide will be very critical.

The area of highest flow activity is generally along the top portion, or "roof," of the port. Injecting from the underside of the port—as is common with hidden systems—will reduce efficiency unless the fuel and nitrous are thoroughly mixed at the point of injection. The only alternative is to aim the injected fuel and nitrous across the port, into the high-flowing area. If this occurs successfully, the fuel and nitrous will be mixed into the inducted fuel-airstream to form a reasonably homogeneous mixture.

Some injection nozzles are designed to inject the flow of nitrous at right angles to the nozzle axis. The injected nitrous is, therefore, generally directed along the same line as the airflow in the port. This can be good or bad. If the nitrous is injected into the lazy part of the port, the pressure of the escaping nitrous may stimulate flow in that area and pull more air into the engine, producing more power. However, if this does not happen and if the fuel and nitrous don't mix properly, which is often the case (due to the lazy airflow), the power increase from the nitrous may be less than expected.

Conversely, injecting into the top part of the port—in line with the airstream—can aid in several ways. Injecting along the line of airflow nor-

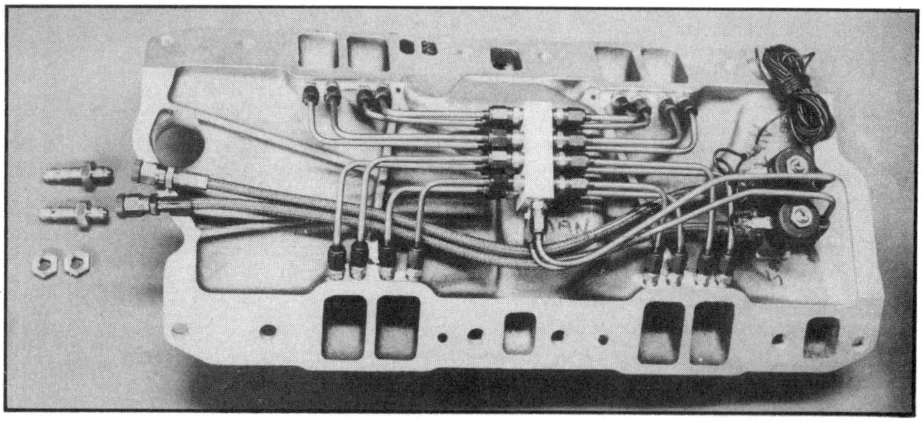

The solenoids and distribution lines of this hidden system are exposed to hot engine oil; as a result, the nitrous boost comes on slowly when the system is activated. The system will not "hit hard" unless the nitrous lines are relatively cool.

mally assists the mixing of fuel and nitrous prior to cylinder entry. The friction between the induction flow and port wall is greatest in the high-speed areas; and injecting the nitrous in line with the airflow, can boost the flow into the cylinder, thus mechanically helping the engine induct more air. This may sound like a minor point, but flow testing has verified that this phenomenon does occur, and the increased airflow can produce more power than would otherwise be expected from the nitrous system.

However, another point to consider is that if the nozzles are located in the top of the port—the area of highest flow—they represent a measurable obstruction to the airflow. As a result, it is best to keep to a minimum the intrusion of the nozzles into the port. And if practical, it's not a bad idea to aim the nozzle straight at the backside of the intake valve.

In the same vein, it is interesting to consider the experiences of Ron Hamell at 10,000 RPM. Ron has devoted many years to developing nitrous-oxide systems, and he has gathered as much dyno data as anyone in the field. First, He has noted that with separate nozzles (i.e., one nozzle for fuel and one nozzle for nitrous) located to allow mixing within the port, as the point of injection is moved farther away from the intake valve, the engine produces more power. However, it must also be noted that his test engines are generally fitted with independent-runner intake system, and they have been either fuel-injected or have employed one barrel of carburetion for each cylinder. This will, unquestionably affect the results.

Second, Ron has noted that when the point of injection is located in the relatively slow flow along the floor of the port the power may drop as much as 20%. Even if the same amount of nitrous and enrichment fuel is injected in the floor area—as opposed to injecting in the roof area—the power will be reduced (in most cases) because the fuel and nitrous do not mix thoroughly when they are injected into the slow-moving air on the port floor.

On the other hand, my own testing with the Alden-Oselli nozzle, which mixes the nitrous and fuel into a fairly homogeneous mixture as close as 0.25-inch outside the injection orifice, has shown that when the point of

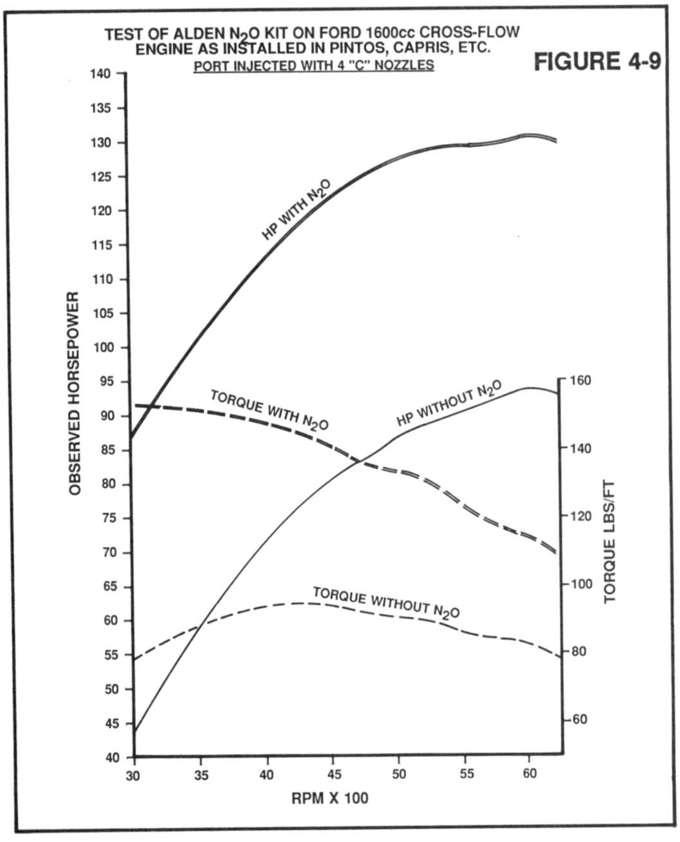

FIGURE 4-9: A port-injection system--especially one with single nozzles and relatively low power boost--produces consistent results, so the nitrous effect is obvious. Note how torque declines progressively as engine speed increases. This seems to substantiate the theory that nitrous gives a constant horsepower increase, regardless of engine speed.

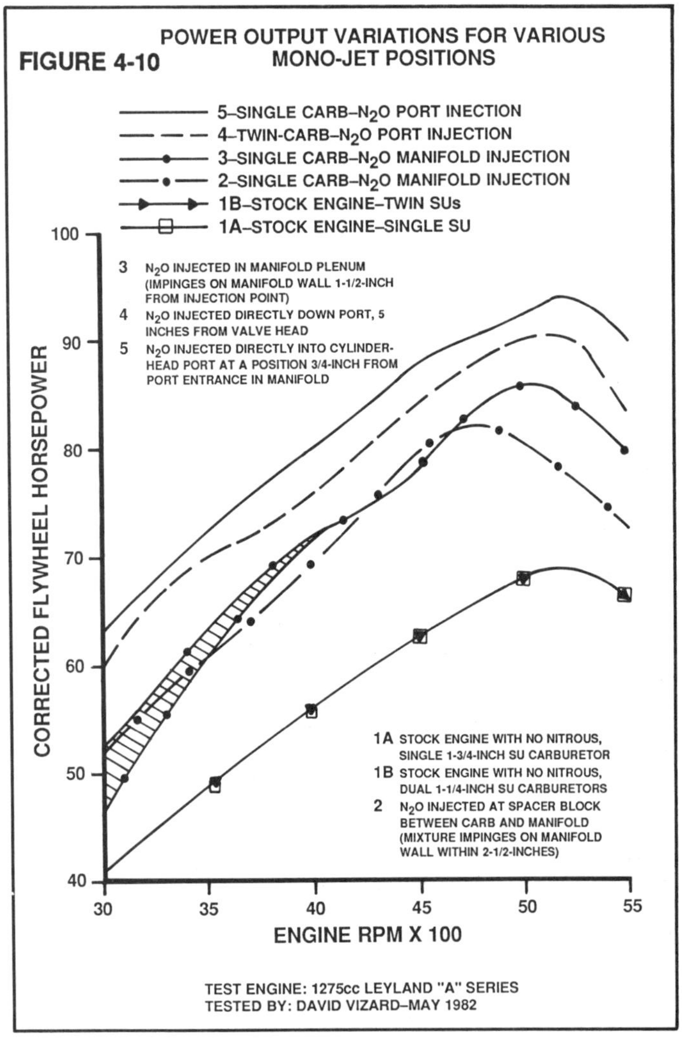

FIGURE 4-10: This is an attempt to verify the effect of nozzle location. Output is constant at low rpm when the nitrous-fuel mixture is sprayed across the path of airflow. Peak power increases somewhat when the point of injection is closer to the intake valve. This superiority is not always evident: Tests with NOS "fogger" nozzles showed a 33hp increase with port-type injection and a 32hp increase when the nozzle was located above the venturi of a Weber 45 DCOE. (Note: the throttle stop of the dual-carb setup was adjusted to give a baseline identical to the single carb; 1A and 1B.)

injection is closer to the intake valve, more horsepower is produced. Of course, there are usually some mechanical limitations and/or space restrictions; but on small 4-cylinder test engines, moving the nitrous nozzle three to four inches closer to the intake valve and giving it a straight shot at the backside of the valve has resulted in, typically, a 5% improvement, and in extreme cases, as much as a 28% improvement.

Figure 4-9 demonstrates the importance of homogeneous fuel mixing and uniform mixture distribution between the cylinders. This power curve shows the effect a port-injection system with Alden-Oselli nozzles has on a cross-flow 1600cc Ford engine. This type of engine was fitted to the 1600 Pinto and is used in Europe in the Cortina and Capri.

On the test engine in Figure 4-9, the four Alden-Oselli C-flow nozzles are rated at 10 to 12 horsepower in each port. These nozzles produced an impressive 42-horsepower increase on the 1600 test engine. Similar tests with the same nozzles in a 2000 Pinto engine showed a power increase of about 45 horsepower.

Again using the Alden-Oselli nozzles, some tests were performed with a 78cid British Leyland 4-cylinder engine. (This was a convenient and inexpensive test engine.) The tests were conducted with two nozzles that were supposedly calibrated to deliver about 12 to 14 horsepower each.

First, these nozzles were mounted into a spacer plate between carburetor and manifold; and, a single carburetor intake manifold was utilized along with water heating on the manifold. By injecting at the plate, an increase of some 18 horsepower maximum was seen from the engine (see Figure 4-10). The low-speed performance was somewhat ragged. This was eventually attributed to uneven distribution of the nitrous mixture between cylinders.

On the next test, the nozzles were mounted in the intake manifold just at the base of the carburetor mount; and they were directed straight toward the backwall of the manifold, as opposed to pointing them straight down the port. This resulted in a maximum increase of approximately 17 horsepower. When the nozzles were mounted in a dual-carburetor installation, with about five inches between the nozzles and the cylinder head, the power increase was raised to 22 horsepower. But when the nozzles were mounted almost flush with the cylinder head on a single-carb manifold, a power increase of 25 horsepower was achieved.

This indicates that if the fuel and nitrous are mixed thoroughly, which can be achieved with a well-designed port-injection system, it is possible to improve the power by moving the nozzles closer to the valve. This gives the nitrous less time to absorb the heat from the surrounding port.

Similar results to those found here can be expected with the NOS "fogger jet." At the time of writing, this appears to be the state-of-art design for single-point injection systems. These nozzles have a self-compensating feature that adjusts flow to allow for fluctuation in storage bottle pressure. This feature can be seen in Figure 4-11.

At this point it should be evident that nitrous-oxide injection has considerable potential to produce substantial horsepower increases. Nonetheless, though it is relatively easy to gain additional power, it is important to remember that utilizing nitrous-oxide to greatest advantage requires a lot more than just "bolting on a kit."

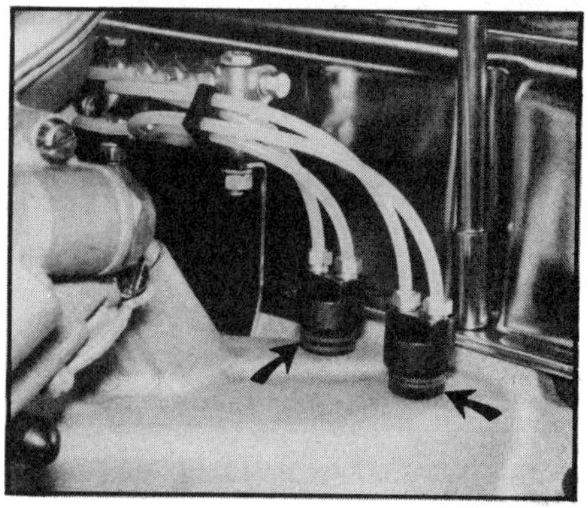

This is a closeup of an Alden/Oselli nozzle. The fiber washers under the base of the nozzle vary the depth that the nozzle protrudes into the port.

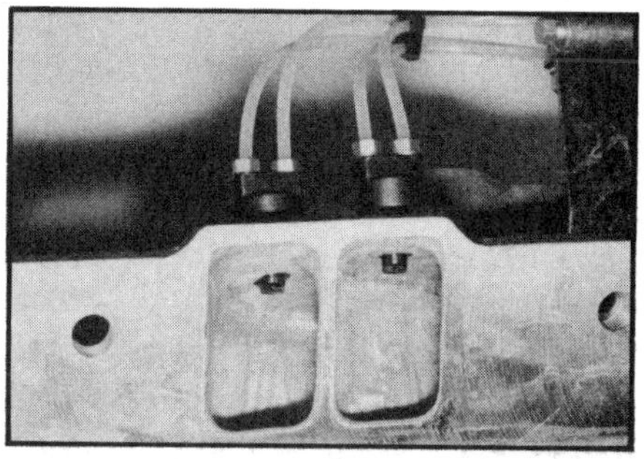

For maximum dispersion, the stream of nitrous exiting the nozzle should point along the direction of airflow through the port.

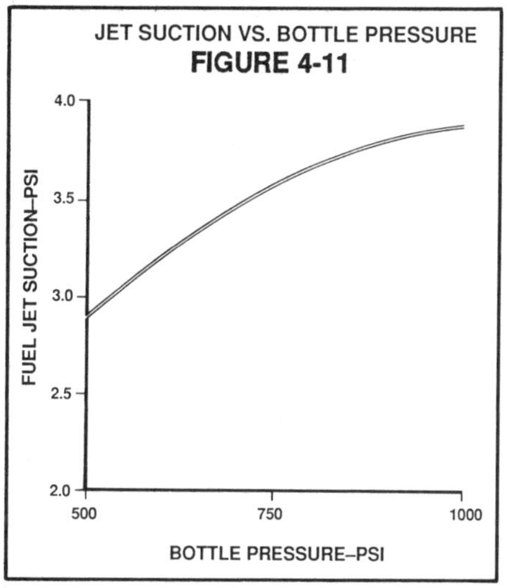

FIGURE 4-11: This graph shows that suction, and therefore the fuel flow, increases with NOS "fogger" nozzles. At higher pressures, slightly more nitrous is delivered into the engine; but this nozzle design compensates and maintains a constant mixture by delivering slightly more enrichment fuel.

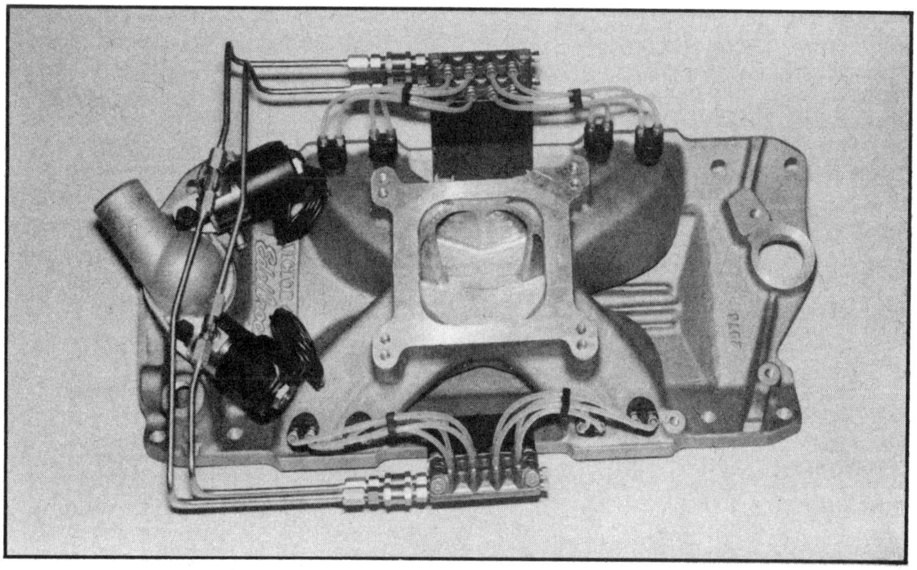

Extensive testing by the author indicated that Alden/Oselli nozzles provide even distribution and quick system response. This system, built by the author, was calibrated to boost peak output by 140 horsepower.

CHAPTER 5

NITROUS COMPETITION SYSTEMS

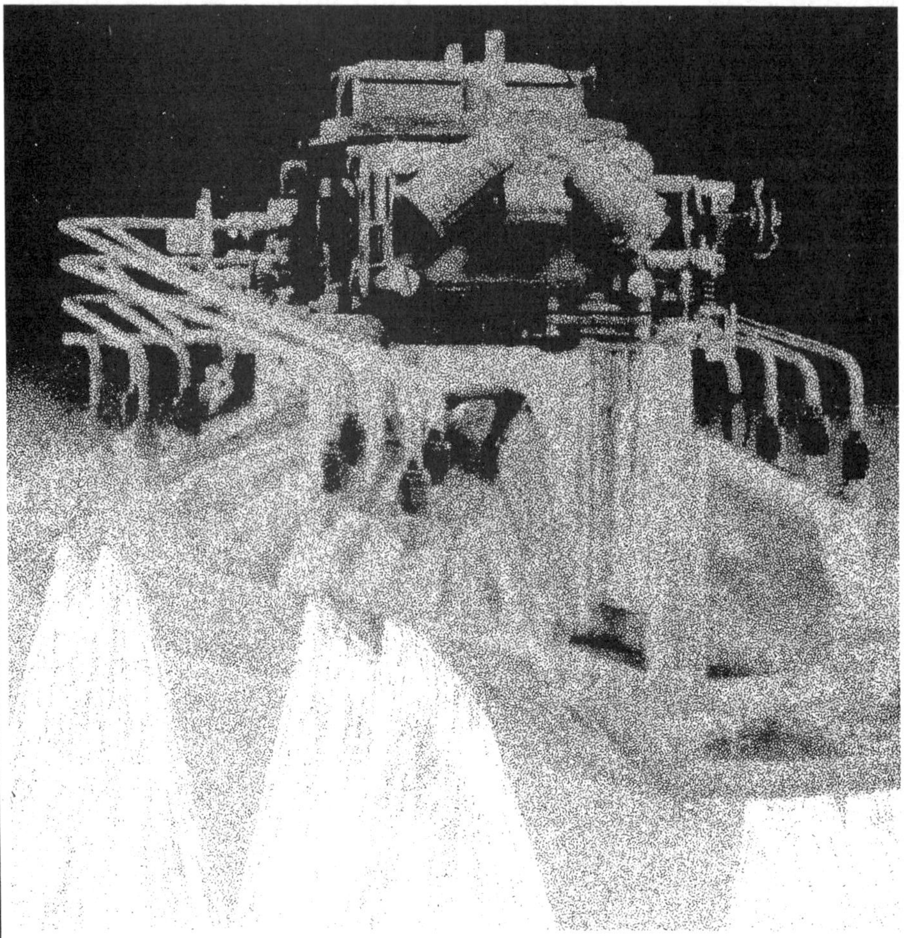

Although we touched on the subject in the last chapter, let's now look at systems that are suitable or designed specifically for racing. Such systems range from the single-stage street systems—which we have already considered—to complex and exotic systems that are suited only for all-out racing.

The most common racing class where nitrous-oxide is widely used is in bracket-type drag racing. To use nitrous effectively the racer must decide whether the system is to be an integral part of the racing package or whether it is to be used as a type of "fail-safe device" that can overcome a slight deficit just before the car crosses the finish. Assuming that the car doesn't break out (record an elapsed time lower than the "dial in"), this will always guarantee a win. It is essential to define the differences between these two approaches because the desired effect and intended usage will to some extent determine the best type of system to buy.

Several factors must be considered. First, if the racer wishes to use a high-power nitrous system and the primary objective is all-out acceleration, it may be necessary to alter the suspension and the overall gearing to cope with the extra torque and power.

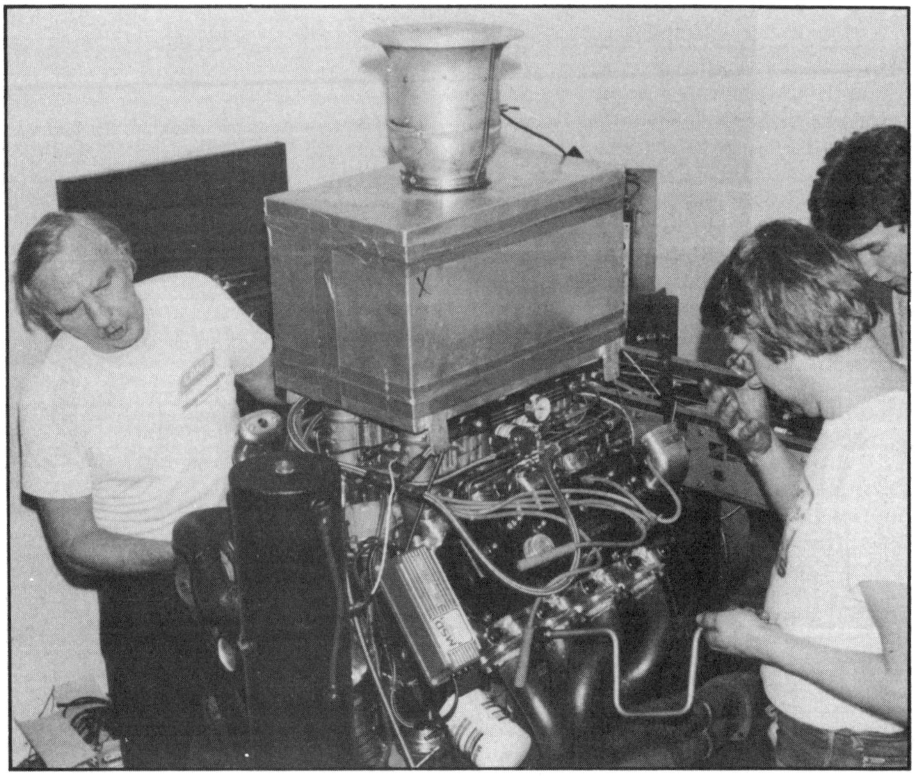

Well-known engine builder Earl Wade puts a 390cid Ford through the paces on the author's dyno. This thundering Ford is fitted with Weber carburetors and a single-stage NOS port-injection system.

If pure top-end speed is the desired effect—whether in drag racing or any other type of application—the same alterations may be required. Of course, if bracket racing is the main goal, the engine and nitrous combination must produce *consistent results* (a factor that we've also discussed previously). However, it is worth restating that since starting-line performance is especially critical when attempting to achieve consistent elapsed times, it is usually best to use the nitrous only in the higher gears. Why? Because too much power off the line can break traction, and this is one of the primary causes of inconsistent ETs.

A good 100-horsepower street system used on a typical 13-second race car can—even if it is only used on the higher gears—typically reduce times by about 0.70 of a second and add about 10mph to the trap speed. With a lightweight racing chassis the reduction in elapsed time will probably be about the same but the trap speed could increase by as much as 20mph. Still, the intent of nitrous-oxide in this particular instance is relatively straightforward: It is used simply to make the car go faster and, possibly, to place the car into a lower/faster bracket.

On the other hand, there are different considerations when nitrous-oxide is intended as a fail-safe to ensure an advantage at the finish line. In this instance it is possible to select a moderate dial-in time and gain a smooth launch (without the nitrous engaged) to avoid wheel-spin. This usually results in relatively consistent start-line performances. The nitrous is used after the shift to high gear in order to gain and hold a slight lead on the opponent until the finish line is crossed.

The lazy start, best achieved by using a relatively high gear ratio, means that the car can be driven very consistently because wheel-spin should not be a problem. Of course this doesn't mean that the driver can fall asleep at the starting line. It is still essential to "cut a good light" or the other driver may simply slip through closer to his dial-in. Nonetheless, many drivers use nitrous to gain a slight lead in the final stages of a close race. This may be the necessary edge to gain an outright win or it may push the opposition to breakout. Either way, it gives a shrewd competitor an important advantage.

Most of the nitrous-injected systems built for street use—and, indeed, some of the moderate competition systems—are built with the idea of adding power to an engine that is well below the ultimate stage of preparation. In other words, nitrous-oxide is often simply a cheap and effective means to increase the peak power output while leaving a wide margin of reliability.

Indeed, if the ultimate goal is all-out power, then a slightly different approach must be taken. Under such circumstances it is not practical to build a maximum-effort normally aspirated engine and then simply add a high-boost competition nitrous-oxide system. Such an engine is not likely to last very long because the nitrous-oxide will thermally or mechanically over-stress the components. It is necessary to look at a competition nitrous-oxide system—at least on an all-out racing engine—as an *integral part of an overall package*. It cannot be viewed simply as a device that, so to speak, adds icing to the cake.

OPTIMIZING NITROUS FLOW

Nitrous flow problems are especially critical in high horsepower racing nitrous systems. To achieve the desired effect—a big boost in horsepower—these systems must successfully transfer large quantities of liquid nitrous from the storage bottle to the point of injection. Under these circumstances it is essential that pressure loss between the supply bottle and the point of injection be minimized.

Starting with the source, we find that many nitrous storage bottles are fitted with an 0.188-inch (3/16) valve orifice. This may be adequate for a

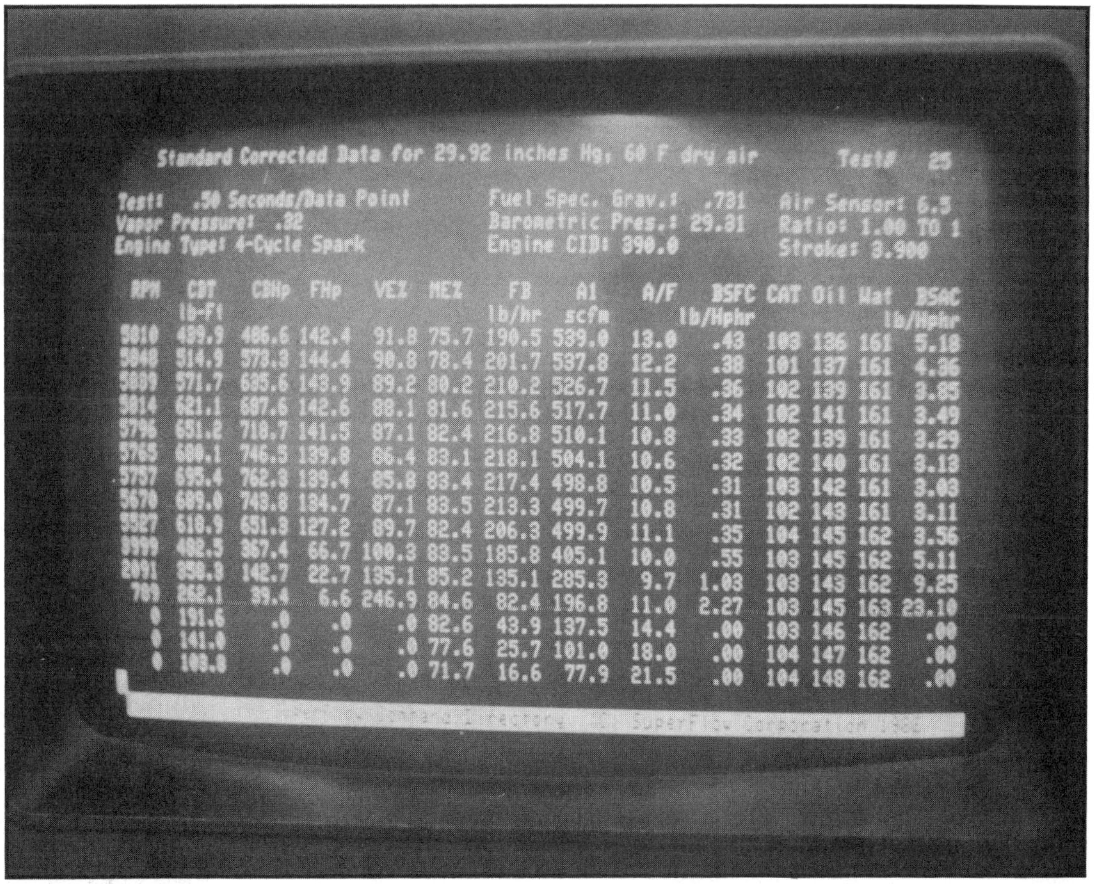

RPM	CBT lb-Ft	CBHp	FHp	VE%	ME%	FB lb/hr	A1 scfm	A/F	BSFC lb/Hphr	CAT	Oil	Wat	BSAC lb/Hphr
5810	489.9	486.6	142.4	91.8	75.7	190.5	539.0	13.0	.43	103	136	161	5.18
5848	514.9	573.3	144.4	90.8	78.4	201.7	537.8	12.2	.38	101	137	161	4.36
5809	571.7	685.6	143.9	89.2	80.2	210.2	526.7	11.5	.36	102	139	161	3.85
5814	621.1	687.6	142.6	88.1	81.6	215.6	517.7	11.0	.34	102	141	161	3.49
5796	651.2	718.7	141.5	87.1	82.4	216.8	510.1	10.8	.33	102	139	161	3.29
5765	680.1	746.5	139.8	86.4	83.1	218.1	504.1	10.6	.32	102	140	161	3.13
5757	695.4	762.3	139.4	85.8	83.4	217.4	498.8	10.5	.31	103	142	161	3.03
5670	689.0	743.8	134.7	87.1	83.5	213.3	499.7	10.8	.31	102	143	161	3.11
5527	618.9	651.3	127.2	89.7	82.4	206.3	499.9	11.1	.35	104	145	162	3.56
3999	482.5	367.4	66.7	100.3	83.5	185.8	405.1	10.0	.55	103	145	162	5.11
2091	358.3	142.7	22.7	135.1	85.2	135.1	285.3	9.7	1.03	103	143	162	9.25
709	262.1	39.4	6.6	246.9	84.6	82.4	196.8	11.0	2.27	103	145	163	23.10
0	191.6	.0	.0	.0	82.6	43.9	137.5	14.4	.00	103	146	162	.00
0	141.0	.0	.0	.0	77.6	25.7	101.0	18.0	.00	104	147	162	.00
0	103.8	.0	.0	.0	71.7	16.6	77.9	21.5	.00	104	148	162	.00

This is the computer screen after a 5800rpm power run of the 390cid Ford at left. The horsepower (recorded under the CBHP heading) jumped from 486.6 to 762.3, a boost of 280 horsepower. Also note the volumetric efficiency under the VE% column. The efficiency of the engine dropped from 91.8 to 85.8%. The computer was set to take readings every 0.5 seconds.

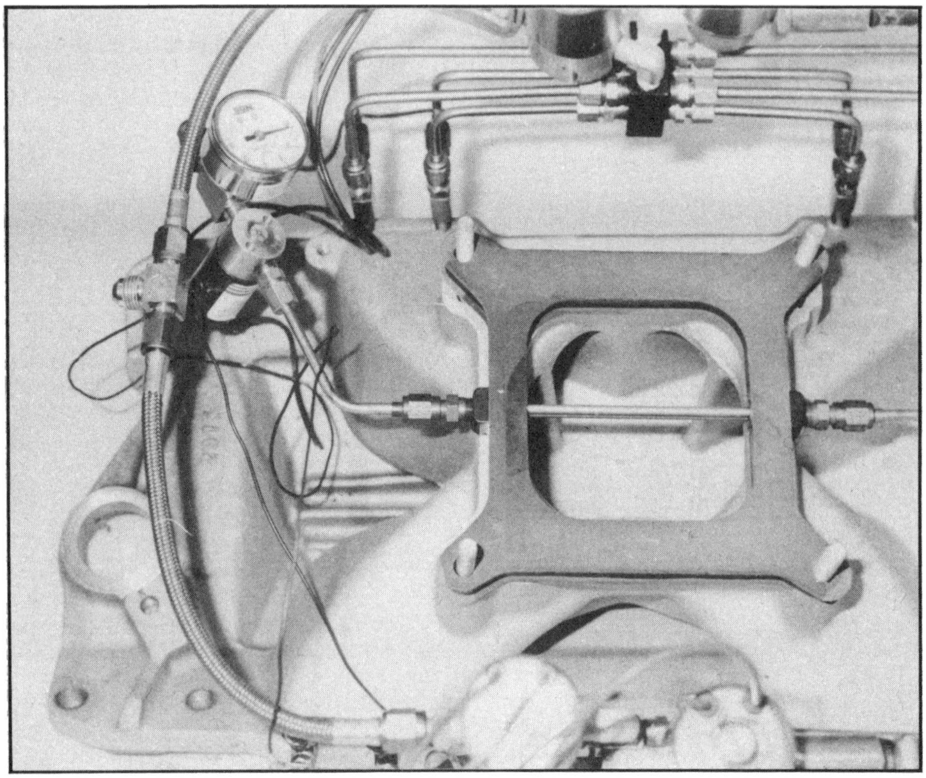

The setup on the author's dyno engine is designed so the flow of nitrous can be directed to the port injectors or to the spraybars in the spacer plate; switching from one to the other allows direct comparisons of the two systems. At low boost levels, the power provided by each system is nearly identical, but at relatively high boost levels the port system is better.

power boost up to about 300 horsepower; but above this level, the nitrous requirements are such that a 0.188-inch orifice can inhibit the flow of nitrous into the system. In 1985 NOS introduced an approved and certified bottle valve with a 0.25-inch orifice. This is a 56% increase in area. Theoretically, the gross nitrous flow through a 0.25-inch orifice should be adequate for power levels up to about 475 horsepower.

When high flow rates are required, it is essential that the inside diameter of the supply line is at least equal to the diameter of the valve orifice. This is especially important in applications that provide 300 horsepower or more. Even though the crosssectional area of the valve orifice and supply line is substantially larger in area than the combined area of the metering orifices (jets), when most systems are activated, it is not uncommon to lose over 100 pounds of pressure between the bottle and metering orifices. This is normally due to restrictions, friction or viscous losses or a combination of these factors. However, for best results, all components of the supply system must be carefully selected and coordinated to eliminate or reduce these losses.

Before moving on we must mention another problem that plagues high-horsepower nitrous systems: bottle "boil off" problems. If liquid nitrous is drawn from the bottle at a very high rate, the contents cannot boil (convert to a vapor) rapidly enough to reestablish the internal vapor pressure. During this occurrence the bottle temperature begins to drop, and when there are uneven temperature gradients throughout the bottle, the pickup point may begin to withdraw emulsified liquid nitrous-oxide that contains bubbles. These bubbles reduce the weight (amount) of nitrous fed to the engine. This causes a drop of peak power.

In one well-documented test Scott Shafiroff experienced these problems with a heavily boosted 427cid big-block Chevy. During max power runs Shafiroff noted that the bottle pressure would drop from 850psi to 750 psi. But when the bottle was heated during the power run—by emersing it in hot water—the pressure climbed back to 850psi and there was a related boost in power output. The higher temperature apparently caused the nitrous to boil off more quickly, thereby maintaining the internal pressure in spite of the high rate at which the fluid nitrous was being withdrawn.

This suggests that when the required nitrous flow rate is very high, multiple bottle systems may be desirable. If a multi-stage system is being employed with expected power boosts in each stage of approximately 200-300 horsepower, it is a good idea to use a separate bottle to feed each stage. At boost levels near 400 horsepower—even with a carefully designed supply system—*the use of a single bottle will almost certainly result in a pressure loss and limit peak power.*

POINT OF INJECTION

Within the circle of nitrous veterans there is a perpetual argument as to whether an under-the-carb plate system or a port jet system is better. No doubt the debate will rage on, but based on personal experience and considerable research gathering data from prominent people in the industry, I believe that an optimized port-located jet system will always produce more horsepower than an optimized plate system. Though we have discussed this in an earlier chapter, it seems worthwhile to restate the two principal advantages of a port system: (1) A port-located jet system does not suffer from distribution problems created by inconsistencies in manifold flow; and (2) The discharge nozzles of a port-injection system can be aimed straight toward the back of the intake valve. This latter characteristic prevents the nitrous from absorbing heat inside the manifold and port—thus more of the nitrous remains in liquid form—and leaves more volume in the intake manifold for the normally-inducted air-fuel charge.

Of course, this argument assumes that the nitrous and enrichment fuel are injected at the optimal point and are thoroughly mixed at the point of injection. If they're not, the performance gain from a port-injection system will be far from the maximum. Unfortunately, it is often necessary to position the discharge nozzles somewhat further up the intake tract than would otherwise be desired. Nonetheless, in the real world, even a less-than-optimal port-injection system will generally have an edge over a typical plate system.

However up to this point in our discussion, the question of superiority has been moot. The horsepower boost levels we have been considering can usually be achieved readily with either a plate or a port-jet system. To put things into perspective, a

350-horsepower increase can be gained with either system; however, an optimized port-injection system could well achieve 375 horsepower on the same amount of nitrous. On the other hand, though it may produce more horsepower, the plumbing of a port-injection system tends to be complex and expensive—because of the numerous nitrous and fuel lines required to feed the individual injectors. In many applications this often makes a plate system a more attractive proposition.

Another factor to be considered—especially with a drag racing engine—is that there are a lot more nitrous lines in a port-injection system to cool. Unless large volumes of nitrous are being used, the supply lines may not cool down until well after the discharge is initiated. This can be an advantage if there is a lot of horsepower available, as it may just "de-tune" the engine sufficiently to allow the car to leave without wheelspin. However, if the chassis hooks well and more power can be used to launch the car harder, the slow boost response may not provide optimum starting line performance.

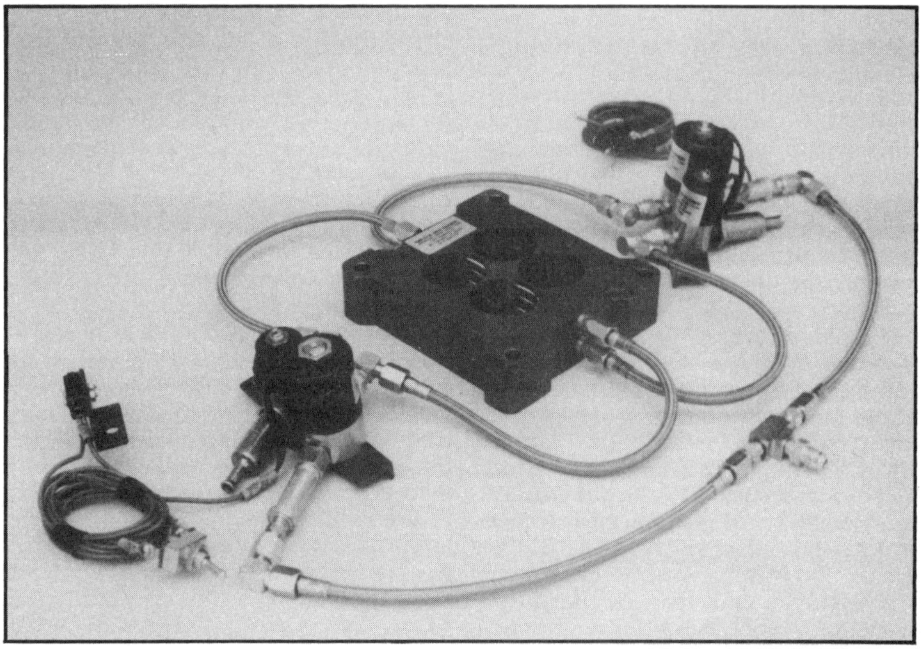

This two-stage high-horsepower system was developed by Ron Hammel of 10,000 RPM Engineering. Incorporating separate spray bars and solenoids for each system, the second stage can be triggered manually, by engine speed, or by throttle activation (see text).

MULTI-STAGE SYSTEMS

For all practical purposes, two major factors determine how much nitrous can be successfully used by an engine. One factor is the compression ratio of the engine. The second factor is the maximum cylinder pressure that the engine can withstand.

In Chapter Four we discussed the basic drawback of all fixed-rate/constant-flow injection systems. When the system is activated, a constant flow of nitrous is delivered to the manifold and drawn into the cylinders by the induction process. And, as engine speed increases, there is less relative time in each intake cycle for the cylinders to take in the nitrous-air-fuel mixture. In other words, it is a little like a supercharger that gives massive boost just off idle and as the engine speed increases, the boost drops off.

The only way to remedy this situation is to increase the flow of nitrous-oxide and enrichment as engine speed increases. Ideally, the flow of nitrous-fuel would be proportional to engine speed and the amount of horsepower added to the engine by the system would rise steadily to a peak at maximum engine speed. This is theoretically and mechanically possible with sophisticated electronics, but the cost would be extremely high. Though somewhat less elegant, a much more practical solution is to use a "staged" approach that simply supplies additional nitrous and enrichment fuel at one or more predetermined thresholds in the engine speed range. This can be readily achieved with one or more coordinated constant-flow systems that operate independently to supply additional nitrous and fuel—in stages—as the engine speed (rpm) increases.

Staged systems are, naturally, more complicated and more expensive. However, for all practical purposes—even with a trick drag-race chassis—it is necessary to consider multi-staging the nitrous system of a small-block engine when the power supplied by the nitrous system exceeds 200 horsepower. On a large displacement big-block engine this level would be in the region of 250 to 300 horsepower. Any time the desired power augmentation nears or exceeds these levels, multi-staging becomes a virtual necessity.

There are currently several multi-stage systems on the market. Most of the reputable companies, such as NOS and 10,000 RPM, have off-the-

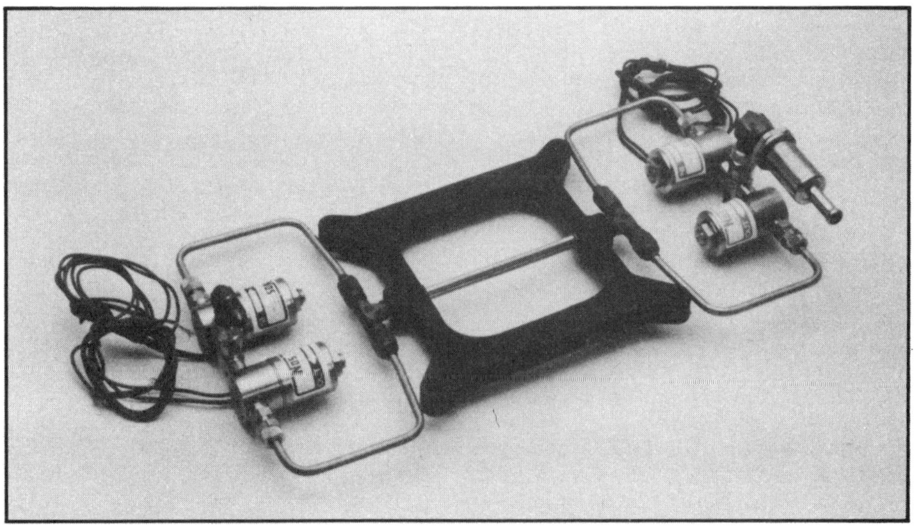

This is about as simple as a two-stage system can be. The routing of the distribution lines indicates that the nitrous and enrichment fuel for both stages of this NOS system are delivered through two spraybars (one for nitrous and one for fuel).

shelf multi-stage systems. Most of these commercially available systems have two stages. Three-stage systems are less common but are not difficult to build (as we will discuss later). Four-stage systems are almost unheard of, but this is not because they are less effective. They are, in fact, rare because such a system is exceedingly complex. But when more racers realize the value of multi-stage system, the tolerance for complexity may increase.

To see why a multi-stage system has so much more potential, we must understand how cylinder pressure relates to power output. Most readers have probably seen the letters "BMEP." They stand for brake mean effective pressure. The torque output of an engine is directly related to the brake mean effective pressure. BMEP is an important aspect of engine performance, and for our purposes here, it is only essential to understand that when the brake mean effective pressure within the cylinders increases (during the combustion process), the overall torque output of the engine increases. (They are linked by the total piston area.) In elemental terms, if the break mean effective pressure increases or decreases by 10%, it is because the torque increases or decreases by 10%.

Now, let's look at an example of how multi-staging can improve the BMEP developed by an engine. Let's consider an imaginary big-block Chevy engine that produces 525 pounds-feet of torque at 4000rpm. When nitrous is added to this engine, let's assume that at 4000rpm the torque increases to 800 pounds-feet. It is also reasonable, given these circumstances, to suppose that this engine may not be very far from the threshold of detonation. The torque output has increased to 800 pounds-feet simply because the pressure (BMEP) generated inside the cylinders has increased.

However, we find that as the engine speed goes up, the torque output drops off. As discussed earlier, this is because the amount of oxygen and fuel inducted to each cylinder during the intake cycle declines as the available time per cycle becomes shorter. In addition, because the proportional flow of nitrous and enrichment fuel in a constant-flow injection system is directly related to intake flow, the percentage of added nitrous-fuel also decreases. This causes a drop in torque. Nonetheless, we know the engine can produce sufficient BMEP to equal 800 pounds-feet of torque. So the trick is to provide enough oxygen—in this case nitrous—and fuel to compensate for the drop off in intake efficiency.

At this point we can activate a second stage that delivers enough nitrous and fuel to boost the torque back up to 800 pounds-feet at 6000 rpm. Under normal circumstances, it would have typically dropped to about 700 pounds-feet at 6000rpm. (Boosting the torque by 100 pounds-feet at 6000rpm represents about 125 horsepower.) However, if the engine speed is raised to 7000rpm, the breathing efficiency of the engine will again drop quite a bit. To compensate, it is possible to activate an additional nitrous and fuel stage to produce another 100 pounds-feet of torque. This will result in 800 pounds-feet of torque at 7000rpm. As the breathing efficiency continues to decline, the torque will probably drop to 700 pounds-feet at 8000rpm and the engine will probably develop about 1100 horsepower at the peak.

In this example about 50% of the power output is being derived from a multi-stage nitrous-oxide system. And though this is entirely possible with existing nitrous hardware, the basic engine need not be sophisticated, other than having a strong bottom end and suitable pistons. The nitrous system, however, is pretty sophisticated and in this case—as with any nitrous system—*all parts of the system must be designed and properly installed to provide optimum nitrous and fuel flow.*

MULTI-STAGE TRIGGERING

Activation of the secondary stages in a multi-stage system should be tied directly to engine speed (rpm). This can be accomplished in a fairly simple and straightforward manner.

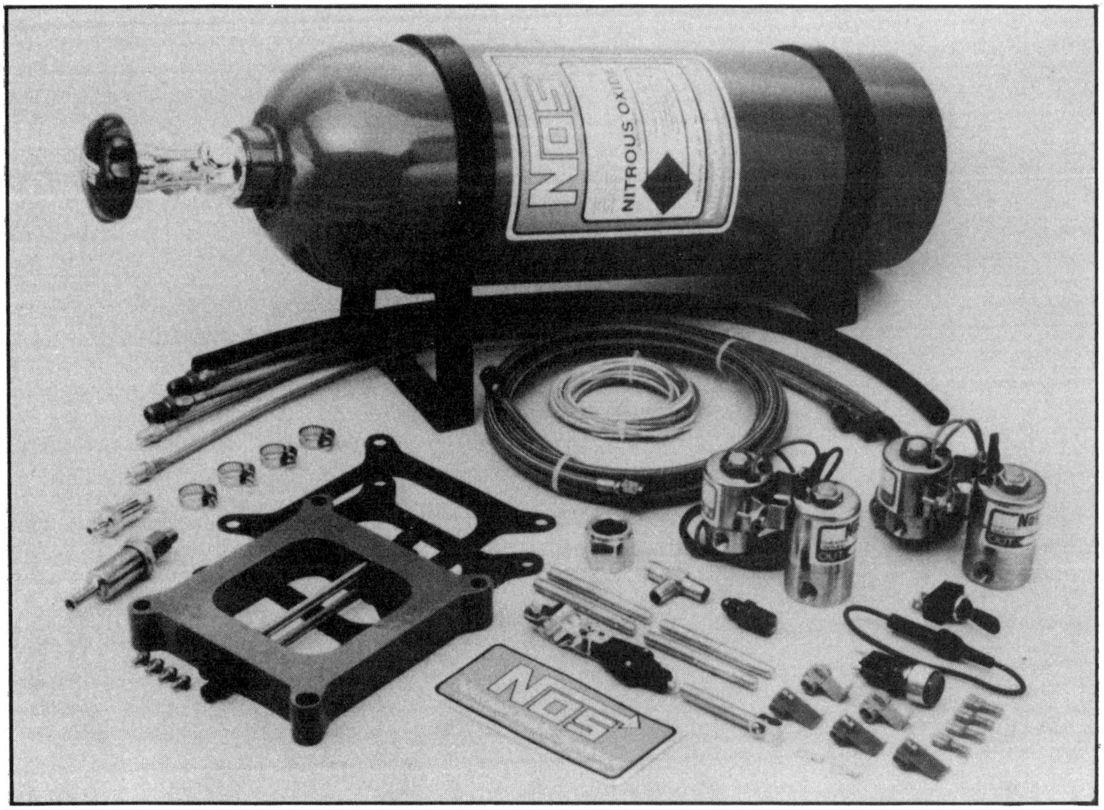

This NOS two-stage system—note the dual solenoids—will provide a "soft" system activation, which is beneficial in certain instances. A system that hits "hard" can cause traction problems at low engine speeds, especially with street tires.

In most cases an rpm-sensing switch is used to activate the control solenoids.

Nitrous Oxide Systems offers an rpm-sensitive switch that can be adjusted to trigger at whatever engine speed deemed necessary. At the present time, one switch is required for each stage. With this unit, it is simply a question of adjusting a knob to set the system to activate at the desired level.

As for the primary nitrous stage, this can be triggered by either a throttle switch or an rpm-sensitive switch. For drag-racing applications a throttle switch is more effective because the first stage generally delivers a fairly modest dose of nitrous and fuel. Most highly developed drag machines have enough power off the line—even without nitrous—and the nitrous is activated after the launch to produce a hard charge from 50 yards out on through the lights.

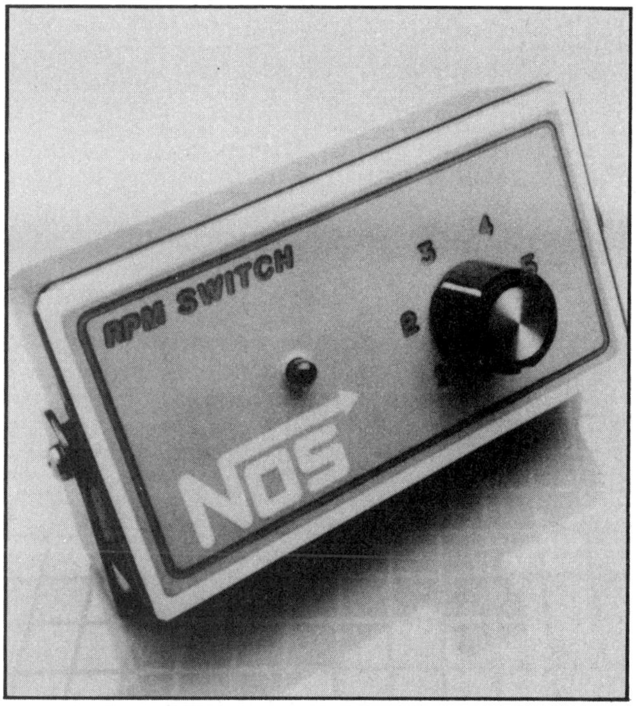

This rpm switch from NOS is used to alter the point at which the nitrous system, or a stage of the system, is activated.

NITROUS & CORNERS

So far we've talked primarily about drag racing. But nitrous also has a place in other types of racing. For instance, any type of racing that places a premium on acceleration—such as autocross or sprints, which involve short, tight courses, and possibly certain types of quarter- and half-mile circle-track racing—may benefit from nitrous augmentation. In every instance, however, the prevailing rules and regulations must be checked to determine if the use of nitrous is precluded.

Many sanctioning organizations disallow nitrous for reasons of safety or economy. The prevalent logic goes something like this: If nitrous-oxide is used by one competitor to gain an advantage—and that competitor most certainly will have an important edge—the rest of his cohorts will almost certainly be forced to eventually do the same thing. And once the nitrous system is installed, it is only (almost) a question of pouring in more nitrous and fuel to gain more horsepower. This leads to greater reliability problems. As the racers push harder and harder for more power, the engine will inevitably reach the point where it cannot withstand the strain. Finally, if everyone is using nitrous-oxide, winning will boil down to the question of who can afford to buy the most engines and who is lucky enough to cross the finish with the engine in one piece. True or not, this scenario is feared by many sanctioning bodies, and currently nitrous-oxide is banned in most forms of organized racing.

Nonetheless, in some forms of short-course racing, i.e., drag racing, sprinting, or serious autocross/gymkhana competition, the question of engine reliability is less critical. Engines are more highly tuned because horsepower is more important than long-term reliability. Let's consider for a moment that we are building an engine for a vehicle that must negotiate corners during the competition. The requirements for the nitrous system are going to follow slightly different lines.

First, it is necessary to make certain that the nitrous is *not used at slow engine speeds.* Most vehicles built specifically for road courses (a course with one or more corners) generally do not have the type of suspension that can readily accommodate the power levels and potential acceleration generated by a heavily dosed nitrous engine. Using nitrous from the start line (with a typical road-type chassis) will usually result in a lot of wheelspin and lost time. However, once the vehicle has reached a reasonable speed, nitrous can be used to gain an important extra measure of acceleration.

In most types of short-course racing a single-stage nitrous system is very effective in conjunction with a manual transmission. In some instances a multi-stage kit can be used effectively. If the particular course has a long fast section, injecting additional nitrous at higher engine speeds—with a second stage—may provide additional power on long straightaways. This can, of course, be an advantage when it is necessary to pass a competitor on the straight sections.

In any type of road event—one where the transmission must be continually shifted up and down through the gears to accommodate deceleration and acceleration in and out of corners—the best choice will be a manual transmission. However, using a nitrous-boosted engine with a manual transmission may substantially affect the driving style. In general, the driver will find that he does not need to make as many gear changes. If nitrous system activation and boost level are properly coordinated with the engine speed, there will be a substantial increase in the available low-speed torque. This will generally allow the car to exit any given corner in a higher gear and with a higher acceleration rate.

With a nitrous-injected engine and properly selected gearing it is possible to attain exceptional acceleration out of even very tight corners. In virtually all cases, this acceleration will far exceed that possible with an equivalent engine of the same power output but without nitrous boost. If the nitrous activation is properly coordinated with the vehicle speed and shift points, this acceleration "boost" can also provide a tremendous edge for passing competitors, especially on a very tight course.

The extra torque may also effectively "cover up" a driver miscue. If the driver has incorrectly positioned the car in a corner, missed a gear shift, or selected the wrong gear, the available power from the nitrous system can pull the car through. However, even though the lap speeds may not show these miscues, repeated use of nitrous boost at very low engine speeds is risky. When the engine is "lugged down" to very slow shaft speeds and

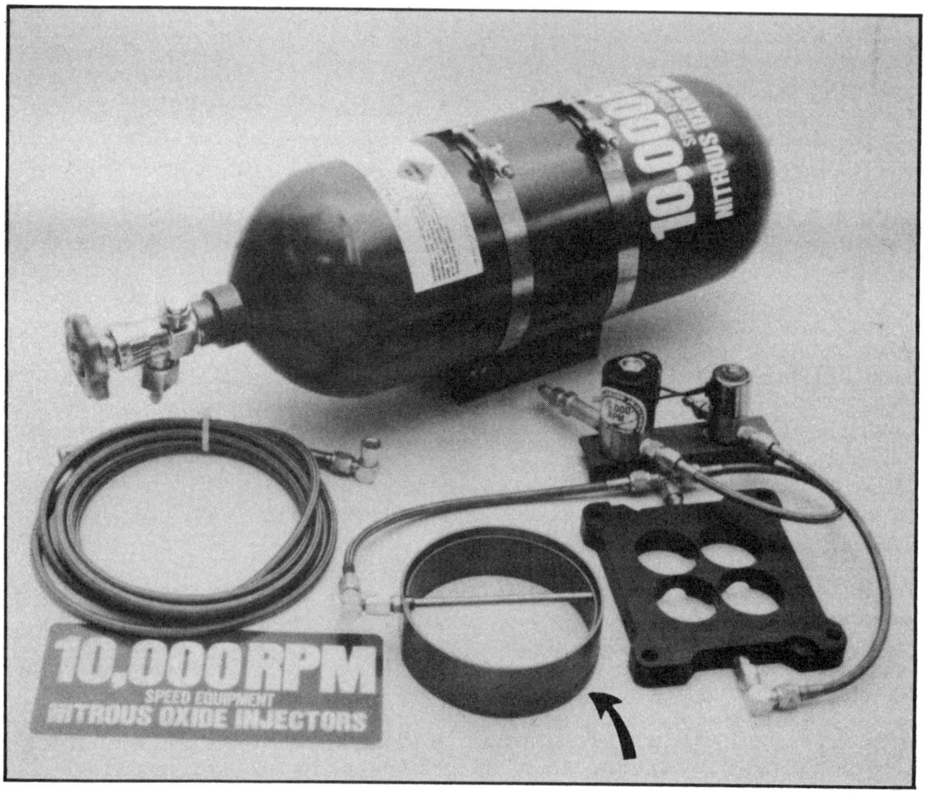

This Power Ring (arrow) from 10,000 RPM is unique. The Power Ring sits on top of the carburetor with the nitrous holes aligned over the booster venturis so that the stream of nitrous is directed through the boosters. This increases the fuel flow from the boosters, thus providing the enrichment necessary for the nitrous.

nitrous is injected to the engine, the combustion pressures can become dangerously high. This can and will eventually lead to mechanical failure, but if the entire racing efforts boils down to one lapse in judgment or one do-or-die effort, the nitrous may well save the day.

However, one additional proviso applies here: If a nitrous-oxide system is used on a car equipped with an automatic transmission, it is important to read and heed the information on nitrous and automatic transmissions presented in the subsequent chapters. Nitrous is not, per se, dangerous, but if the transmission is not able to withstand the potential power levels generated by a nitrous-boosted engine, a dangerous situation may develop.

10,000 RPM POWER RING

Though it is applicable to any form of racing where top-end power is needed, this is as good an opportunity as any to mention 10,000 RPM's "Power Ring." This is a nitrous distribution device that installs on top of the carburetor. Two spraybars span the mouth of the carb—currently models are available for either a Holley or Q-Jet—and orifices are positioned on the underside of the bars to direct small amounts of nitrous through the booster venturis.

The stream of nitrous produces a significantly higher "signal" in the booster—just as if a much larger volume of air was being drawn into the engine—and the carburetor responds by delivering more fuel into the airstream. Also, the nitrous tends to cool the air in the vicinity of the carburetor, which increases the density, to some extent, of the air passing through the most restrictive part of the induction system—the carburetor.

In effect, the Power Ring makes the carburetor believe that the engine is drawing in more air than it actually is. Although very little extra volume of air is passing through the carb (the air is somewhat cooler and more dense, but the effect is relatively modest), the increased flow through the venturi—due to the Power Ring injection—"fools" the carburetor metering system into delivering more fuel to the engine.

Typically, the quantity of nitrous used by the Power Ring would only generate an increase of about 20- to 25-horsepower if it were delivered by a conventional spraybar or nozzle system. But by injecting what is, in essence, a small amount of nitrous-oxide into the booster venturis, about 50 extra horsepower can be generated on a typical race-prepped 350cid engine.

Coincidentally, if something like the Power Ring is used with a two-stage system, the effect is similar to a three-stage system, without necessarily adding vastly to the consumption of nitrous or the complexity of the system. The third stage—the Power Ring—can be triggered to activate at an engine speed of 5000rpm or higher.

From the discussion so far we can see that it is relatively simple to boost the output of an engine by as much as 300 to 400 horsepower with a well-engineered nitrous-oxide system. Developing this much power, of course, requires high-quality engine components and meticulous assembly procedures. But it is not beyond the realm of practicality to build a 650- to 700-horsepower smallblock or a 950- to 1000-horsepower big-block. No matter what type or brand of engine you prefer or what type of racing you're considering, this is pretty potent power.

NITROUS & ALCOHOL

Up to now we have talked only about the use of nitrous with gasoline. If nitrous is used with alcohol in a properly prepared engine, there is the potential to produce even more power. There are some wrinkles to be ironed out when they are paired together, but the subject deserves to be explored in greater detail because carbureted alcohol engines are now very popular in some drag racing classes.

The anti-detonant and cooling qualities of alcohol prevent many of the heat problems associated with extreme-output engines. As a general rule, using alcohol along with a typical nitrous system designed for a smallblock V8 engine will give an additional power boost of about 50 to 80 horsepower, and on a big-block the additional boost can equal as much as 80 to 100 horsepower. As has already been suggested, however, to get these results it's not simply a question of changing fuels.

Alcohol and nitrous are, in many respects, made for each other. Because of the lower nitrogen content, nitrous-oxide tends to make any fuel detonate more readily. On the other hand, as many readers are no doubt aware, alcohol has a very high resistance to detonation. In fact, the resistance of alcohol to detonation is so high that it can afford to "give away" some of that detonation resistance when it is used with nitrous-oxide.

Under most conditions, the combination readily demonstrates an advantage over other fuels—such as gasoline—in a normally-aspirated engine.

The detonation resistance of alcohol is very dependent on temperature. When alcohol is heated, the detonation resistance diminishes quite rapidly. However, with the cooling effect of nitrous-oxide, the detonation resistance of the alcohol increases to the point where it largely counteracts the detonation-inducing effects that nitrous-oxide has inside the combustion chamber. The net result is that theoretically we can use larger amounts of nitrous-oxide in an engine when it is fueled with alcohol.

Also, the latent heat of evaporation (cooling due to evaporation) of alcohol is very high, so the density of the induced air charge is increased. Couple this with the cooling effect of nitrous-oxide, and we have a considerable potential to increase the volumetric efficiency of the engine.

If we used the same absolute quantity of nitrous-oxide, but switched from gasoline to alcohol, it would be necessary to make fuel flow adjustments to get the correct nitrous-to-fuel ratio. But, when the ratio has been corrected, theoretically the engine should produce about 8-10% more horsepower. In actual practice, though, when a nitrous-boosted engine is switched from gasoline to alcohol, the measured horsepower gain is almost always less than this theoretical projection.

The discrepancy is not really understood, but some results from informal testing by Ron Hamell are worth noting. Ron dyno tested an engine with different combinations of fuel, nitrous and enrichment-fuel. The most revealing of these tests indicated that an engine running a base fuel of alcohol would produce more peak power if, in place of alcohol, racing gasoline was used as the enrichment fuel in the nitrous system.

(From a purely practical viewpoint, this sounds complicated, but in fact, It is not difficult to use gasoline in the nitrous system of an alcohol racing engine. An auxiliary pump, a small motorcycle battery and a one-gallon fuel tank can readily be used to deliver the enrichment gasoline.)

A detailed study to determine and measure the effects of nitrous and different fuels would probably clear up many of these uncertainties. Unquestionably one of the highest priorities in this effort would be to establish why heavy loads of nitrous and alcohol don't deliver as much power as a combination of alcohol, gasoline, and nitrous. The best theory to date seems to be that the straight alcohol-nitrous combination may be "too cold" to burn effectively in an unsupercharged motor. The dissociation of the nitrous into base compounds of oxygen and nitrogen occurs very slowly at lower temperatures. The gasoline could be the ingredient that boosts the combustion temperature to the point where expected gains are realized.

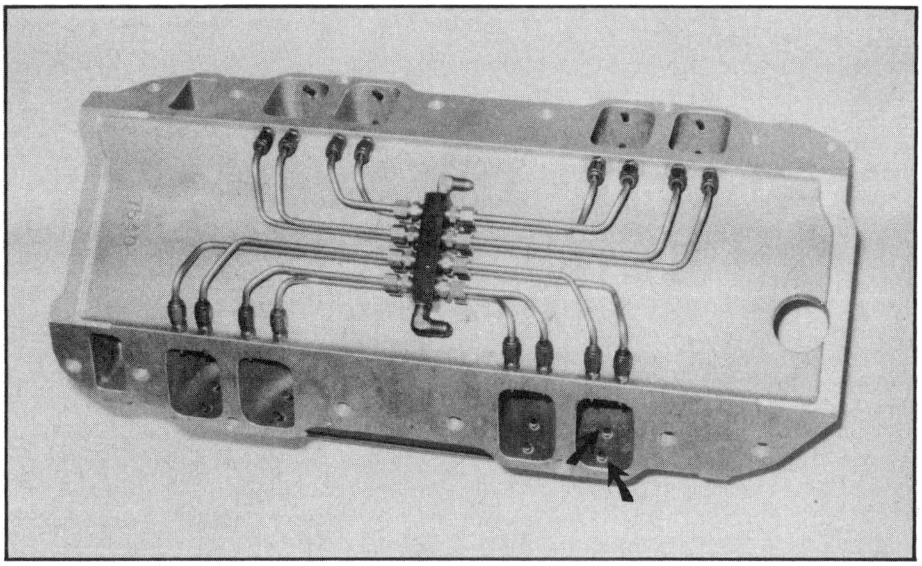

From the bottom, this under-the-manifold port system looks pretty conventional. But notice the extra pair of nozzles protruding through the roof of the port. A multi-stage port-injection system can potentially yield a power boost of 400 horsepower.

It would also be very interesting to study in greater detail what effect a nitrous-alcohol boost mix might have on a gasoline-fueled engine. A few years ago the author saw a *nearly stock* 427cid big-block Chevy with a single 4-barrel on an open-plenum intake manifold equipped with three stages of nitrous—two plate and one port injection—develop in excess of 800 horsepower. In this case the engine was fueled with gasoline while alcohol was used as enrichment fuel for the nitrous system. Each stage of the boost system should have produced about 100 to 110 horsepower, totaling about 330 horsepower; but in this instance, the three stages combined to produce 375 additional horsepower. It is also impressive to note that this power was produced at relatively low engine speeds (rpm). During drag runs the shift point was only 6500rpm and the engine still propelled a heavy race car into the low 9-second category.

ALCOHOL MIX RATIOS

As most racers are aware, the

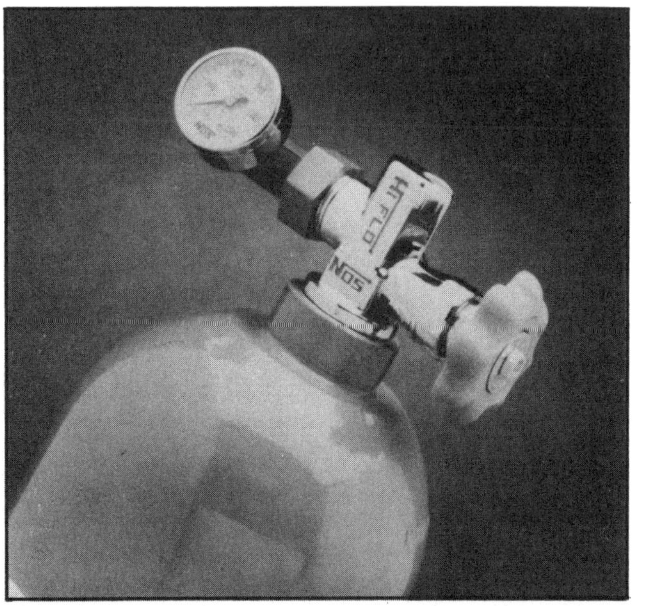

If the system is designed to produce high horsepower with alcohol, exceptionally large quantities of nitrous and enrichment fuel must be delivered to the engine. A high-flow bottle valve is essential and the lines from the bottle to the solenoid must be large enough to flow sufficient quantities of nitrous.

amount of alcohol required to produce the optimum mixture—with either alcohol and air or alcohol and nitrous—is substantially greater than that required for gasoline. As far as the nitrous system is concerned, there are two ways to achieve the desired delivery: increase the size of the jets or raise the fuel pressure.

Let's assume that we are converting a typical nitrous kit from gasoline to alcohol. If the original calibration for gasoline is correct, about 230% more fuel flow will be required for methanol. In other words, the volume of enrichment fuel supplied by an alcohol system must be 2.3 times greater than the volume originally supplied by the gasoline system. This will require jets or flow restrictions that are 52% larger *in diameter* than the originals.

This, of course, presumes that if the jets are drilled oversize, the flow efficiency of the drilled orifice is not adversely affected. In reality, there is no guarantee of this. A dull drill or small burr can easily produce a variation or imperfection that may disrupt flow through the orifice. The interior wall of the redrilled orifice must be smooth and if there are approach or exit ramps to the original orifice, the redrilled orifice must have ramps that duplicate the original. Don't dismiss this as a minor factor. A 0.002-inch burr in a small orifice can affect flow by as much as 20% or 30%. This is only barely within the range of flow variation that can be tolerated for safe engine operation.

Without question, drilling flow restrictions or jet orifices is a touchy game. However, it is important to remember that alcohol engines can tolerate a rich mixture to a much greater extent than gasoline engines. So to be on the safe side, it might be wise to allow an extra margin and enlarge the orifices to 60% oversize.

All of the foregoing assumes, of course, that the jets are the only calibrating restrictions in the system. When especially large jets are required—as is common with alcohol—it is possible that the flow area of the orifice in the solenoid may be smaller than the combined area of the jets. If this happens, the solenoid orifice becomes a significant restriction to flow and, in effect, the solenoid orifice becomes the calibrating point of the system (preventing sufficient flow through the jets). As mentioned earlier, this is not acceptable, and to insure proper system functioning with large jets, it may be necessary to use replacement solenoids with a larger flow capacity.

It is also important to use the right type of solenoids. When alcohol is used as an enrichment fuel, Bill Wheatley of ICE suggests using only solenoids with Teflon-coated plungers. Solenoids that have Viton or Neoprene plungers should be avoided as these materials swell when they come in contact with alcohol and may seal improperly or inhibit flow through the plunger orifice.

The best way to insure against flow difficulties is to actually measure the effective flow of the system. The easiest method is to place the nitrous system in a bucket, activate the fuel system at the working pressure for 30 seconds, and measure the amount of fuel emitted by the system. After completing the conversion to alcohol, the same test is performed and the orifices are carefully enlarged until the volume of fuel trapped in the bucket (within an identical time period) equals 2.3 to 2.4 times the original volume.

If the vehicle has a high-pressure fuel system, the problem can be approached in another way. Many nitrous systems are designed to run at four, five or, at most, six psi of fuel pressure. However, some fuel pumps will deliver as much as nine or ten psi. And some fuel pumps—especially those used in racing fuel-injection systems—will deliver as much as 100 psi. Usually a regulator valve is used with these high-pressure pumps to reduce the delivery pressure to the required level. If, in fact, the pump can produce excess pressure (and it will maintain the pressure at the flow rate required), the delivery volume can be increased by simply raising the pressure.

To get the correct mixture ratio, the fuel pressure must be increased by a factor of 5.3. For instance, if the system is operating at 5.0psi on gasoline, when it is converted to alcohol, the pressure can be increased to 5.3 times 5.0, which equals 26.5. If the fuel pump can deliver enough pressure, the regulator can be readjusted to 26.5psi, and the delivery volume should be approximately correct for alcohol.

One aspect that needs careful attention is the matter of gross fuel flow. Large amounts of alcohol are required to maintain the proper air-fuel mixture in a racing engine running at wide-open throttle. When the nitrous system is activated, the fuel demands are even higher—provided the system uses alcohol as the enrichment fuel—and the total alcohol requirement can be exceedingly high. In fact, the required amount of fuel

If you're looking for maximum horsepower, remember that a clandestine system hidden under the intake manifold will not—all things being equal—produce as much the power as a conventional exposed system.

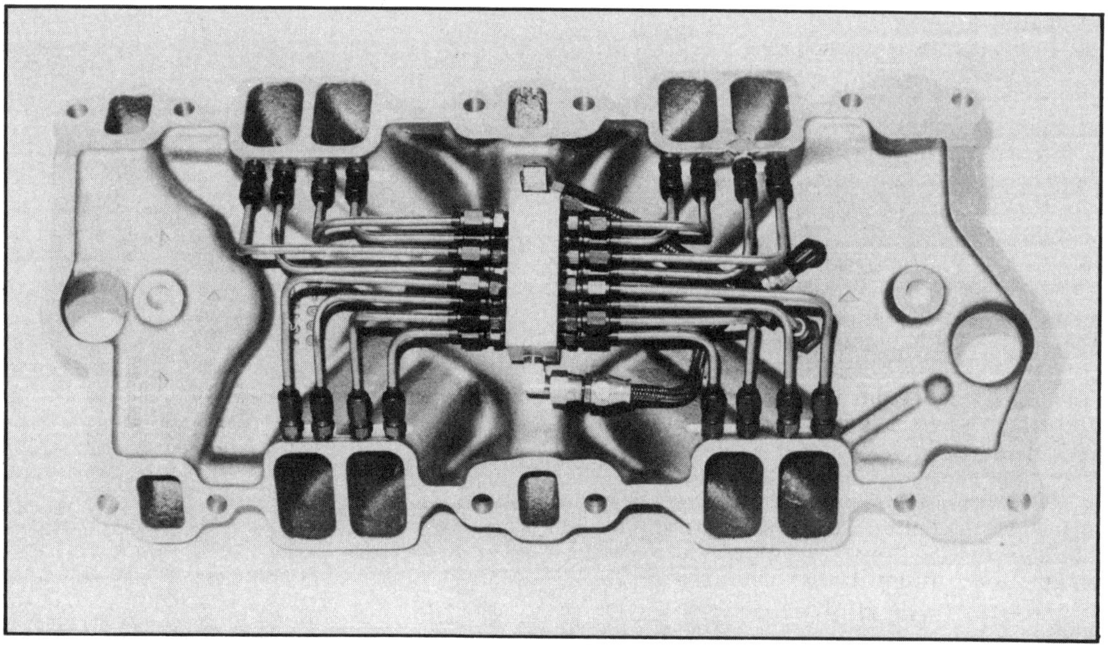

can easily exceed the capabilities of a single pump. To attain adequate flow volume, it is usually necessary to use more than one pump. And some large-displacement, nitrous-boosted alcohol engines need as many as three high-capacity pumps to maintain a correct fuel balance.

In many cases electric pumps are used to deliver the fuel to the the engine. This type of pump is relatively inexpensive and readily available, but the use of multiple pumps places a high demand on the electrical system. When this requirement is added to the current draw required by a two- or three-stage nitrous system, the total electrical load will be considerable. It is essential, therefore, to carefully maintain the battery fully charged—and in race cars that do not have a charging system it may be necessary to use multiple batteries to ensure adequate capacity—otherwise the fuel flow may decline simply because the electrical system is loaded beyond capacity. In the worst case, this can be fatal to the engine. There may be enough potential to hold the nitrous-fuel control valves open—so the flow of nitrous to the engine will continue—but there may not be enough potential to keep the fuel pump(s) operating to full capacity. This, as has been stated many times before, will result in a lean fuel mixture, excessive combustion temperatures and catastrophic engine damage.

With some racing engines the electrical problem can be avoided by utilizing a mechanical engine-driven pump. The most common example, of course, is the Hilborn or a similar fuel-injection pump. These pumps usually have more than enough capacity for a typical high-output nitrous-boosted engine.

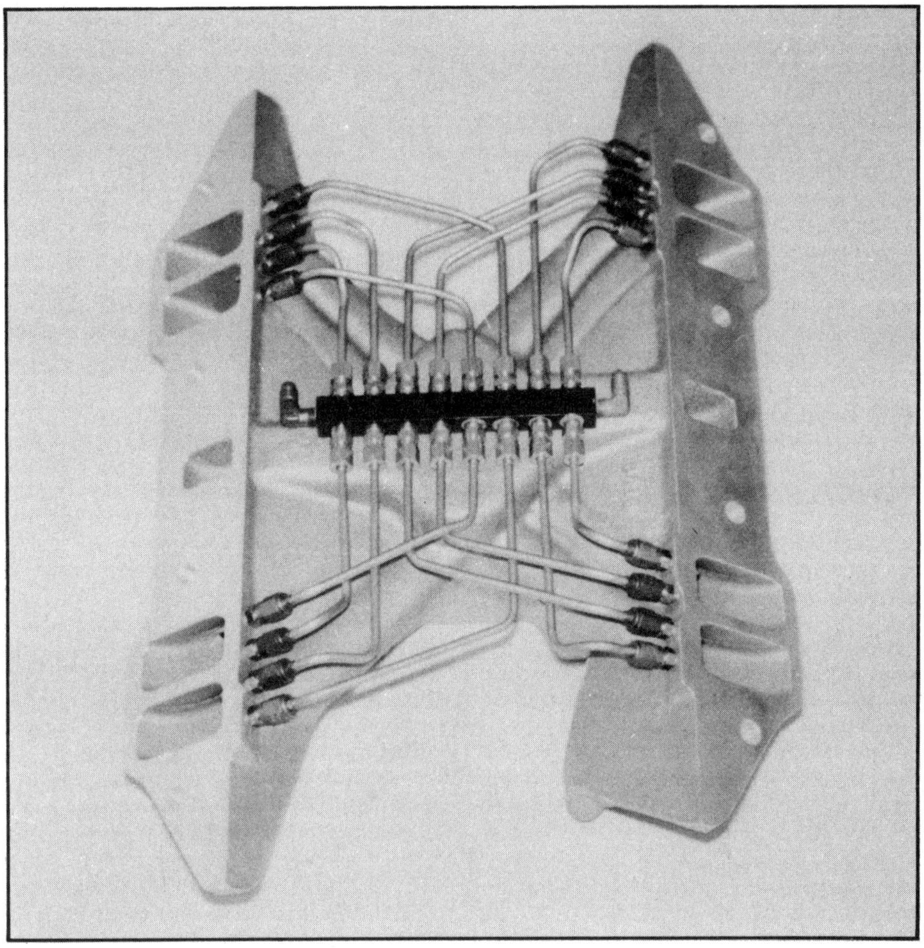

Because of the quantities of nitrous and fuel required, a port injection system will produce better distribution and higher peak output from an all-out alcohol engine.

ENGINE REQUIREMENTS FOR NITROUS-ALCOHOL

If the intended goal is to boost the output of an alcohol engine by 100 to 150 horsepower, the engine need not be altered significantly from normal alcohol specifications—i.e., use high compression. Commonly available V8 cylinder heads are designed for relatively low compression ratios—they are generally intended for passenger-car engines—and it is difficult to obtain actual mechanical ratios much higher than about 12 or 13:1. In many cases this is the practical upper limit, even with modest nitrous assist. However, when the nitrous power boost exceeds approximately 20% of the total output, the compression must be progressively reduced as the proportion of nitrous-assisted output is increased. When the nitrous augmentation produces approximately 50% of the total output, the mechanical compression ratio should not exceed 9:1.

With sufficient preparation, a racing engine with extremely high nitrous boost should produce—with the nitrous in operation—a peak output of 2.2 to 2.5 horsepower per cubic inch of displacement. If specific power levels higher than this are desired, the compression ratio will have to be reduced even more. Specific power levels as high as 3.5 horsepower per cubic inch are possible, but for reliable operation, the compression ratio must be restricted to about 8:1.

Output levels of 3.5 horsepower per cubic inch might seem like a pretty tall order, even for a nitrous-injected engine, but if the nitrous is supplied to the engine in the correct proportions—and within the right engine-speed range—such power levels are theoretically possible. Mechanically supercharged engines fueled with alcohol currently develop specific power outputs near this level, so why not add some nitrous just to make up the difference?

NITROUS AND SUPERCHARGING

Readers who follow drag racing probably know Dale Armstrong as a long-time proponent of nitrous-oxide injection. He has successfully used nitrous on many record-holding blown-alcohol funny cars and dragsters. It would appear that Armstrong typically adds 200 to 300 horsepower to his alcohol motors by utilizing nitrous in the higher rpm ranges—just as the breathing efficiency of the engine begins to decline—to produce a boost in torque and horsepower. The nitrous is activated only after the car is well down the strip and the engine speed is relatively high.

One of Armstrong's crew members had an interesting comment about the importance of coordinating nitrous operation with engine speed: Hit the nitrous too close to the start line and you will drive over the crankshaft! Of course, very few vehicles in this type of racing have what can be termed "insufficient power" at the start line. Through the first 100 yards most dragster develop more power than the tires can effectively handle,

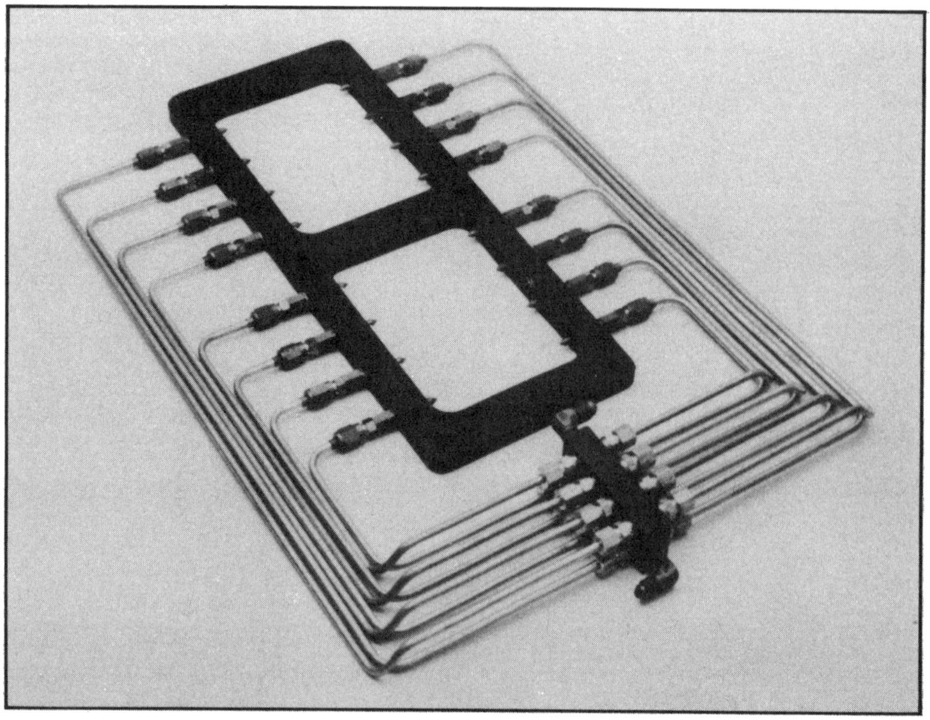

This is a nitrous system sandwiched between the supercharger and the fuel-injection system of a Top Fuel engine (much like a spacer-plate system on a conventional engine). When the engine is boosted by both a blower and nitrous injection, the bottom end better be strong because the peak power potential is awesome.

but past the 100-yard mark, the name of the game is pure horsepower. This is where nitrous-oxide is typically used to advantage, but there are other possibilities that can be explored.

First, we must consider why and how an engine is supercharged. In simplest terms, a supercharger "packs" more oxygen into the engine. The typical supercharger is a pump that is powered by a mechanical link to the engine. A typical Roots-type supercharger is big and heavy (weighing at least 80 pounds), and at maximum engine speed, as much as 300 horsepower is required to drive this relatively large pump. Naturally, the 300 horsepower drawn from the crankshaft to drive the supercharger is power output that cannot be used to drive the flywheel. But, of course, on the credit side, since the supercharger delivers more air—and consequently, more fuel—into the engine, the cylinder pressures developed during combustion are much higher. In our example, the higher pressures can equal as much as 800 horsepower. So the net result is the difference between the gain and the loss—in this case about 500 horsepower.

Now consider this. What would happen if the supercharger did not have to be driven by the engine? Suppose we could attain the same amount of boost and cylinder pressure and all of the additional output was delivered straight to the flywheel: an instant 300 extra horsepower. Let's also assume that it is not necessary to carry the weight of the supercharger. Instead, the air normally supplied by the supercharger is compressed, stored in cylinders weighing about 25 pounds, and delivered to the engine as needed. If this were possible, the engine would be lighter, simpler and more powerful.

Taking this another step. Instead of compressing air, let's compress something that contains more oxygen. Air, after all, is only 23% oxygen. Nitrous-oxide, on the other hand, is 36% oxygen (by weight). If we use nitrous in our theoretical supercharging system, there will be 50% more available oxygen from the same relative volume. As a bonus, our "boost oxygen" can be stored as a liquid. Under these conditions, the oxygen within the nitrous-oxide molecule is bonded to the nitrogen, and the container does not have to withstand extreme internal pressure. Theoretically at least, all of the "supercharging" in this system is accomplished apart from the engine. In other words, the vehicle carries cylinders of "pre-supercharged" oxygen and power does not have to be withdrawn from the total output to accomplish the supercharging task.

This appears too good to be true, but if it were possible, we have to wonder why the weight and complexity of a mechanical supercharger is necessary when the function of a supercharger is available within the contents of a simple nitrous-oxide bottle. The answer is obvious: What is needed is a system of nitrous metering that can deliver the nitrous-oxide in a manner that emulates a supercharger—i.e., in progressively increasing amounts as engine speed increases.

This all sounds a lot easier than it actually is. We must remember the two deadly engine killers: (1) excessive cylinder pressure and (2) exces-

Initial experiments with nitrous and blowers have left many questions unanswered. The nitrous can be helpful to "clean up" the idle qualities of the engine, but few racers have been able to find the proper "balance" between blower and nitrous boost.

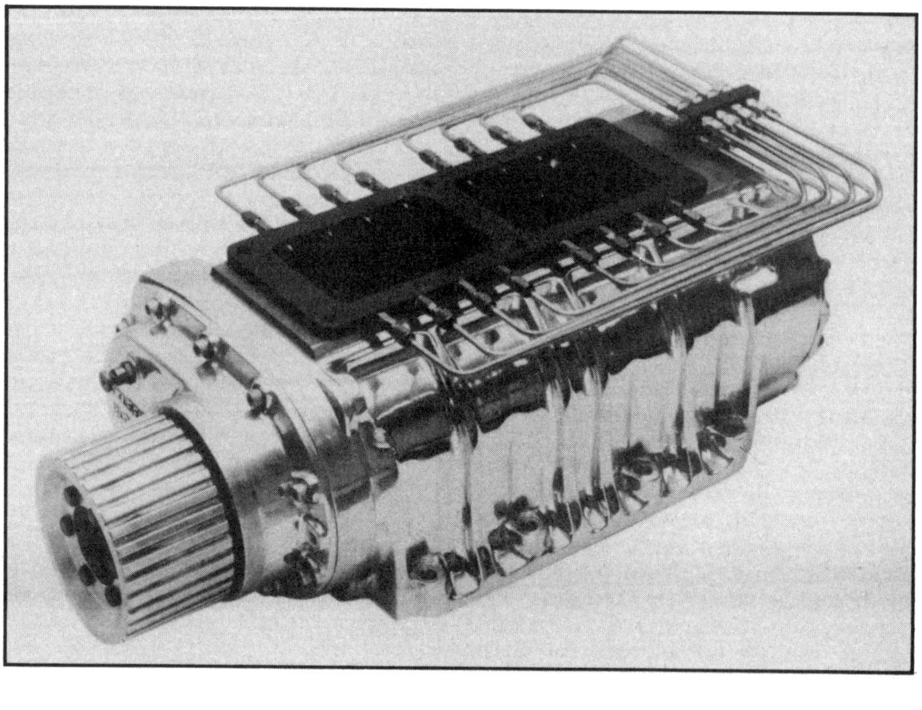

sive engine speed. A high-output constant-flow nitrous-oxide system can produce excessive cylinder pressures at low engine speed. This is a primary reason for multi-stage systems. As more carefully coordinated stages are added to the system, the problem of excessive cylinder pressures becomes less and less likely.

Given these conditions, the ideal extreme-output nitrous engine would endure very high engine speeds and utilize some form of metering system that can deliver nitrous-oxide and fuel in sufficient quantities to hold the cylinder pressure just below the point of ultimate failure. If this were possible, a nitrous-injected engine would theoretically produce more horsepower than a conventionally supercharged engine. However, at the time of this writing, very few developers (if any) have tried to develop a non-supercharged nitrous engine that will produce super-high horsepower.

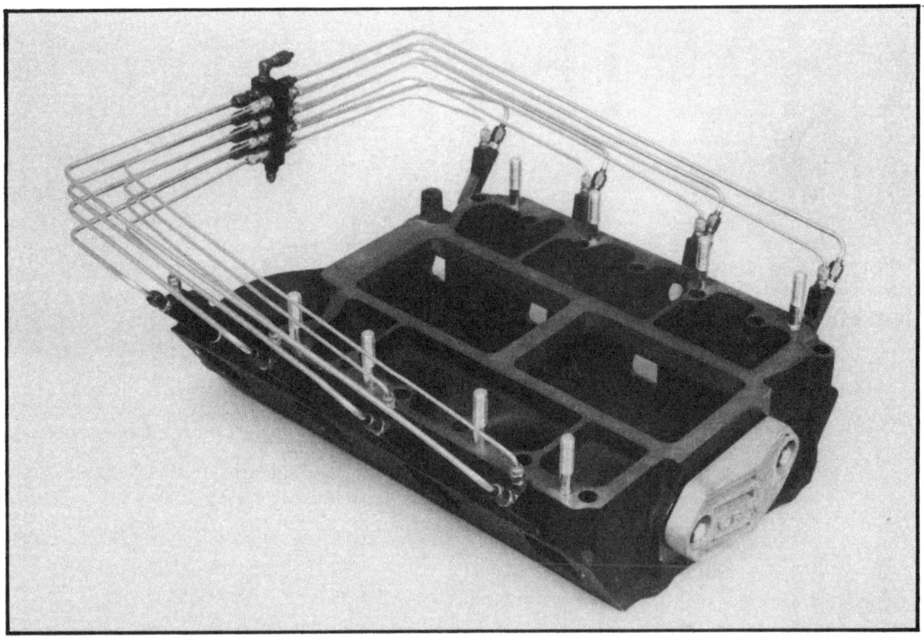

This system is more like a conventional port system, but very little documented research has been undertaken to compare this type of system with one that injects the nitrous above the blower (like a spacer system on a conventional carbureted engine).

NITROUS AND NITROMETHANE

It is not likely that many readers are involved in Top Fuel or Funny Car drag racing, but the effects of nitrous-oxide and nitromethane are unique and interesting. To date, nitrous has been disappointing as a power augmentation device for Fuelers. And basically, for a very good reason: nitrous-oxide and nitromethane are not extremely compatible.

Nitromethane is not a very good fuel; it has a very low calorific heating value: it is only about a quarter as powerful as gasoline. Alcohol—to name just one example—is a much more powerful fuel than nitromethane. However nitro is useful as a racing fuel because it is 53% oxygen (by weight). But during combustion, the oxygen content of the nitromethane is not used entirely within the cylinders. Nitro decomposes in two stages. The second phase does not occur until a lot of heat has been absorbed by the nitro, so the decomposition is usually still in progress as the nitro passes into the exhaust pipe. (This decomposition in the exhaust pipe is what makes exhaust flames and noise associated with fuelers.) So a portion of the oxygen content of nitromethane is wasted.

Nitrous-oxide is, obviously, also rich in oxygen. However, since nitromethane is already well-laden with oxygen, the effects of the oxygen content in nitrous are not as pronounced as with gasoline or alcohol. And though this area is largely unexplored, if nitrous-oxide is to be used with nitro, then the nitromethane has to be proportionately reduced because nitrous-oxide increases the sensitivity to detonation—and nitro, itself, is very sensitive to detonation.

As of 1986, some sanctioning bodies allow blown-alcohol cars with nitrous augmentation to run in Top Fuel classes. And aside from the mechanical questions, a comparative look at the cost of nitromethane and nitrous-alcohol is interesting. Most fuelers currently run mixtures of nearly 100% nitromethane (small amounts of alcohol are usually blended with the nitro), and nitro is very expensive. On the other hand, nitrous-oxide is relatively cheap. One way to view this comparison is to take the price of one pound of nitrous and divide by 0.36 (nitrous is 36% oxygen) and compare this result to the price of one pound of nitromethane divided by 0.53 (nitro is 53% oxygen). Of course, the two compounds are consumed at different rates, but some calculations by Bill Wheatley of ICE showed that, at the time of this writing, a competitive Top-Fuel nitromethane engine consumes about $300 of nitro on a single run. A comparable engine, augmented with nitrous, would only consume about $30 of nitrous-oxide.

So why aren't all Top Fuel racers using nitrous? I am not certain of the answer to this question. However, it seems to be a matter of priorities and limited resources. Most professional fuel racers are very busy keeping their engines and teams together as it is, much less committing the time and effort required to properly research an unproven technology.

On the other hand, with suitable research, nitrous-oxide could represent a viable alternative to nitromethane and the 8-71 Roots-type blower. It is entirely possible to build a 3000-horsepower turbocharged engine for drag racing. After all, the Cosworth engines used for Indy-style racing can, with only 132 cubic inch, top the 1100 horsepower mark with ease. And remember, these aren't "hand grenade" engines; Indy engines have to last 500 miles and are usually raced in "mild" tune. Rumor has it that with maximum boost these engines produce over 1500 horsepower. If such an engine had a broader power range—and turbo lag could be eliminated—there would be more than sufficient power output per cubic inch to make a successful Top Fuel engine.

In theory, a nitrous-injected Top Fuel engine—using alcohol as the principal fuel—seems to be viable. However, the change is likely to be slow. Nitrous has been banned from fuel classes because in the past some engine builders have had bad experiences with nitrous.

This does not mean, though, that nitrous-oxide has not found a place in Top Fuel racing. Some engine builders have found that the engine idles better and is a bit more responsive off the line when a small quantity of nitrous-oxide is injected at idle. Some prefer to inject the nitrous as a gas and some prefer to inject it as a liquid, but according to many professional racers, the net effect is to "clean up" the idle and prevent the spark plugs from fouling as readily. As a result, the engine generally "runs nicer."

CHAPTER 6

HIDDEN NITROUS SYSTEMS

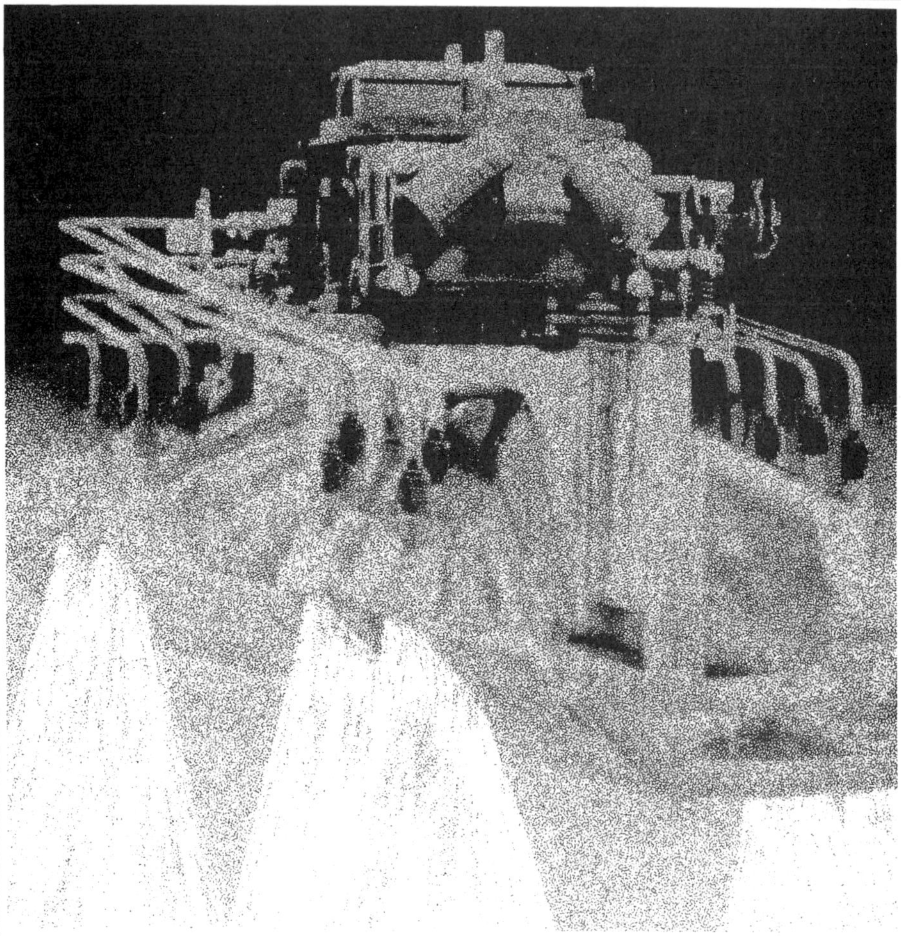

So far we have discussed nitrous-oxide systems that are plainly in view. However there is another aspect to nitrous, namely systems that, for one reason or another, are hidden.

In the early days, nitrous injection was used by clever "informal" racers to make an innocent-looking machine that could lure an unsuspecting victim into a big-money race. This type of racing had no formal rules, so

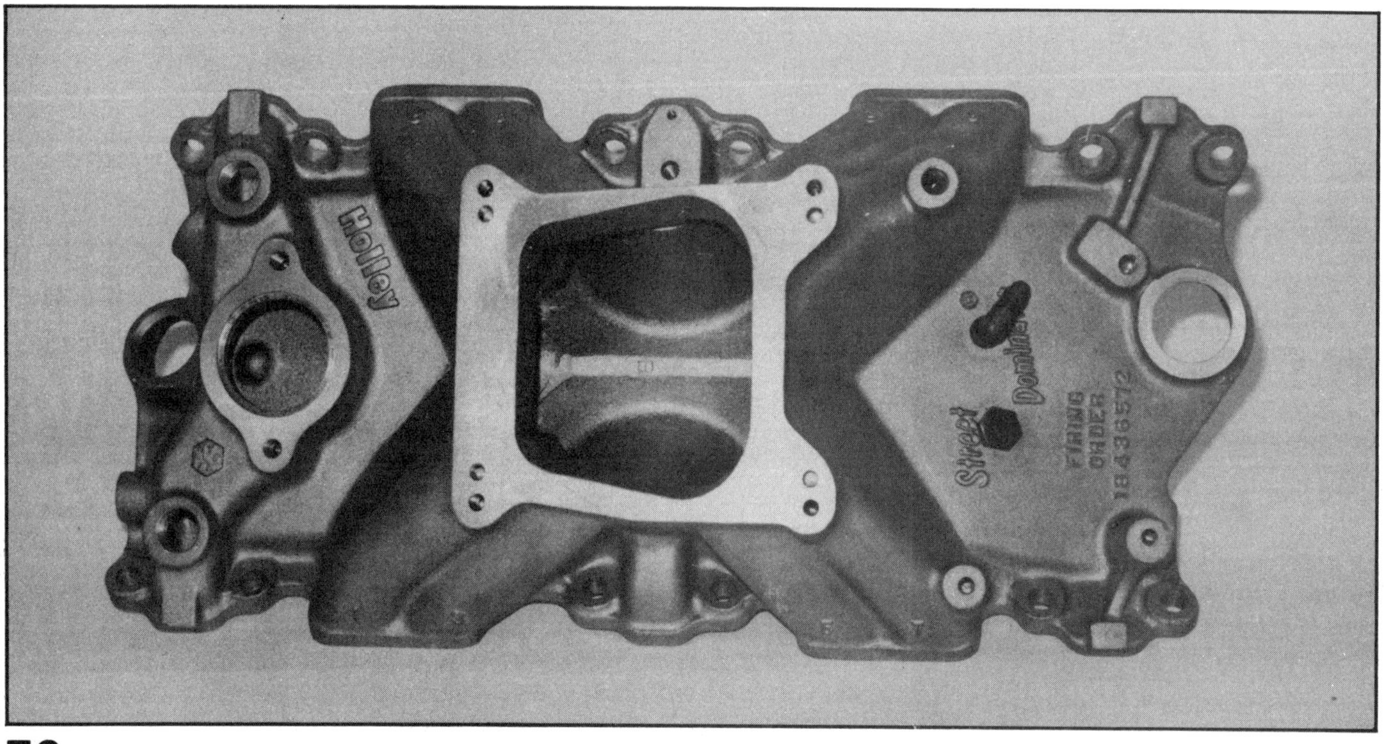

If you don't notice the hose fittings protruding from the end, this manifold looks relatively innocent. However, there is more than meets the eye.

it was a matter of "survival of the baddest." But if a car looked too "bad," it was difficult to entice prospective opponents to the challenge. So the most successful money racers went to great lengths to make their cars look innocuous on the outside, while using every available trick under the hood to make as much horsepower as possible.

For instance, if a modest-looking car is equipped with a well-hidden nitrous-oxide system and a puny-looking 2-barrel carburetor, any opponent—if he has a similar car, but with a 4-barrel or dual 4-barrels—is likely to believe he can win some easy money. Experience has shown, however, that a moderate nitrous system can produce more raw horsepower than even the best multiple-carburetor inductions. In this instance, all else being equal, the nitrous-injected 2-barrel engine will walk away from the more complex, but less effective, multiple-carburetor engine. The bottom line here is to remember that "all's fair in love, war *and street racing*."

Another obvious reason that a racer may want a hidden system is, in plain language, to cheat. Whatever the reasons or motivations, it is not our purpose here to argue ethical questions. Instead, we will deal strictly with the mechanical practicalities of running a hidden nitrous system.

Most hidden systems are installed through the underside of the intake manifold, and for all practical purposes they operate just like a conventional exposed port-injection system. The accompanying photos show typical installations. Some of these examples are early installations that appear very simple, but many of the latest hidden systems are extremely sophisticated.

On the face of it, a system hidden under a manifold that injects through the floors of the ports should present no more problems than building that same system on top of the manifold. However, it is not that simple when an entire system is situated, for the most part, completely inside the operating engine.

Most importantly, the system is subjected to more heat. If the correct type of solenoids are selected, they will be impervious to the oil mist inside the engine, but these valves will be heated by the oil, which is generally around 210 to 220 degrees during engine operation. This will unquestionably influence system operation.

When a "hot" system is initially fired, there will usually be a notable hesitation before the engine reacts. During this period, the fuel supply system delivers a relatively full dose of enrichment fuel, despite the fact that it is heated by the hot engine oil. However, the heat—from hot engine oil—soaked up by the nitrous supply system initially causes the nitrous flowing through the system to convert to a gas, and as a result the nitrous flow is reduced until enough heat is soaked out of the system—by the nitrous—and a full liquid flow is established. As a result, with most hidden systems, the engine runs "rich" for about a second before the nitrous-fuel balance stabilizes and the engine develops full power.

Of course, when the supply system is cooler, this problem is less pronounced. The easiest solution, therefore, is to bleed some nitrous into the system by "burping it" before full activation. This initial shot of nitrous will effectively cool the nitrous supply system so that full nitrous flow can be achieved more quickly. This is, in fact, common practice among experienced nitrous users.

Hidden systems generally fall into one of two categories. When a hidden system is used for street racing, the required power boost may be as high as 80 to 100 horsepower. But these high horsepower nitrous-oxide systems require a large storage bottle and relatively bulky solenoids. Also, fairly substantial supply lines are needed between the bottle and the solenoids. These systems are difficult to hide completely. At best, they are usually just "inobvious."

On the other hand, for close competition—where a clandestine system is used—only small amounts of nitrous are needed to tip the scales. During a competitive race only 20 or 30 horsepower is needed for a critical passing move or to record an unusually fast qualifying lap or just for knocking off a tenth of a second in a tight drag race. With some ingenuity, this type of minimal system can be hidden entirely from view.

Not all racers feel inclined to cheat. But those who don't—and the officials who govern events—must be

A view of the underside reveals a potent nitrous-oxide system. This system boosts engine output by 150 horsepower.

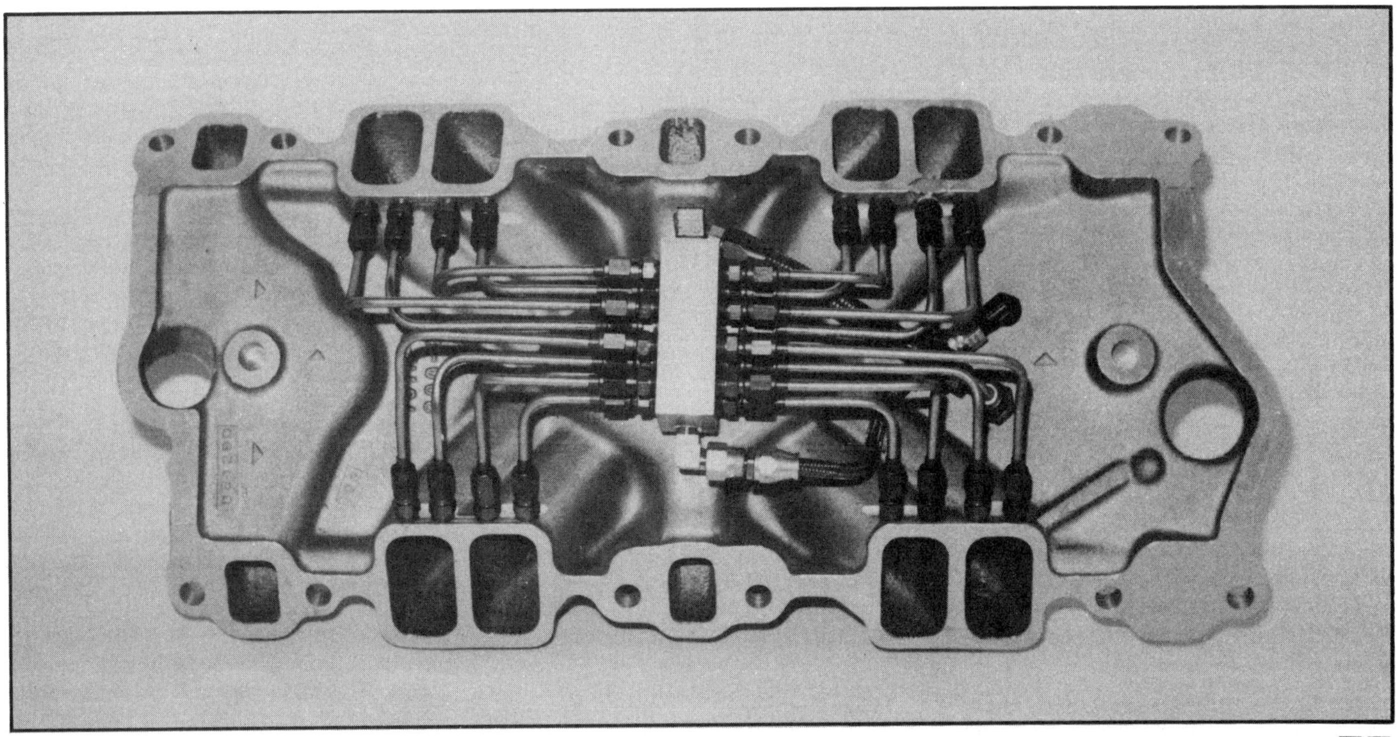

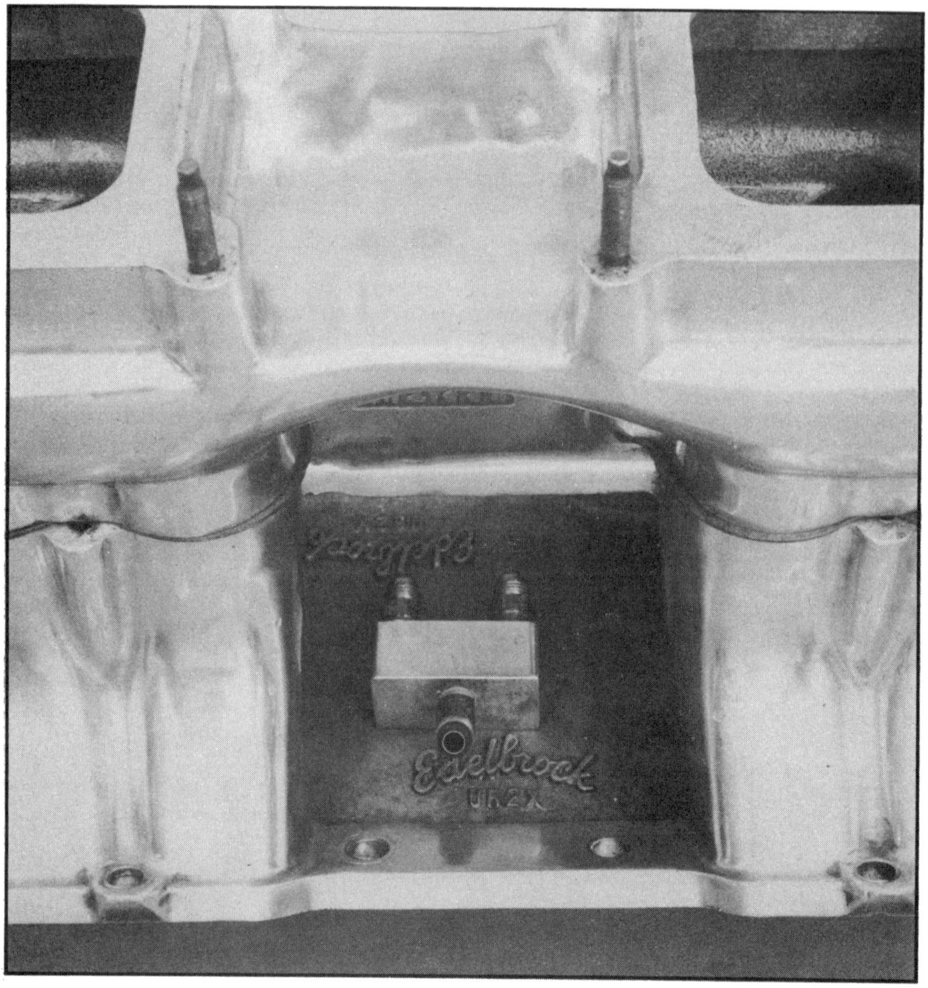

To the untrained eye, the purpose of the fittings in the bottom of the plenum is not obvious, but they serve a useful purpose.

able to spot those who do! This is not an easy task. For every method of hiding a system that is known to tech officials, there's sure to be one that is not. The bottom line is that the ingenious cheat is usually one step ahead of the tech inspector.

In the early days, cheating was pretty simple because very few people knew about nitrous. Since tech inspectors didn't look for it, the nitrous equipment was not seen for what it was. Even high-horsepower systems weren't so much hidden as just inobvious.

In general, the biggest problem was—and still is—finding a place to hide the nitrous storage container. For instance, what easier way to carry nitrous-oxide than in a fire extinguisher bottle? And it only seems logical to have a lot of plumbing running from the fire bottle to various parts of the car—including the engine and carburetor. This trick was common for several years, but is now well known. Today, the first thing a tech inspector checks is the fire system to see if any suspicious components are routed too near the engine.

The tubes of the roll cage are also excellent camouflage for a liquid nitrous-oxide container. And if the car is a sedan, the number of hiding places for a tiny storage cylinder are almost countless. Just consider some of these: underneath the driveshaft hump, underneath the seat, behind the back seat, behind a false back in the trunk, behind the inner fenderwells, between any double skinning of the body work—and how about inside an air scoop.

This last bit of ingenuity surfaced a few years back when a *fairly* competitive Pro Stocker suddenly became *very* competitive. According to trackside rumors, the newly acquired stature was achieved in the following ways: (1) The air scoop was molded directly to the hood, but the outside length of the air scoop was longer—about six inches—than the inside length of the scoop; (2) A small nitrous cylinder and solenoid was concealed inside a false wall of the scoop; (3) The wiring for the solenoid was fed through two Dzus fasteners, and the circuit to the solenoid was made when the hood was clipped down; (4) Tubes molded into the surface of the scoop directed most of the nitrous into the mouth of the carburetor and a small amount into the float chamber—to pressurize it slightly; (5) This pressurization increased the fuel flow to the engine to maintain the nitrous(oxygen)-fuel balance; (6) An inconspicuous pushbutton inside the car activated the system.

Whenever the car was inspected at teardown—which was pretty often, because it won numerous events—the tech inspectors would watch complacently as the crew innocently removed the hood and carried it into their transporter. Thus removing all evidence of the nitrous system.

Long-time practitioners of nitrous injection have an almost endless number of tales to tell about various ways they have seen or heard of people cheating. (Tech officials often ask well-known kit manufacturers to assist in locating hidden systems.) Ron Hammel of 10,000 RPM could tell enough tales to fill the pages of this book; but a few of the most interesting will serve our purpose.

Veteran Nascar fans will remember that some years ago the displacement limit for Grand National cars was 427 cubic inches. This limit was subsequently reduced to 350 cubic inches, but during an interim period, both 427-inch and 350-inch engines were allowed to race. To even the odds, the bigger engines had to use restrictive carburetion that could flow no more than 390 cubic feet per minute (at wide-open throttle), and the smaller engines were allowed to run a much larger carburetor. This would, theoretically, put the two engines on a par. However, not everyone felt that this was the case; and most of the 427-inch engines ran slower than the 350's.

It was during this changeover period that Ron Hammel built a kit for a Nascar driver, who obviously wishes to remain nameless. This driver was consistently competitive with a 427-inch Chrysler Hemi—until the displacement change. He then found that he was consistently one or two places off the bump spot. So Ron built a special Holley carburetor for this racer. While he has built many similar setups, this particular "cheater carb" was ingenious because it was, at that time, practically impossible to spot.

Ron began with a Holley carburetor that had an unused and unthreaded inlet on the rear float bowl. Here he installed an additional "fuel" line that actually carried a hidden nitrous line within it. Inside the carburetor, he directed this nitrous into the airstream by plumbing it to the throttle bores just below the butterfly. This system added nitrous, but the real ingenuity was shown in his method of adding enrichment fuel. Ron also directed the

Once the manifold is turned over the hidden nitrous system is exposed. A racer equipped with this advantage is going to be hard to beat.

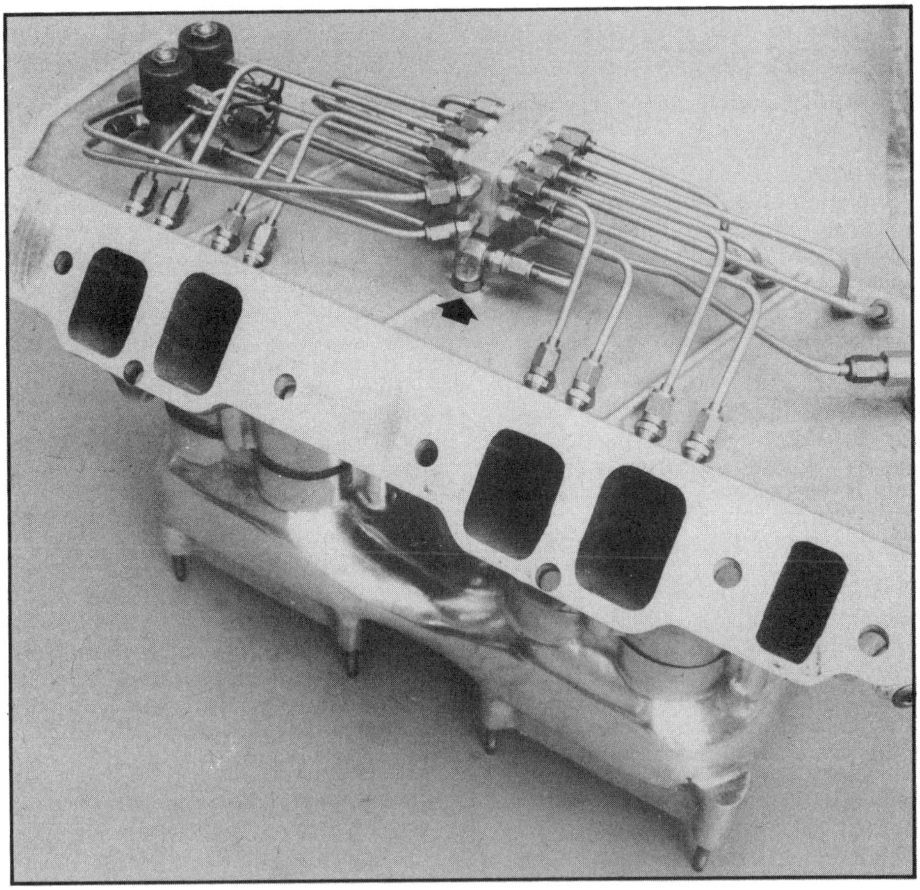

nitrous to the power-valve chamber which pressurized a specially modified power valve that added extra fuel when nitrous was being injected while maintaining the correct air/fuel ratio when no nitrous pressurized the valve. On this system, when the bottle pressure dropped to zero, no extra fuel flowed, so there was no engine bog. The nitrous for this system could be housed either in a tank under the seat (so that it could be taken in and out) or in the roll cage.

At the next race, the car ran a legal qualifying lap that would have placed it 38th on the grid; but when the nitrous was used for a "hot lap," the speed increased sufficiently to move the car up to 4th spot. Needless to say, many of the other drivers felt that a 427 Hemi on a 390cfm Holley had no right to be so high on the grid. It was faster than Richard Petty's 340-inch car, and Petty, who knows a thing or two about Chrysler Hemis, was immediately suspicious. As a result of a protest, the car was impounded, given a four-hour tech inspection, declared legal, and returned to the driver.

This is but one of several known cases where nitrous has been used illegally. Even though it seems obvious now, we must remember that nitrous "cheater systems" were a well-kept secret for many years, and most tech inspectors would not have known what to look for, even if they did see something that was a little suspicious. In those bygone days, a "special power valve" could be justified as exactly that—a special power valve. The question of legality would only arise if the carb was actually disassembled and all internal components checked individually. Even then, power valves were not covered by existing regulation, and a tech inspector would have no reason to suspect foul play.

It was several years before the capabilities of clandestine nitrous systems was understood and outlawed. For instance, in 1977 a speed-equipment dealer from Texas phoned Ron Hammel of 10,000 RPM to suggest that he exhibit his nitrous-oxide kit at a local tractor pull. Ron took his suggestion and went down to the Texas meet with some samples. While watching the contests, he noticed that several of the winners were also long-standing customers of his. Since Ron's nitrous-oxide kits were displayed for all to see, it wasn't long before some of the competitors spotted

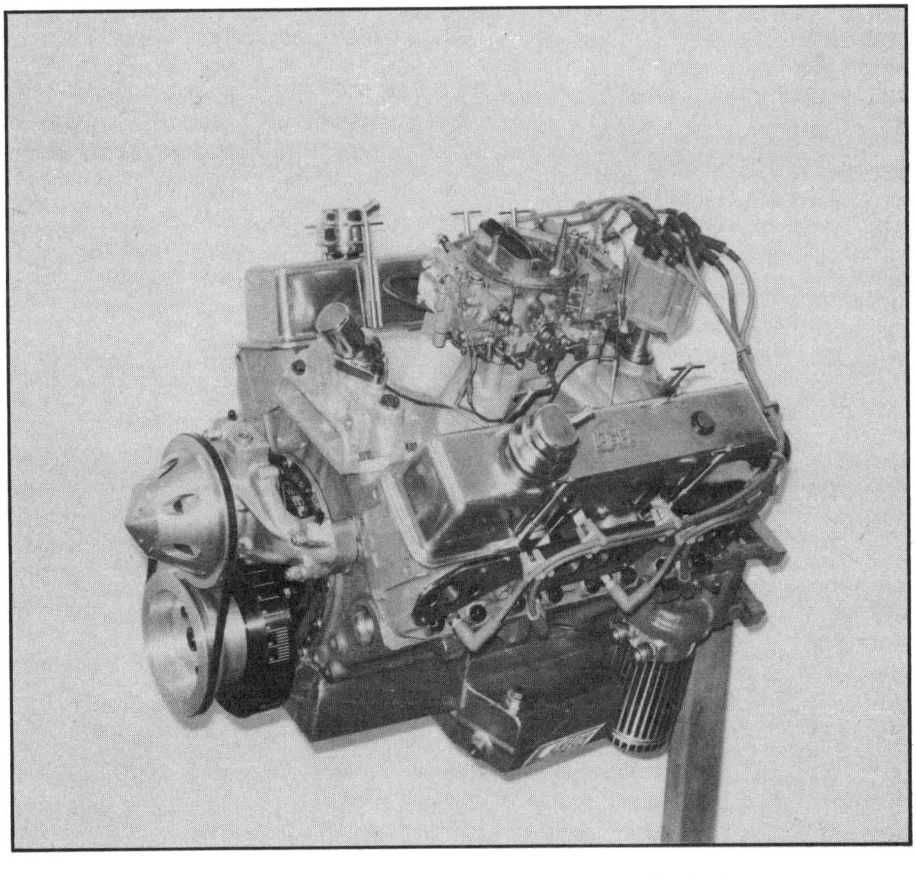

The author built this circle-track engine to test under-manifold nitrous systems. These installations boosted the power output by 80-150 horsepower. Such an increase could make an average engine into a front runner.

the link, which led to an on-the-spot ban of nitrous-oxide in the contest. However, Ron recalls that at least one of the contestants had a very well-hidden system. He escaped the howling protests and quietly went on to win his class.

Unfortunately, this is one example of sound technical innovation that has been thwarted by self-serving dullards. Prior to this particular contest, tractor-pull regulations did not specifically refer to nitrous-oxide as illegal. Nonetheless, when less-informed contestants finally discovered that some of their competitors had been using an effective—and legal—"competitive edge," they forced the sanctioning officials to immediately ban nitrous use. This attitude has repeatedly plagued and limited the development of nitrous-oxide.

Admittedly, early nitrous users discovered the value of nitrous and most of them went to great lengths to keep it a secret from other competitors. However, the search for any and every technical edge seems to be part of the very nature of competition. This raises a pertinent question. Should technical advancements be banned simply because some racers use them more effectively, or should the bleating outcries of less-informed competitors—usually the majority—be recognized and legitimized? Since the technically competent are usually in the minority, the sway is almost always against technical innovation. However, people who participate in any form of motorsports should realize that innovation is part of the game.

Of course, the prevailing attitude to ban anything that is out of the ordinary contributes to a sense of paranoia shared by most successful racers. Ron Hammel can readily attest to this. One of his favorite tales is about how Tom Jenning challenged the land speed record for full-size trucks at Bonneville. A Detroit diesel held the record of about 131mph. It had taken the Detroit team five years of development to get their vehicle up to this speed. Jenning decided to go after the record, and talked to Ron about using nitrous. Ron had built a nitrous system for Tom, who raced his truck on circuit events. With one of Ron's custom 10,000 RPM nitrous system installed, the diesel produced 650 horsepower at 3000rpm, with the nitrous contributing 185 pounds-feet to the total torque output.

Nitrous-oxide was—and at the time of this writing, still is—legal for this class. But Ron advised Tom to hide the system. With some experience in these matters, Ron reasoned that while nitrous might be perfectly legal when Tom pushed off for the run, if he broke the record, nitrous could be "illegalized" by the time he returned to the pits.

Working together, they designed a system and camouflaged it in two redundant pressure tanks normally used for the pneumatic brakes. They cut the tanks open and installed a 20-pound nitrous bottle in each one. An inconspicuous opening in each tank allowed access to turn on the nitrous valve. On the first attempt, Tom Jenning set a new record (two-way average) of 141.506mph! And there was no furor over the use of nitrous-oxide.

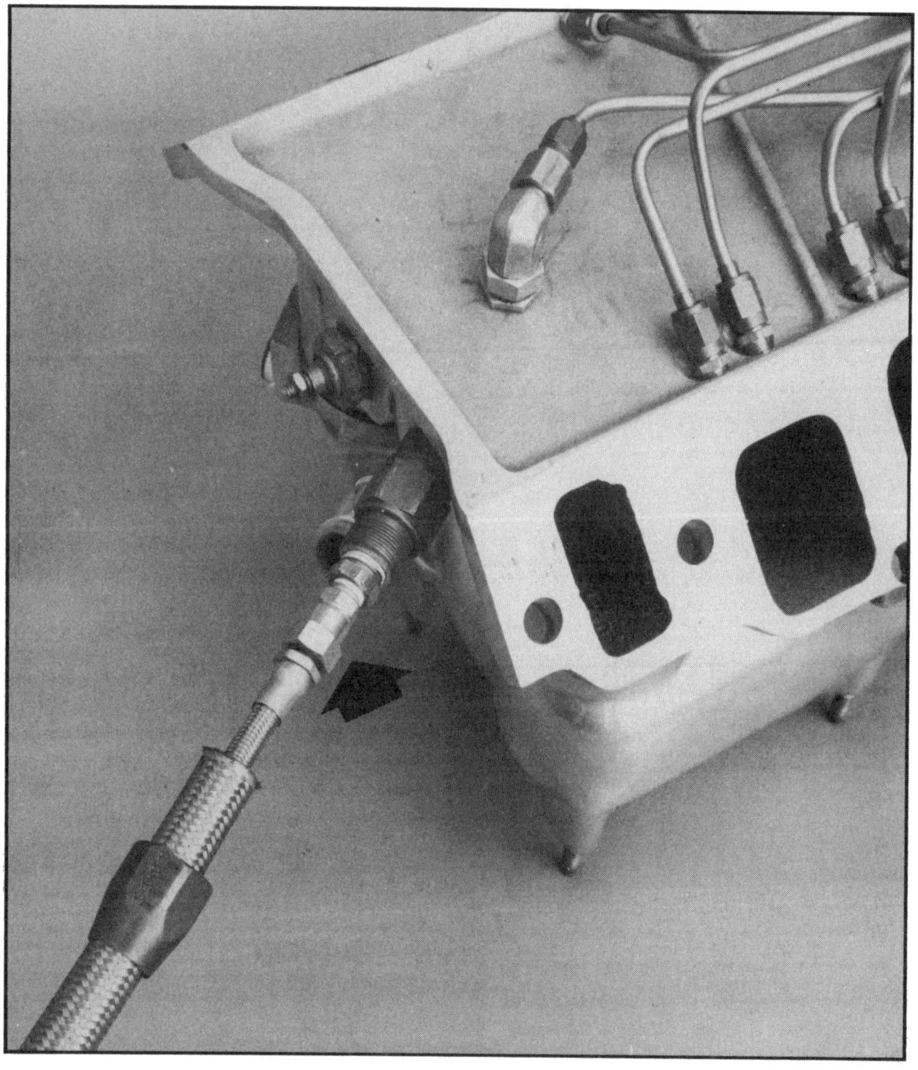

The nitrous has to get from the bottle to the engine, even in a hidden system. An innocent water hose could camouflage a line that feeds nitrous to a clandestine system.

SPOTTING A CHEATER

The list of ways to hide a nitrous system is virtually endless. So our concern will be aimed toward finding nitrous where it is specifically banned from certain vehicles and types of competition.

The first step is a simple visual check. Tubes or electrical wires that appear to go nowhere are obvious, but often overlooked, tipoffs. Wires must go somewhere—usually to solenoid valves and switches—and nitrous supply tubes must eventually lead to the induction system. Don't take anything for granted. If a system is hidden, there are numerous ways to make you think that tubes and wires serve a useful, innocent function.

In one instance, a nitrous bottle tucked under the dash fed nitrous into the engine via a tube leading to the carburetor float chamber. Inside the car, a fuel pressure gauge was attached to the line from the float bowl. For some time, it apparently didn't occur to tech inspectors that this setup—which appeared to be an innocent fuel pressure gauge—was not. After all, the actual fuel pressure in the float bowl will be about zero (ambient)! The float-bowl inlet valve effectively isolates the fuel inside the bowl from the high pressure fuel delivery line. Any meaningful fuel pressure measurement must be taken prior to the bowl inlet valve. This example highlights an important point: Be suspicious of any and every tube or wire leading to any part of the engine.

The hardest systems to find are those using a very limited amount of nitrous. Due to the close competition in most racing classes, the amount of power—and nitrous-oxide— needed to move a car to the front of the field is quite small. It would only take 20 or 30 extra horses to move a professional Pro Stocker from bottom qualifier to national champion. A clever competitor will not use obvious methods—just remember the example where electrical contact was made through commonplace Dzus fasteners in a fiberglass hood.

On the other hand, nitrous is easier to spot if it is being used to considerably bump the power. Let's assume some nerd is racing with an illegal nitrous setup that boosts 100 horsepower into the engine. This will be easier to spot because of the way the car reacts on the track. Since most nitrous installations are calibrated on the rich side, the engine inevitably produces a burst of black smoke when the system is initiated. A careful eye can spot this as a dead giveaway. Nitrous will also change the exhaust characteristics of the engine; the exhaust note becomes notably harsher and deeper.

A sudden increase in performance would also be good cause to check a car very carefully. If a car is pretty evenly matched to the rest of the opposition for a substantial portion of the race and then at a crucial juncture it suddenly pulls in front with ease, be suspicious. Nothing puts a good boost in the torque curve like a small dose of nitrous. This is not to say that all winners are cheaters, but a suspicious boost in performance should be viewed as just that—suspicious!

Finally, a nitrous system may be harder to detect if the system is used cleverly and consistently in every race. This situation is most likely to occur in drag racing competition, and is very difficult to uncover. If a car fails to "launch" hard at the line but charges exceptionally hard at the topend, be suspicious. As discussed earlier, the torque boost produced by nitrous can most effectively be used at the finish line. Here again, a black puff of smoke and/or a sudden deepening of the exhaust note may also be a tipoff. In drag competition, any car that leaves soft and charges hard at the finish should be checked carefully.

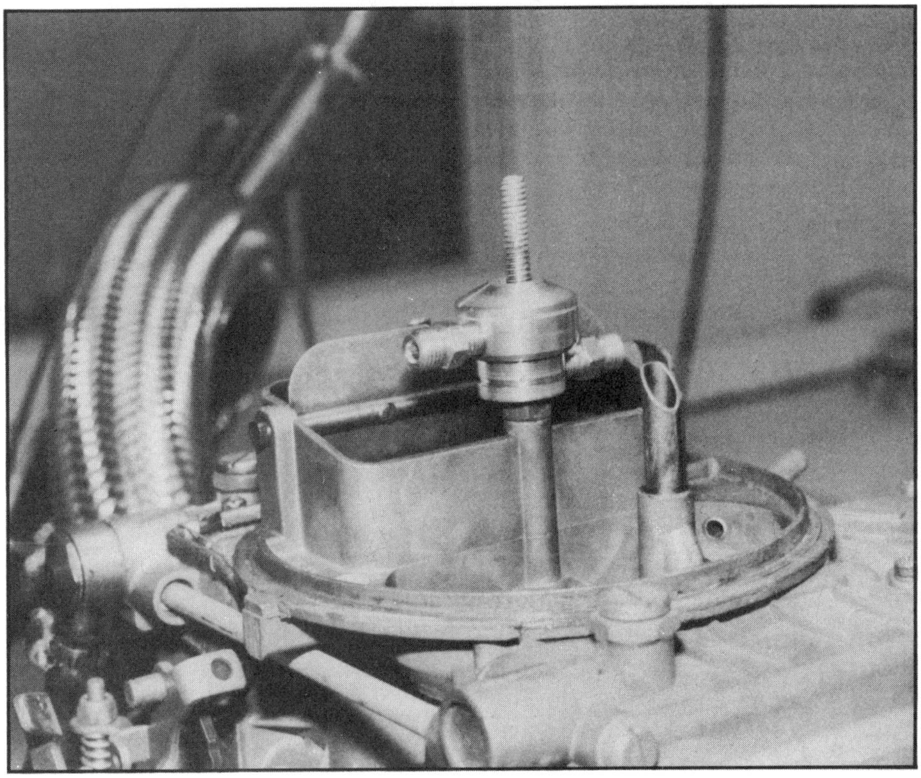

This simple and effective injection system developed by NOS mounts on the air cleaner stud of the carburetor and sprays nitrous through the primary venturis of the carburetor.

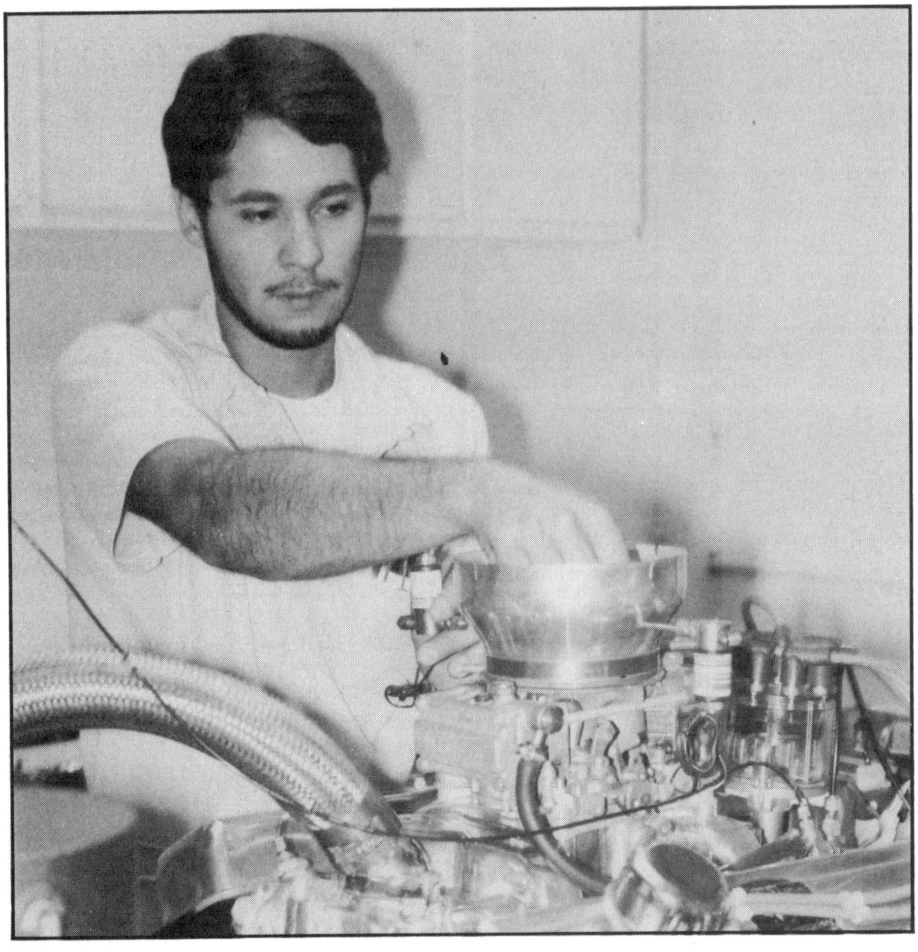

On the NOS dyno the carb-mounted system boosted power about 80-100 horsepower. This system can be completely hidden inside the air cleaner, and the nitrous line can be disguised as a fuel or vacuum hose.

CHAPTER 7

NITROUS & TURBO-CHARGING

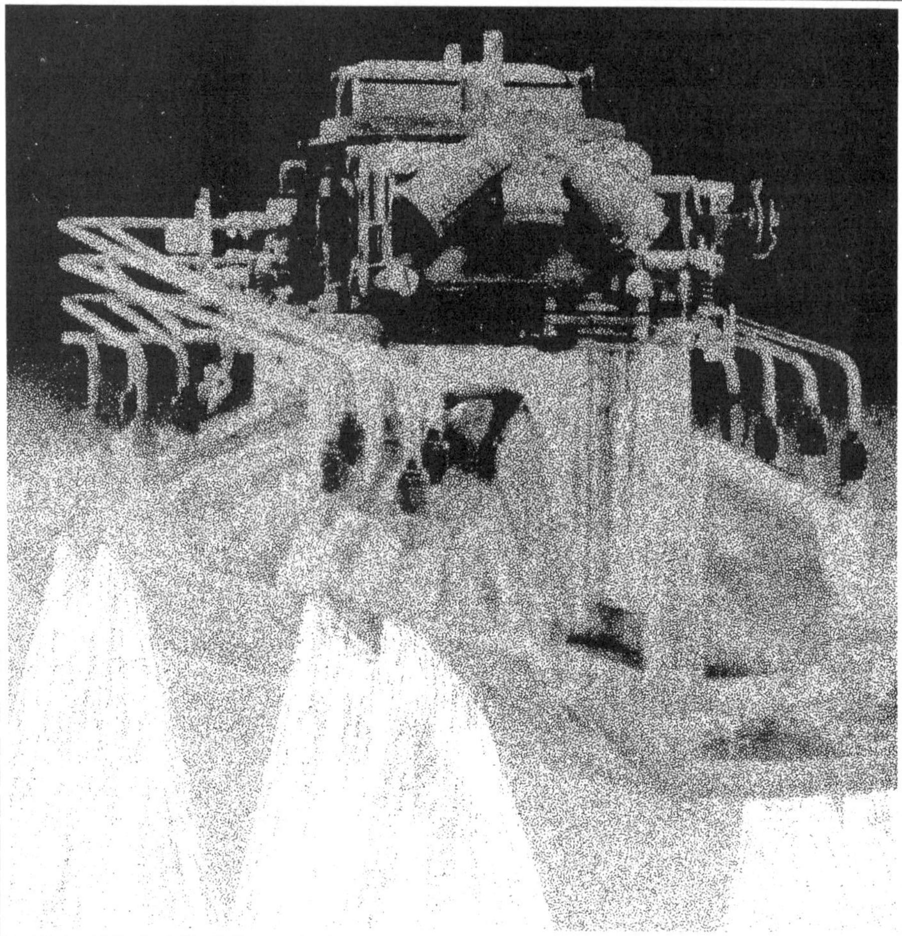

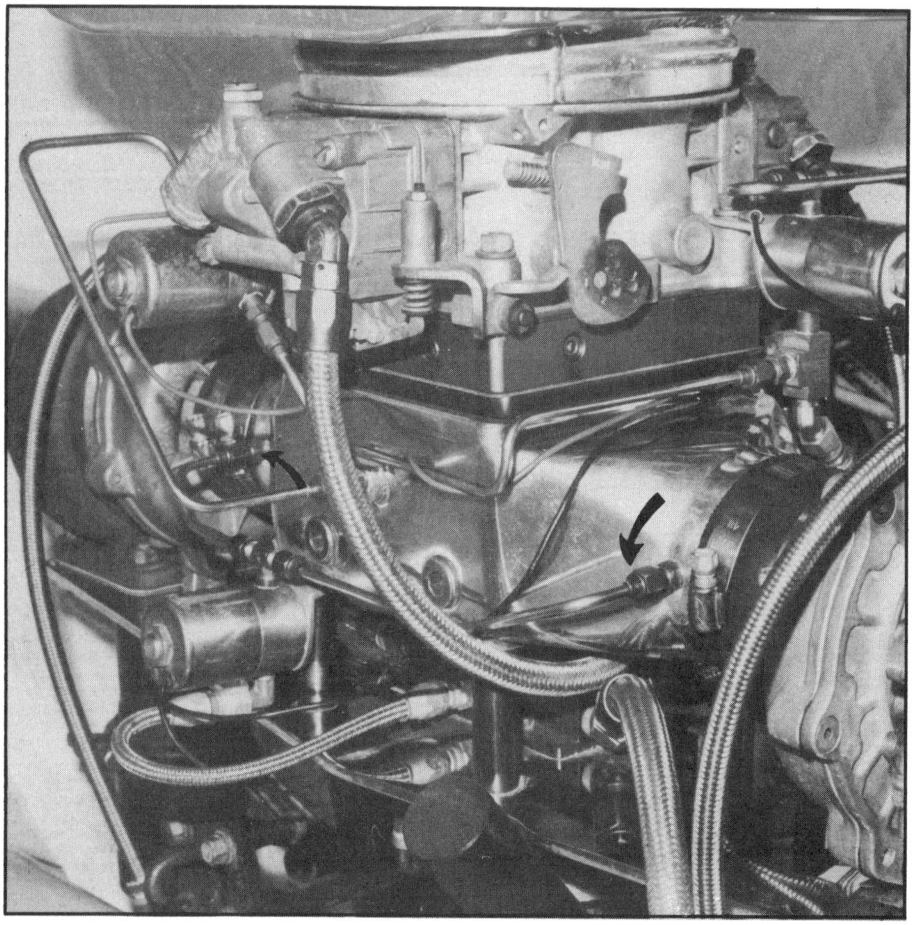

The two lines (arrows) on this turbocharged big block feed nitrous to the intake of each turbocharger. Enrichment fuel is added under the carburetor.

Occasionally two performance systems work so well together that the combined results enhance the best features of each individual system. This effect is rare, but the combination of nitrous-oxide injection and turbocharging is an excellent example of two systems that are totally suited to each other.

We know that nitrous can produce a substantial power, but when nitrous is used to augment peak power for relatively long periods the rate of nitrous consumption is very high. Obviously, if power augmentation is desired for extended periods, very large quantities of nitrous must be available. The size and weight of the high-pressure storage bottles required to store this amount of nitrous are prohibitive. In addition, there is the relatively high recurring cost of refilling. These are very real limitation in certain situations and types of racing.

Turbosupercharging can also produce impressive power levels. An excellent example is the 1000-plus horsepower developed by 90cid Formula One engines. In fact, current turbocharging technology produces more specific horsepower (power compared to displacement) than nitrous. This is due, no doubt, to the vast amounts of time and money recently devoted to research and development of racing turbocharger systems. (Although, I believe that it is theoretically possible for a similarly developed nitrous system to produce short-term specific power levels equal to those of turbocharging.)

As is typical with all types of superchargers, turbochargers boost horsepower because they pump copious quantities of air (oxygen) and fuel into the engine. However, the major limitation of most turbocharged engines is a lack of low-speed torque resulting in sluggish low-speed acceleration. This problem is usually called "turbo lag," but in point of fact, it should be more correctly described as boost lag. When the throttle is floored at low engine speeds there isn't sufficient dynamic flow through the engine to accelerate the exhaust turbine and, consequently, produce sufficient compressor speed to develop a high level of boost. Some street-oriented turbo systems overcome this boost lag by using a relatively "tight" exhaust turbine. This means the turbine will accelerate more readily at slow engine speeds, and as a result, the turbo will "spin up" faster and develop boost relatively quickly. This approach usually results in better low-speed boost response; however, the top-end power will be limited because the restrictive turbine element will choke exhaust flow and reduce maximum boost.

Nitrous-oxide is ideally suited to overcome this problem. One of the attributes of nitrous-oxide is that it considerably boosts torque in the lower speed range. In fact, nitrous actually produces a relatively greater torque boost at lower engine speeds than at higher engine speeds. In effect, then, the two systems ideally complement each other. The nitrous can effectively boost torque at low engine speeds and the turbocharger(s) can boost power at high engine speeds.

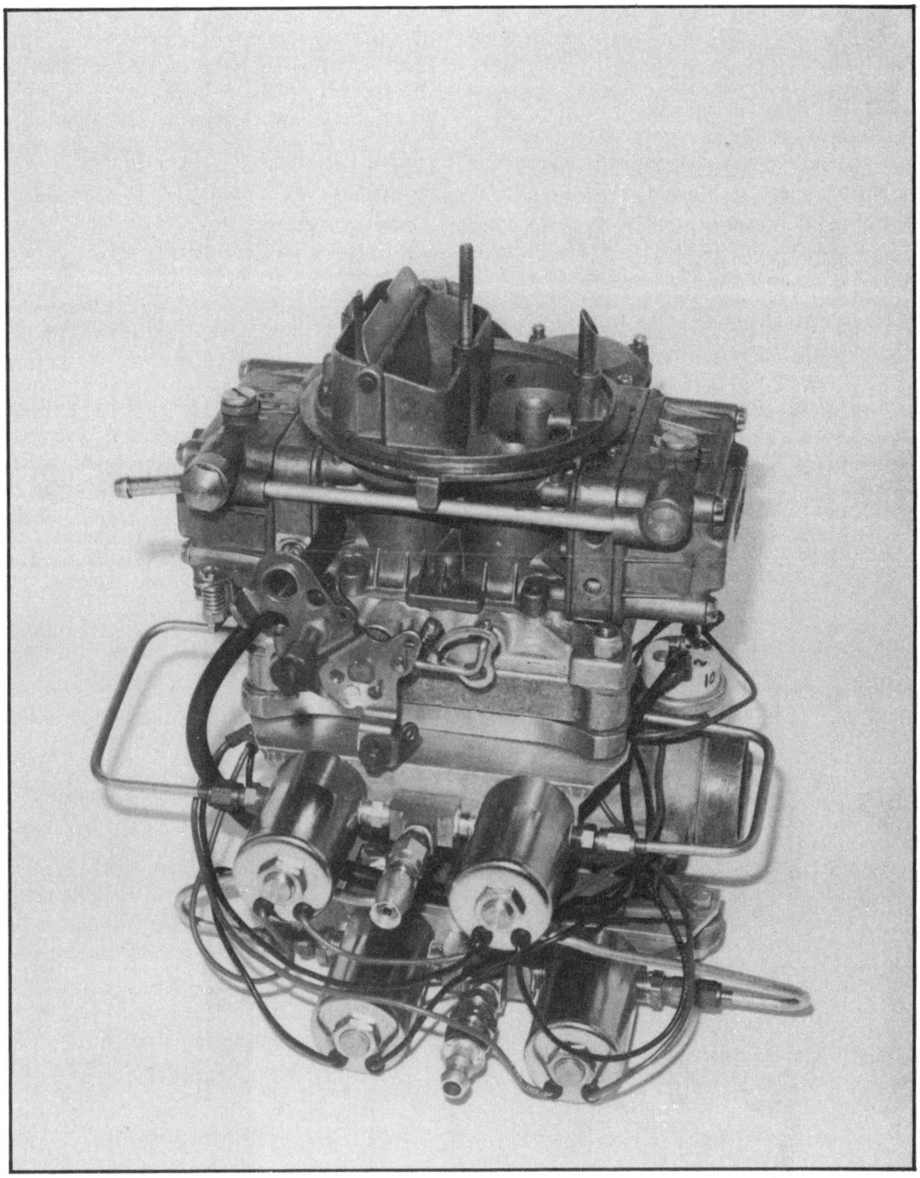

This cleverly designed nitrous system serves multiple purposes. During normal acceleration it delivers a small shot of nitrous to reduce turbo lag. During hard acceleration a low-power stage boosts the low-speed torque and as engine speed rises a second stage adds more nitrous to enhance top-end power. In addition, the system is an effective intercooler.

To see how this might work, let's imagine a turbocharged-nitrous engine running at cruise speed. When the driver floors the throttle at this relatively low engine speed, there is insufficient dynamic flow through the engine to develop a rapid boost response in the turbo system. But when the throttle reaches wide open, it triggers a nitrous system. The nitrous/enrichment fuel is injected into the engine, and there is an immediate boost in torque. This, of course, provides the desired acceleration. But there is another effect. The activation of the nitrous system also generates a considerable and immediate increase in the exhaust flow exiting the engine. This, of course, accelerates the turbocharger, which produces a corresponding increase in manifold pressure. To complete the system, a pressure switch monitors the intake manifold, and as soon as the manifold pressure (boost) reaches a prescribed level, the nitrous system is deactivated.

The nitrous system required for this type of application need only be capable of relatively modest boost. A typical V8 street nitrous kit—which produces a total boost of about 100 to 150 horsepower)—is more than adequate. A nitrous shot at low engine speed equal to about 15 or 20 horsepower will usually overcome any significant boost lag in the turbo system. And a system that provides a 20-horsepower increase (at about 1500rpm) will boost the total engine torque output by about 75 pounds-feet. On a 350cid turbocharged engine that typically develops about 200 to 225 pounds-feet of torque (unboosted), this additional 75 pounds-feet of torque will very significantly affect low-speed acceleration.

The nitrous system on this type of setup will typically be in operation for approximately three-tenths to, at most, one second. During this time the boost will climb very quickly because of the large volume of exhaust flow generated by the nitrous. However, on some engines it is possible for the boost level to fall significantly when the nitrous system is deactivated. This occurs when the turbocharger design is not well-coordinated with the engine, and the engine fails to generate enough exhaust flow to maintain the boost level. However, the type of nitrous system described here is, in effect, self-compensating. When the boost level drops below the preset threshold of the system deactivation switch, the nitrous will switch on briefly until the manifold boost again climbs above the preset threshold.

Figure 7-1 demonstrates the combined effects of well-coordinated turbo and nitrous systems on a 350-inch smallblock Chevy. (Note: Due to the injection of the nitrous, the boost equivalent—i.e., the amount of oxygen that the engine perceives as passing into it—is very high, even at low engine speeds.) The success of a combined system depends a great deal on the design of the turbo system and the specific turbocharger(s) used. If the application emphasizes low-speed acceleration, the maximum effect will be achieved if the turbocharger develops considerable boost at low engine speeds. In this respect, a modern turbo system can produce as much as 5psi of boost at crank speeds as low as 2000rpm. If high-speed power is desired, the turbocharger should be selected to develop peak boost at relatively higher engine speeds.

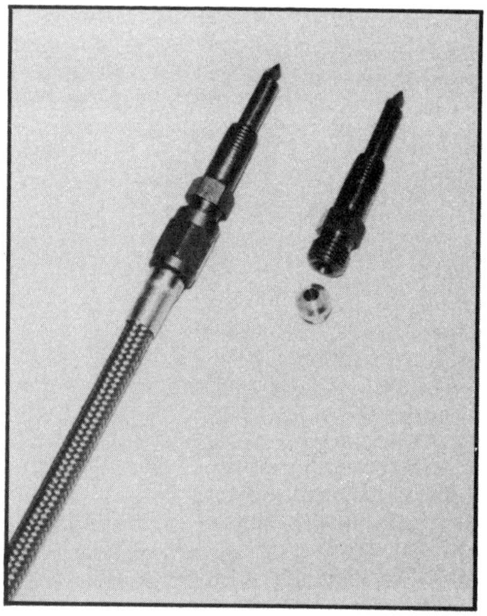

These simple jets from NOS can be installed into the intake manifold of a turbocharged or carbureted engine to calibrate the flow of nitrous and fuel.

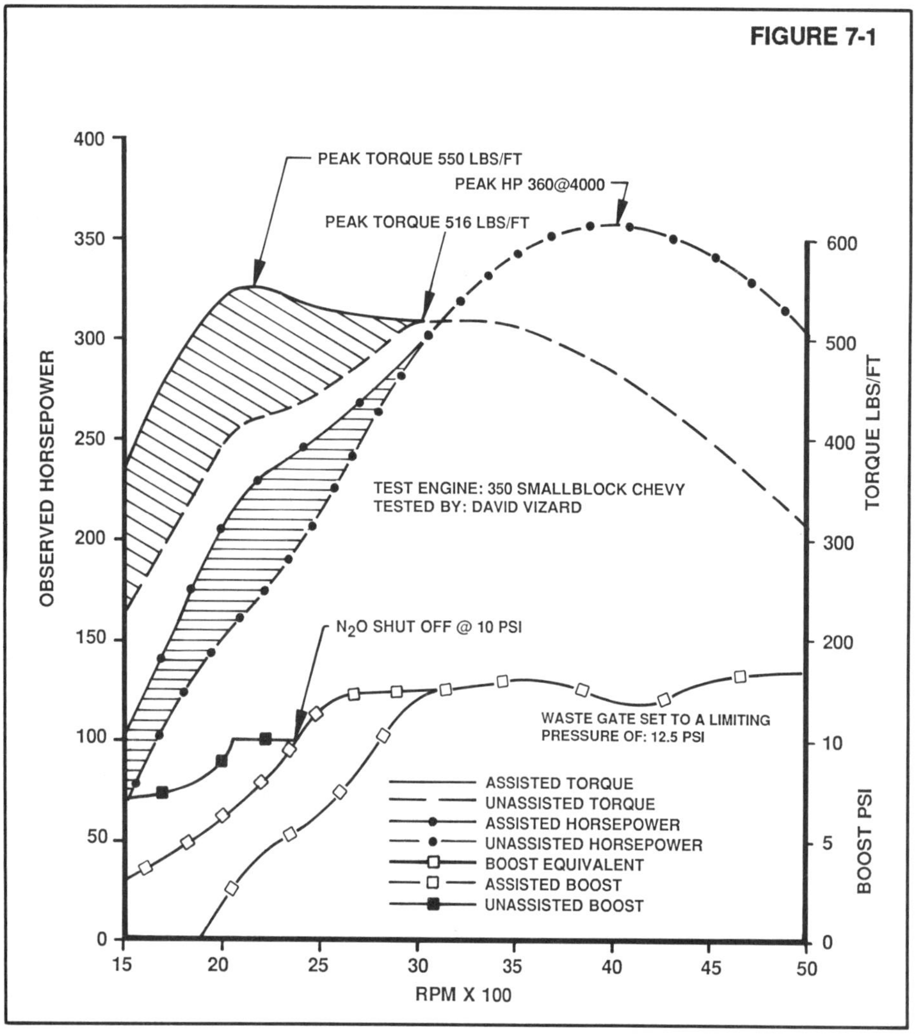

FIGURE 7-1: The low speed torque of a turbocharged engine is substantially improved with nitrous injection. Even though the nitrous flow is modest (about two pounds per minute), the elapsed time will be lowered approximately 2-7 seconds due to the better launch. The "assisted boost equivalent" is a representation of the amount of oxygen available due to the nitrous injection. This is a theoretical figure based on the equivalent amount of conventional supercharging the engine would require to obtain the same amount of additional oxygen.

This type of system produces impressive performance, especially in a street machine. The nitrous augmentation makes even a modest turbocharged engine feel like a large displacement, long-stroke normally-aspirated engine. And since the nitrous is only activated briefly during the initial stage of acceleration, the onboard supply of nitrous will last for a considerable period. Of course, this depends on the weight of the driver's foot, but experience with this type of system has shown that a typical 15-pound bottle of nitrous will last up to 10 times longer than with a conventional nitrous system.

SYSTEM LAYOUT

In general, there are two types of turbocharger systems. In a draw-through system, the turbocharger "draws" air through the carburetor, where it is infused with air. Then the mixture passes through the turbo and is directed into the engine through an intake manifold. In a blow-through system, the turbo "blows" pressurized air into the carb, where fuel is infused into the airstream. Then the air-fuel is delivered directly to the engine through an intake manifold. There are important functional differences between these two approaches, and in each case, the addition of nitrous boost will be somewhat different.

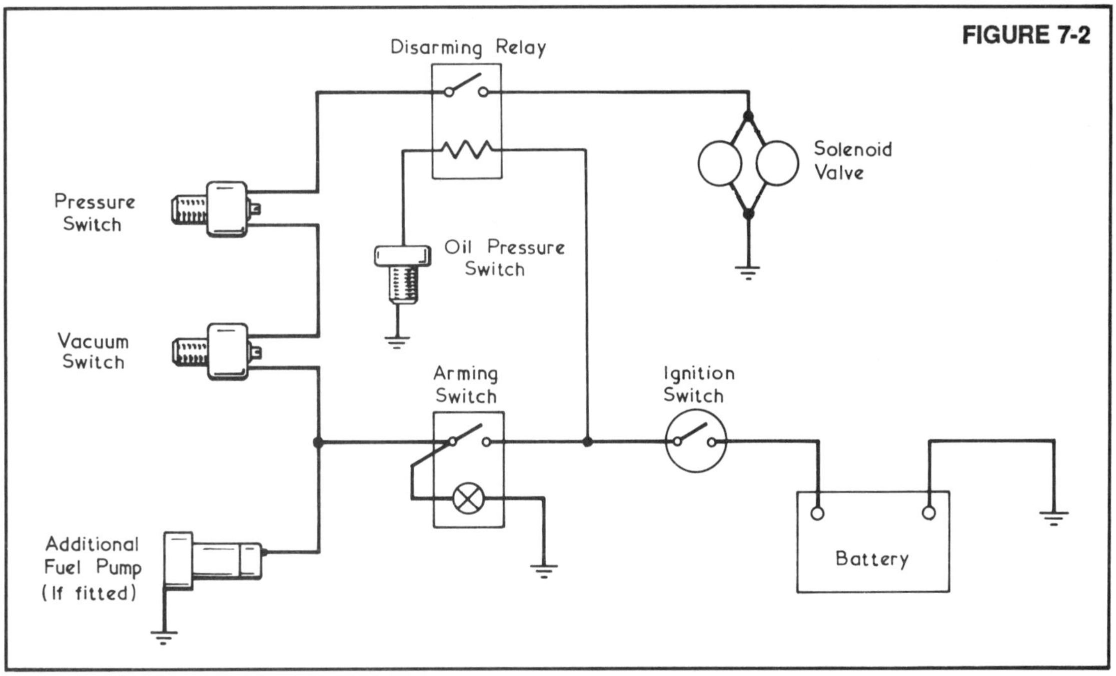

FIGURE 7-2: This is the typical layout of a nitrous system designed to reduce the low-speed boost lag of a turbocharged engine. Note the safety features—especially the disarming relay.

Figure 7-2 shows a typical schematic wiring diagram for a system designed to eliminate turbo lag. When the driver wants complete control over nitrous activation—such as in racing—the vacuum activation switch can be replaced by a throttle-operated switch. In fact, the throttle switch is much better in most situations. A vacuum switch may activate the nitrous even when the throttle is not wide open. Under some circumstances, this could unexpectedly drive the engine into boost. A throttle switch will only activate the system when the driver pushes the throttle wide open.

Irrespective of whether the turbo is of the blow- or draw-through type, a pressure-sensing switch may be used to deactivate the nitrous when the relative manifold pressure reaches a preset level. The best type of switch for this, or almost any pressure-sensing application, is a Hobbs adjustable switch. An adjustable switch allows the nitrous deactivation point to be tailored to suit the specific characteristics of the engine. Typically, a setting of 3-4psi is adequate. However, if the engine is fitted with a long-duration cam—resulting in relatively low manifold vacuum conditions—the deactivation point may have to be as high as 10psi.

In this system a safety device has been incorporated into the system to prevent nitrous flow when the engine is switched off or if the engine accidentally stalls. In most instances, an oil pressure-sensing switch is used to disable the nitrous actuating system whenever the oil pressure drops below a preset level—usually 10 or 15psi.

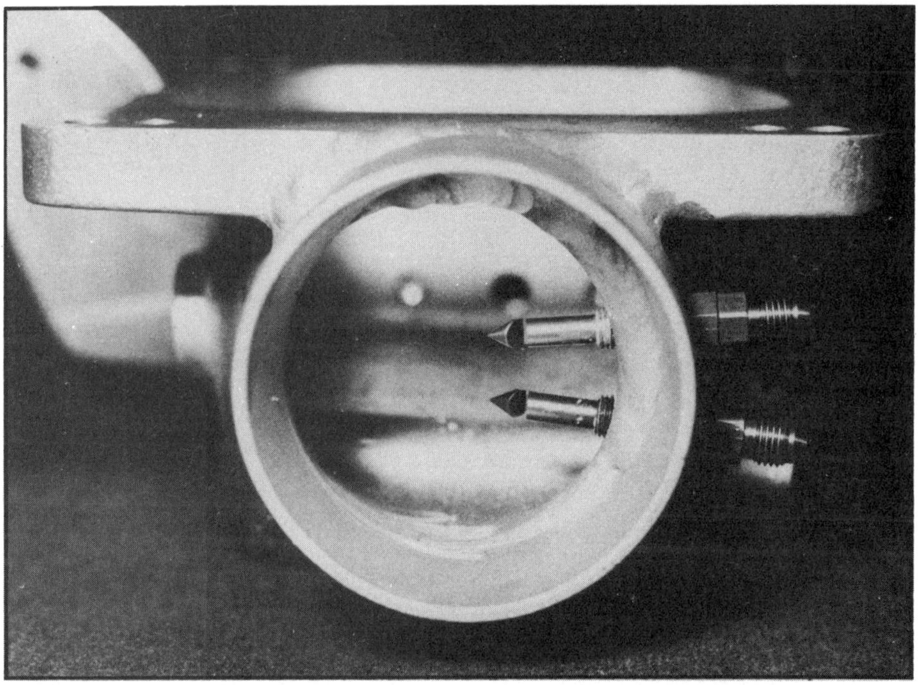

Careful calibration of the nozzles to optimize fuel and nitrous flow can not only eliminate turbo lag, but also can substantially lengthen the amount of time the system will operate on each refill of the nitrous bottle.

Another feature to note is the addition of a suitable high-volume fuel pump. If the fuel is being injected downstream of the turbo, the fuel will be injected into manifold with high relative pressure. Under these conditions, a high-pressure fuel pump will be needed to insure proper fuel flow.

Now, let us look at the detailed differences between draw-through and blow-through turbo installations. Figure 7-3 shows a typical draw-through installation on a turbocharged 4-cylinder engine (the installation will be similar on 6- or 8-cylinder engines).

The most efficient method to inject nitrous into a turbocharged system is to use a combined fuel and nitrous nozzle—like the NOS calibratable nozzle. Failing this, the conventional nozzles produced by most nitrous companies can be used.

In a draw-through system the

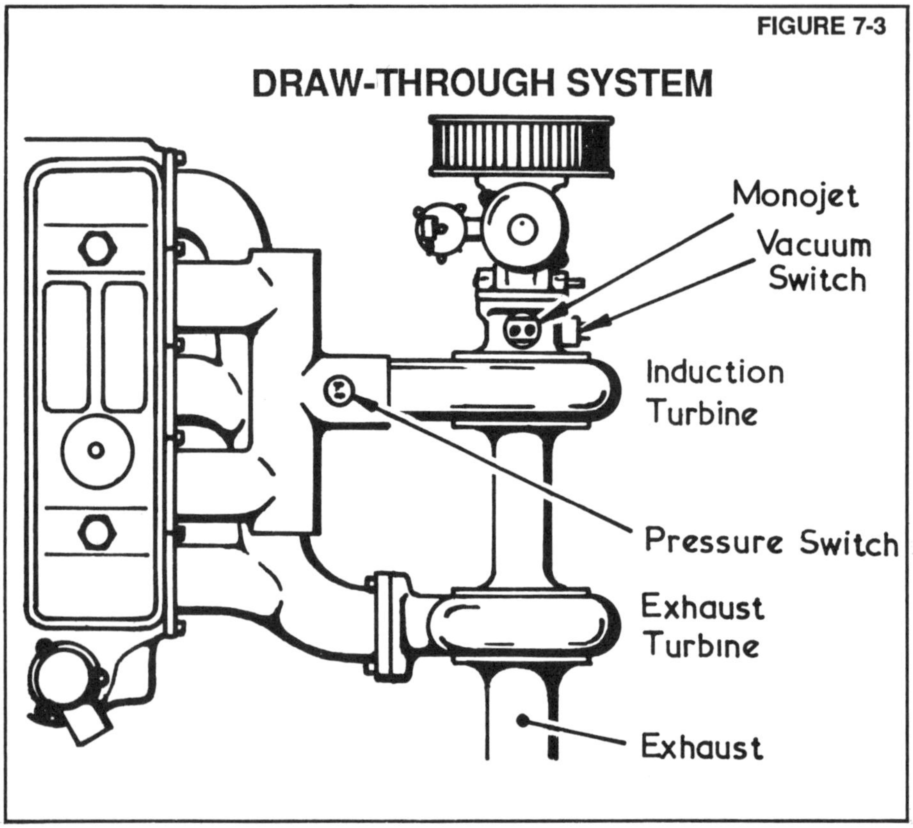

FIGURE 7-3: In a draw-through turbocharging system, the carburetor or injector nozzle introduces fuel into the airstream before the mixture reaches the turbocharger. A vacuum sensing switch must be placed at the tubo inlet and a pressure switch should be located in the intake manifold.

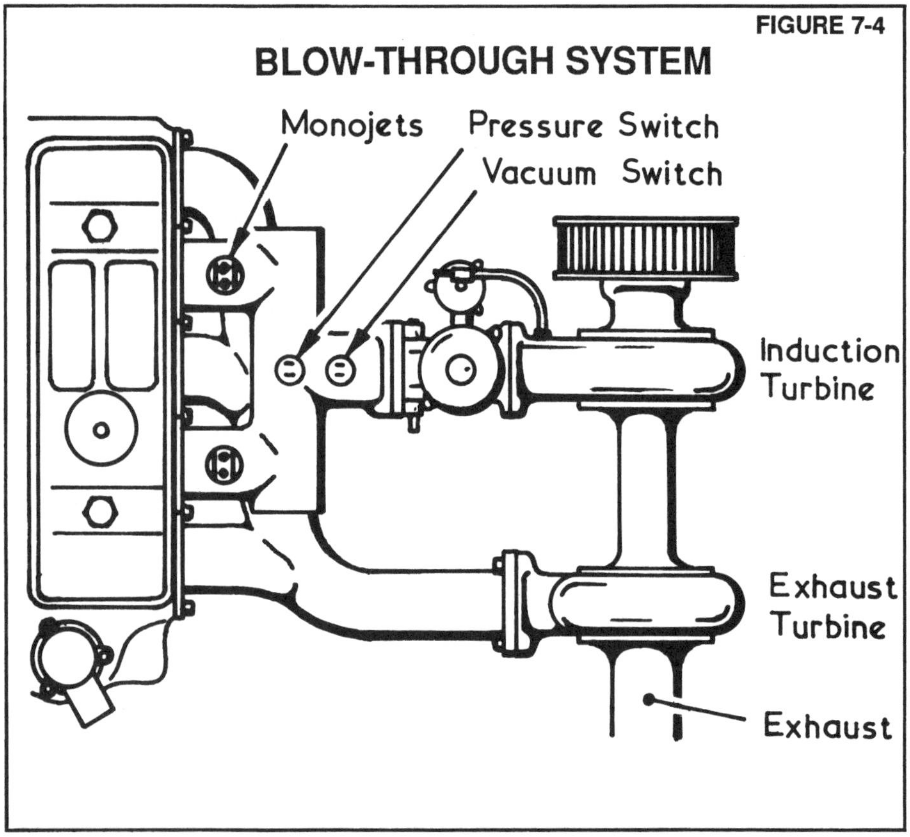

FIGURE 7-4: A blow-through turbocharging system forces pressurized air into a carburetor or injector body. When using this design, install both pressure and vacuum switches in the intake manifold plenum.

pressure-sensitive activation switch should be positioned downstream of the carburetor and upstream of the turbo. This switch can be replaced by a throttle switch, if so desired. The deactivation switch, of course, must be situated in the intake manifold; and the simplest place to inject the enrichment fuel is straight into the intake of the turbo. Tests have shown, however, that slightly better results can be obtained by injecting the fuel downstream of the turbo. (If this arrangement is desired, a high-pressure fuel pump is essential.) Nonetheless, the difference is usually quite small, and it is much simpler to inject the fuel into the turbo intake.

The situation is slightly different when nitrous is used with a blow-through system. The schematic in Figure 7-4 shows the layout of a typical 4-cylinder engine (the arrangement would again be similar for a 6- or 8-cylinder engine). In this particular system, the pressure and vacuum switches are both in the intake manifold. Once again, the vacuum switch can be replaced by a throttle switch, if desired. And once again, we must remember that anytime the point of injection is on the pressure side of the turbo *the fuel pressure must be kept above boost level.*

In the diagram, nitrous and fuel are distributed through monojet nozzles in a port-injection arrangement. This looks simple enough, however there are some difficulties. When the amount of nitrous to be injected is relatively small—as is typical in a system designed strictly to reduce boost lag—it is impractical to make the orifice in the nozzle small enough to properly meter the nitrous. The practical low limit is an orifice that produces about seven or eight horsepower. This low limit must be multiplied by the number of nozzles (usually one per port/cylinder) to determine the lowest practical performance boost available from the system.

Although the illustration shows individual fuel and nitrous nozzles, it is also possible to use a spacer plate—sandwiched between the carburetor and the manifold—to inject the nitrous and fuel. The distribution orifices in this plate must be recalibrated for the required modest flow rates (the orifices in most plates produce 100 horsepower or more). A plate-type injector usually distributes fuel and nitrous through a series of orifices—four to eight—so it is relatively simple to restrict the nitrous flow by simply reducing the number of orifices. Using this technique, a spacer-plate system can easily reduce the low-speed nitrous boost to as little as 25 horsepower.

SYSTEM EFFICIENCY

When a nitrous system is properly integrated into a well-engineered turbo system the results can be truly astounding. However, for maximum effect the turbocharger components must be selected with an understanding of how nitrous-oxide injection will alter engine performance. The details of turbocharger system design are beyond the scope of this book, but a simple discussion of these matters may help the reader understand the overall goals.

We touched on this briefly, but at this point we must again emphasize that a turbocharger is effective over a relatively limited operational range. An analysis of this mechanical limitation is fairly straightforward but very lengthy, so we won't attempt to look at this in detail. Fortunately, though, the results are easy to explain. It is simply not possible to bolt a turbocharger to an engine and expect to produce massive horsepower from 1000rpm all the way up to an upper speed limit of, say, 7500rpm. If the turbo is designed to produce a maximum effect at lower engine speeds, it will respond quickly to acceleration demand and produce relatively high boost. But at higher speeds, it will "choke" the exhaust side of the engine and limit high-rpm boost and performance. On the other hand, if the turbo is designed to produce maximum effect at high engine speeds, it will produce maximum boost and performance within a relatively narrow range, high in the engine-speed range. But in this instance, the turbo will not produce boost at low engine speeds, and it will respond sluggishly to acceleration demands.

The designers of modern high-tech turbo systems reduce this inherent design limitation by using intercoolers and boost controllers. However, The effect of these components will be altered when nitrous-oxide injection is used to augment the performance of the engine.

INTERCOOLERS

The peak output of an engine is ultimately limited by detonation. This is true of all spark-ignited engines, but detonation is really a big problem with turbocharged engines. A turbocharger is a pretty simple air pump, and a properly designed turbocharger or multiple turbochargers can be used to pump tremendous quantities of air (and fuel) into an engine. This inducted air, in effect, is compressed by the turbocharger, and because of various physical principals, the air also becomes a lot hotter. In addition, as the air moves through the turbocharger, it picks up heat because of the proximity of the hot exhaust gases passing through the exhaust turbine of the turbo. Add to this the accumulated heat in the engine compartment, and the net result is that the inducted air inside a turbo system becomes very, very hot before it reaches the combustion chambers. And at the bottom line—within the combustion chambers—heated air detonates more readily than cooler air.

Various types of intercooling systems have been devised to reduce heat buildup in the intake tract of turbocharged engines, but if the engine is nitrous-injected, the nitrous also becomes a form of intercooler. When pressurized liquid nitrous is released through a nozzle, the nitrous converts to a gas and the temperature drops to about -128 degrees. Therefore, as nitrous is discharged into the intake tract, the temperature within the tract is reduced considerably. Consequently, nitrous injection of a turbocharged engine delivers many advantages. First, the extra oxygen (and enrichment fuel) provided by the system increases the torque output. Second, the nitrous boost causes the turbocharger to accelerate very quickly and reach the maximum boost level more rapidly. Third, the nitrous cools the intake charge and allows the turbocharging system to produce a relatively greater boost level before the detonation limit is reached.

Because of this three-fold enhancement, the combined effects of nitrous and turbocharging can be spectacular. In fact, the nitrous-oxide injected into a turbocharged engine actual-

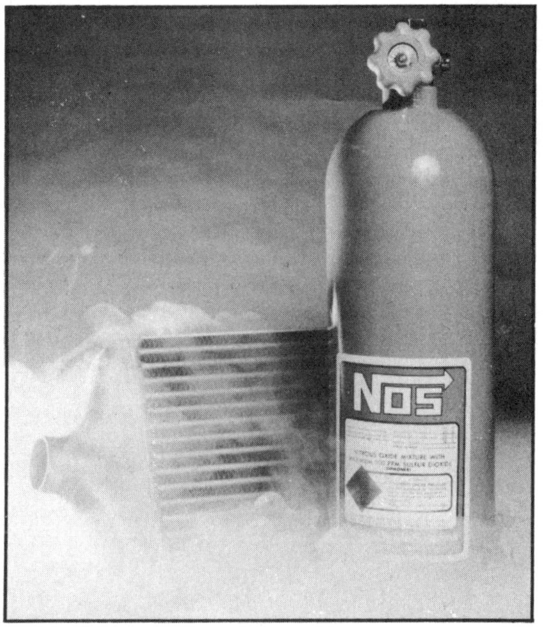

Nitrous-oxide can help turbocharged engines overcome detonation by substantially cooling the intake charge. This cooling is accomplished without the added weight or cost of an intercooler. Properly designed nitrous and turbocharging systems can work together to build exceptional horsepower while overcoming both boost lag and detonation.

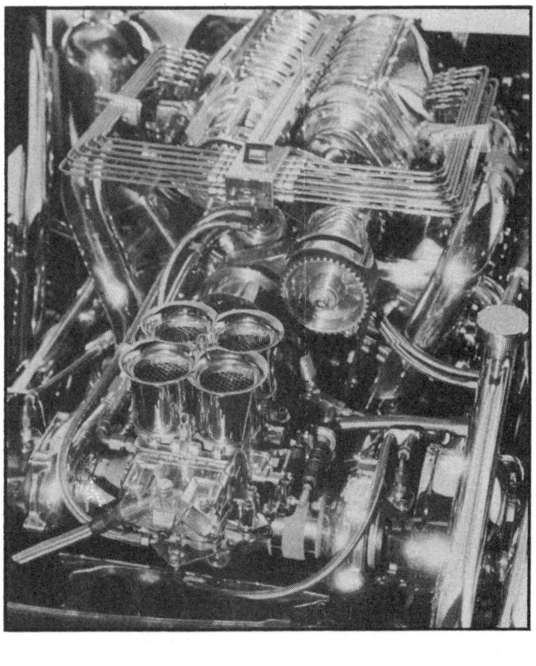

This is Rick Dobbertin's awesome Pontiac J-2000. It's equipped with a smallblock that has been supercharged, turbocharged and, of course, nitrous-oxide injected. Believe it or not, it's street legal and driveable!. This extraordinary project car was recently named Hot Rod Magazine's Street Rod of the Year.

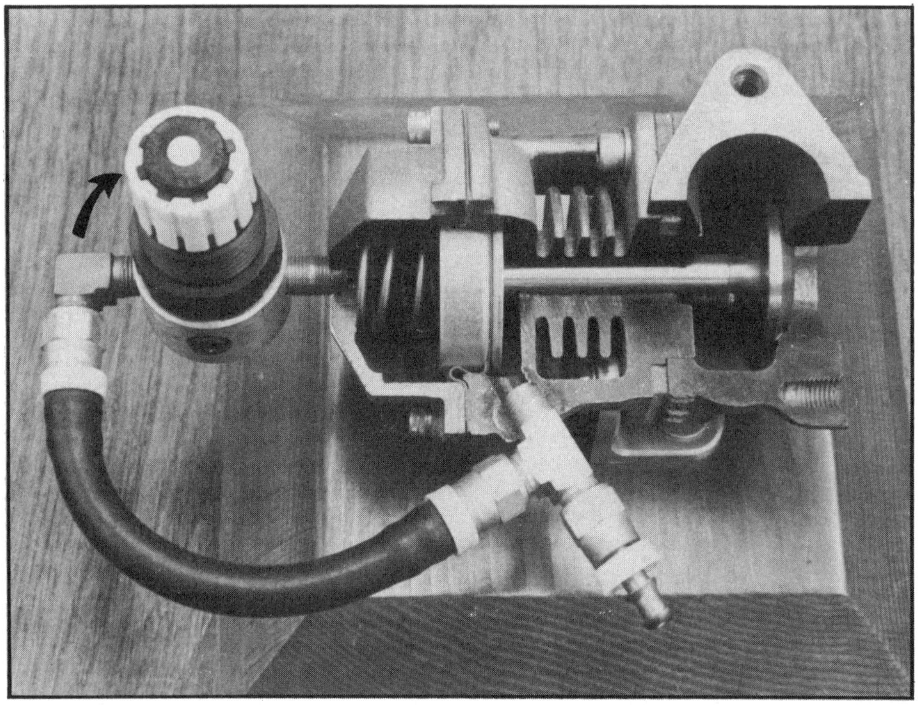

A pressure activated "wastegate" valve is the most efficient method of limiting turbocharger boost. This cutaway view shows the spring loaded diaphragm connected to a special high-temperature valve. This wastegate is adjusted by the knob on the pressure regulator attached to the pressure chamber.

ly creates more specific horsepower than a comparable amount of nitrous injected into a normally-aspirated engine. It is not unusual for a nitrous delivery rate that produces a 50-horsepower boost in a normally-aspirated engine to develop as much as 100 or, in optimal conditions, 150 extra horsepower in a turbo engine.

BOOST CONTROL

There are several methods available to "control" turbo boost, but the wastegate is among the most efficient and most reliable. In effect, the wastegate is a "limiter" that controls the maximum amount of exhaust gas delivered to the exhaust turbine of the turbo. The wastegate is located in the exhaust system, between the exhaust port(s) of the engine and the turbine of the turbocharger. When a predetermined level of boost is reached—through a simple mechanical arrangement the wastegate "monitors" the pressure conditions in the intake manifold—a vent port in the wastegate opens and excess exhaust pressure is dumped from the exhaust system before it reaches the turbine. This effectively prevents the turbo from spinning faster and developing more boost.

The wastegate is very effective because it does not restrict mid-level performance and, of course, it is easily adjustable. During low- and mid-level performance (boost) conditions the wastegate allows the full volume of exhaust gas to reach the turbo turbine. If the turbo is properly sized to the performance requirements, this unrestricted flow of exhaust through the turbo should result in excellent turbo efficiency and good engine response. However, as the performance requirement (boost) rises, the exhaust flow also increases. Until, at a preselected "boost limit" level, the wastegate opens a port in the exhaust system allowing excess exhaust pressure to vent away before it reaches the turbine. (This boost limit is usually preset at a specific level by the adjustment of a mechanical screw on the wastegate, but in some racing engines the limit may be variable and is adjusted by a remote valve controlled by the driver.)

Not all turbo systems use wastegate(s)—some designers simply produce a system that is effective in a narrow rpm range—but when a wastegate is used, the design of the turbocharger(s) is generally optimized to produce maximum boost pressure at low engine speeds. However, when a wastegate, or some similar limiting device, is used to restrict high-rpm boost, the turbocharger is less efficient. Due to various effects, a turbo is most efficient when it produces maximum boost at approximately the peak point in the engine speed band.

Nitrous-oxide injection can largely overcome this compromise. When nitrous is used to boost low-speed performance, a large turbocharger can be selected for maximum efficiency at relatively high engine speeds. Generally, the turbo size—the so-called A/R ratio—can be increased by one or two steps, sometimes as much as three steps. On a typical turbocharged V8-type engine this may increase peak output by 50 to 100 horsepower!

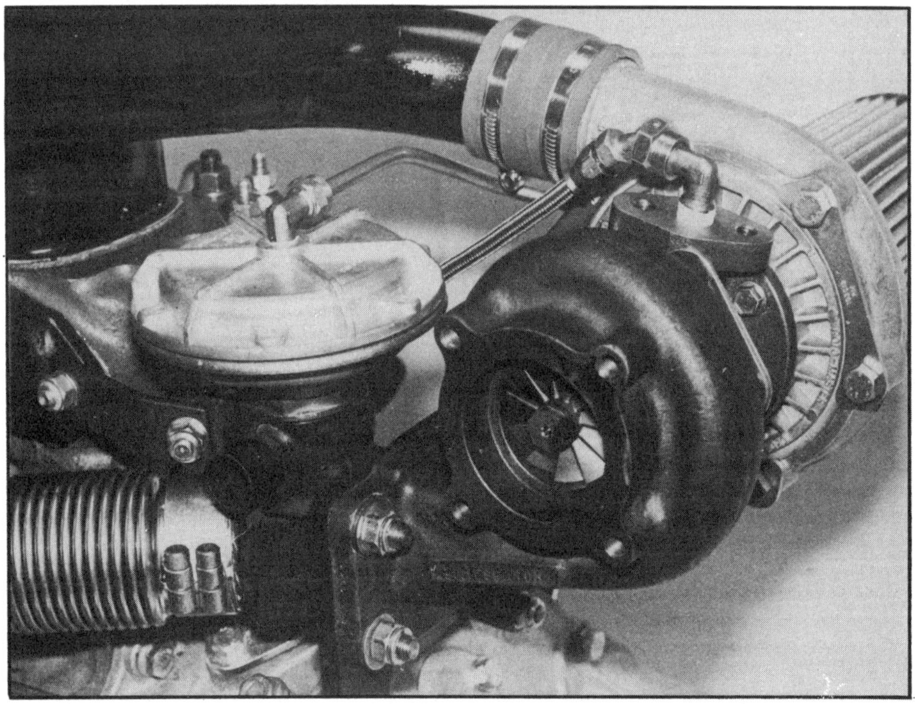

If nitrous is used to boost low-speed torque, the turbocharger can be selected to maximize mid-range and top-end horsepower. The net result will be more horsepower, reduced turbo lag, and in most cases, the heavy and expensive wastegate(s) can be eliminated.

In addition, the need for boost-limiting device(s) is eliminated. As we have mentioned, most racing turbo systems use wastegates to control boost, and reliable, high-quality wastegates are expensive. In general, the out-of-pocket expenses for a nitrous system will be greater than the money saved by eliminating one or more wastegates, but the resulting system should produce more horsepower throughout the engine-speed range.

ENRICHMENT FUEL

Whenever nitrous-oxide is injected it must, of course, be accompanied by a properly proportioned amount of enrichment fuel. In some of the systems discussed here the point of injection for the enrichment fuel is downstream of the turbo. Therefore, the fuel is discharged into the pressurized portion of the intake tract. This means that *the pressure in the enrichment fuel system must be maintained at a level above the boost pressure.*

It will be necessary to use a fuel pump, or a multiple-pump arrangement, that is fully capable of delivering the *required maximum fuel volume* (at wide-open throttle) at a fuel pressure that exceeds the manifold boost pressure by at least three pounds. For instance, if the turbo system can develop 15 pound of boost, the fuel pump(s) must be able to deliver the required fuel volume at a line pressure of at least 18psi. This is an absolute minimum, and if at all possible, it is better to maintain the fuel-delivery pressure at five pounds above the manifold pressure.

A good fuel pump for this type of system is the Walbro roller pump. This design is capable of fuel pressures—at typical flow rates—of up to 100psi. It has ample pressure in reserve, and of equal importance, I have found the Walbro pump to be very reliable.

The most effective way to maintain the required pressure and fuel flow is to use a pressure-sensing fuel regulator. This type of regulator is used in some blow-through turbocharger systems. It is very handy because it can be adjusted to maintain the fuel pressure at the desired level *above* the manifold boost pressure.

SYSTEM COORDINATION

If the nitrous is used to augment top-end power, as well as to eliminate boost lag, the delivery rates and actuation mechanism must be matched to the specific engine and operational requirements. This is, more than anything, a matter of trial-and-error, and will require a lot of development effort. With proper turbo selection, the wastegate(s), or similar boost-limiting devices, can usually be eliminated. This will often improve top-end power, but for maximum effect, the A/R ratio of the turbo should be selected to provide peak boost at the max crank speed (rpm) of the engine.

When the goal is to produce maximum horsepower, the question of balancing turbo boost and nitrous boost inevitably arises. As far as this author has been able to determine, there is no definite answer to this dilemma. Very little research has been completed on max-effort turbo- and nitrous-boosted engine. However, these general (unsubstantiated) guidelines may be helpful as a starting point. Maximum turbo boost on gasoline should be limited to about 30 to 35psi. On alcohol, the turbo boost limit could be raised to about 45 to 50psi.

Additional max-power augmentation can be gained from nitrous injection, but any increase in nitrous-fuel delivery should be undertaken with care. When the nitrous delivery is not correctly balanced, the gross power level may drop off, even when the turbo boost is increased. Current thinking points toward injecting nitrous at a rate of approximately 3.0 pounds per minute for every 15 pounds of boost—this assumes the use of high-octane gasoline or alcohol. These figures apply to a typical smallblock engine in the 300- to 370-inch displacement range. If the engine displaces more than 370 cubic inches (up to a typical practical limits of about 550 inches), the amount of nitrous used can be increased somewhat. In fact, on very large engines I believe it may be possible to deliver as much as 6.0 pounds (per minute) of nitrous per 15 pounds of turbo boost. *These are only general guidelines and are based on the very limited knowledge available in the area of max-power nitrous augmenataion.*

For most street-driven engines the turbo boost level will be relatively conservative and the rate of nitrous delivery will be very modest. Indeed, if the delivery rate is too high, there will be a problem with detonation (due primarily to the low octane and anti-knock properties of conventional pump gasolines), even though the induction temperature is reduced by the nitrous.

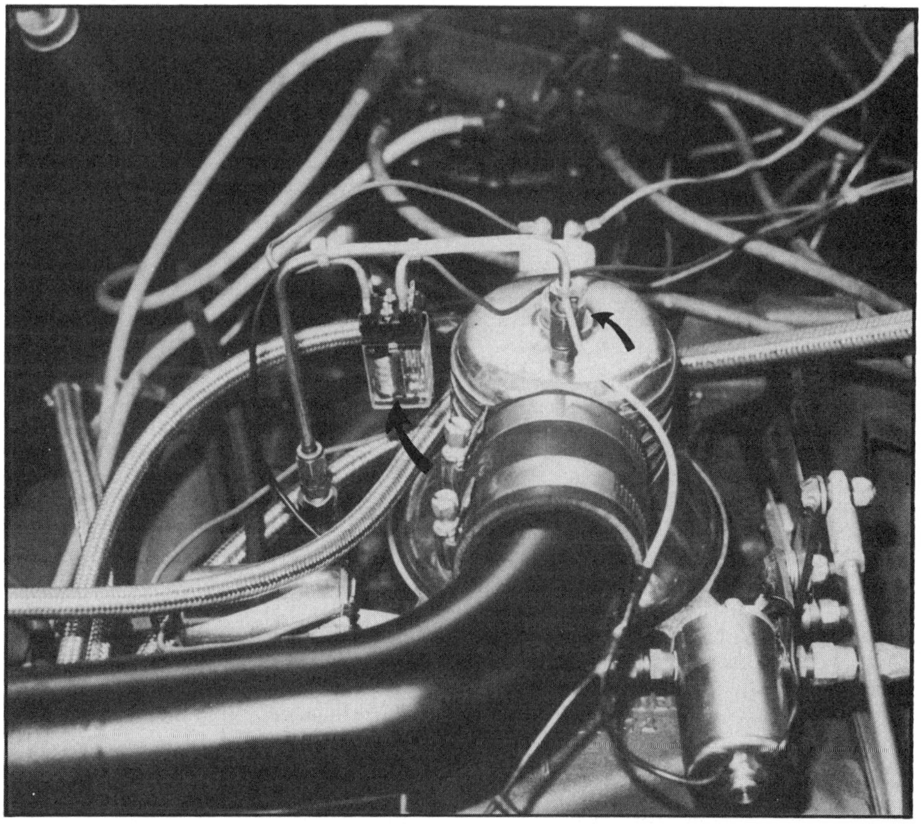

Note the relay and the injection lines. The relay is controlled by an oil pressure switch, which deactivates the nitrous system when the oil pressure drops below a preset limit. This prevents the nitrous system from activating when the engine is not running. Also note that the nitrous and fuel lines inject directly into the plenum.

CHAPTER 8

INSTALLING AND REFILLING

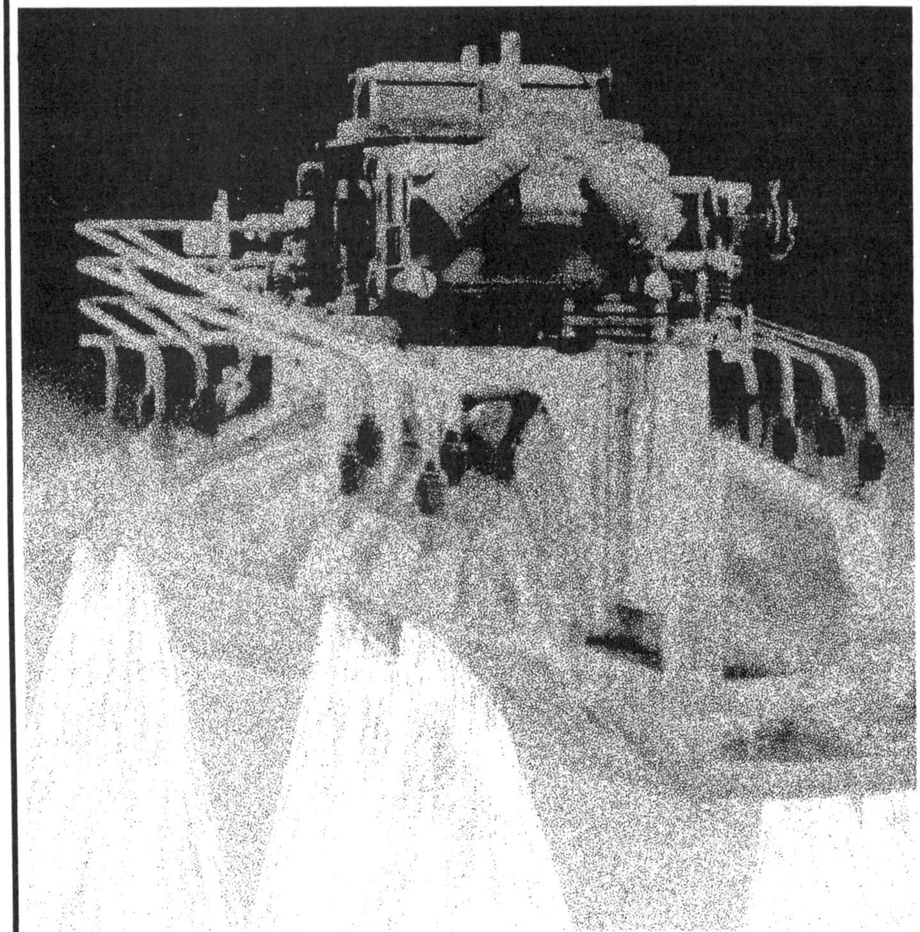

Previous chapters have discussed the design and development of nitrous-oxide systems, but in this chapter we will look at the "nuts and bolts" of installing a typical nitrous system. Currently at least 90% of the installed nitrous systems utilize plate-type injectors, so we have included a step-by-step photo essay of a typical installation.

This type of system is overwhelmingly popular because the location and installation of the injectors and/or feed orifices is extremely simple. As the name implies, the point of injection in this type of system is located in a plate positioned between the carburetor and the intake manifold. This eliminates the need for complicated machining procedures —required to insert individual injectors into the manifold—and in most cases, a typical plate-type system can be installed in a relatively short time, using only ordinary handtools.

Although this installation specifically covers a plate-type injection system, with the exception of the individual port nozzles, the installation of most port-type systems is very similar. It must be remembered, however, that in a port-injection system, the location of the injection point—relative to the intake valve—will greatly affect overall engine performance. The guidelines in Chapter Five concerning the placement of nozzles may be helpful. It is important, though, to follow the recommendations and specific instructions provided by the kit manufacturer. Modifications may have unexpected results and should be undertaken with considerable care.

PORT SYSTEMS

As we have mentioned, a port-injection nitrous system is more complex than a plate system, however, the basic installation procedures are quite similar to a plate-type system. The primary difference involves the installation of the individual nozzles and the extensive plumbing required to connect the nozzles to the solenoids.

Nitrous-Oxide Systems has recently developed a new monojet port injector—NOS calls it a "fogger nozzle." The NOS fogger nozzles usually improve nitrous performance somewhat—because of the increased mixing of nitrous and fuel—but for all practical purposes, this system is similar to conventional port systems that utilize individual side-by-side or inline nozzles for the nitrous and enrichment fuel.

The location of the nozzles is important. If a conventional-style injection system with separate nozzles for fuel and nitrous is used, the system will generally produce more power boost when the point of injection is moved away from the intake valve. This, of course, provides more time for the nitrous and fuel to mix together. If mixing nozzles are used—like the NOS fogger nozzles—the results will generally be better when the point of injection is located closer to the intake valve.

However, there are times when convenience may dictate the position of the nozzle. For instance, successful results have been obtained by positioning NOS fogger nozzles to inject directly into the carburetor mouth. This will probably reduce peak power slightly, but at moderate power levels the loss is minimal. For instance, a setup that produces a 100 horsepower increase when injected through the ports may only produce 92-95 horsepower at the mouth of the carburetor. The word *may* here is very important. These are fairly representative numbers, but individual circumstances can cause considerable variation in peak power.

REFILLING

One of the facts of life about nitrous injection is the periodic requirement to refill the storage bottle or tank. The easiest method is to rely on a local performance shop that sells nitrous equipment or a commercial gas supplier—companies that sell industrial gases and/or welding equipment—to refill the bottle. But if the system is used a lot, the trips to a local supplier will become a bit of a nuisance. It is practical and not very difficult to set up a small refilling station that will allow a user to store convenient quantities of nitrous-oxide in his or her own garage.

It is usually possible to buy or rent a large reservoir tank that will easily hold 60 or 80 pounds of nitrous-oxide. A local supplier of commercial gases can usually provide such a bottle. If this is not practical, large storage tanks can be purchased from some manufacturers of nitrous kits. This is probably the best source, because the manufacturer can also supply a suitable stand that will hold the reservoir in an inverted position so that liquid nitrous, instead of gaseous, is transferred to the on-board bottle.

Though the process is simple, certain basic facts must be remembered when the small, on-board bottle is refilled. First, the transfer of the nitrous can only take place *from a high-pressure source to a low-pressure receptacle*. And, for all practical purposes, the relative temperatures will determine the pressure differential between the on-board bottle and the main reservoir. For accurate and efficient nitrous transfer, the reservoir tank (i.e., the large bulk-storage bottle) needs to be relatively warmer than the small on-board bottle being refilled. If at all possible, the pressure in the large (warm) tank should be 100psi above the pressure in the small (cool) bottle. This much pressure differential is not absolutely necessary, but the differential should be at least 80 to 90psi.

It is not practical, therefore, to remove a nitrous bottle directly from the hot trunk of a car and refill it from a cool storage reservoir. The best approach is to remove the bottle and place it in a freezer overnight to reduce the temperature and, consequently, lower the internal pressure. In most cases this is not a problem, but some users find it convenient to have two bottles. While one bottle is used in the car, the other can be cooled, conveniently refilled, and transferred immediately to the car as soon as the on-board bottle runs low.

It is not necessary to freeze a bottle before it is refilled; it just helps. If the bottle is cooled, the internal vapor pressure is lower, and the nitrous will flow relatively quickly from the large reservoir into the cool bottle. It is important to remember, though, that it is possible to "overfill" the typical on-board bottle. A full nitrous bottle does not contain 100% liquid nitrous. If it did, the slightest temperature rise would cause the internal pressure to rise dangerously high. In reality, a properly filled bottle contains about 32% free space above the liquid. Even a slightly overfilled bottle can cause a problem. Under certain conditions (when the temperature rises) a pressure rise may cause the safety vent to blowoff.

During the refilling operation, the bottle should be placed on a set of scales. To fill the bottle properly, it is necessary to know the capacity and weight of the empty bottle. The weight of an empty bottle is called the *tare weight*. This weight is stamped somewhere on the bottle—usually near the outlet.

It is not likely that the bottle will be completely empty. Some nitrous inevitably remains in the bottle. To determine the amount, weigh the bottle and subtract the tare weight. If only a pound or so is left, it is best to discharge this remainder. Point the nozzle to a safe area, open the valve and vent it to open atmosphere. Leave the valve on the tank open.

Next, with the reservoir tank inverted, take the transfer line—which must have a filter in it—point it in a safe direction, and vent a small amount of nitrous through the line to purge it of dirt or sediment. Then, loosely install the transfer line to the bottle to be filled. "Loosely" means that the fitting will require about one more complete turn before the line fitting is completely secured to the bottle valve. At this point the fitting must be able to leak a bit.

Now slowly turn on the control valve at the reservoir. Crack it open just enough so that liquid nitrous eventually escapes from the loose fitting. When this happens, tighten the fitting. This operation purges the air from the filling line, leaving it full of liquid nitrous. While the bottle to be filled is still on the scales, fully open the tap on the supply reservoir. Note the weight reading and continue to watch the scale as the bottle fills.

The maximum weight reading should equal the *rated weight plus the tare weight*. In other words, if the bottle has a tare weight of 12.5 pounds and a capacity of 10 pounds, the bottle is "full" to the rated capacity when the scale reads 22.5 pounds (12.5 plus 10.0 pounds). *Do not under any circumstances attempt to overfill the bottle.*

Once the bottle has been filled to the specified weight limit, close the bottle valve and then close the reservoir valve. Carefully loosen the transfer line fitting at the bottle valve and *safely vent the liquid nitrous remaining inside the line* and remove the transfer line.

Remember, the liquid nitrous remaining in the line will be very cold and *can cause freeze burns if it comes into contact with skin.* BE CAREFUL.

HOW TO INSTALL A TYPICAL INJECTOR-PLATE SYSTEM

The motivation to install a nitrous-oxide system on a street machine generally falls into one of two categories: (1) to boost the performance of a sluggish late-model car, or (2) to add more performance to a vintage "musclecar." The installation shown here falls in the latter category, but the installation procedures are approximately the same no matter what the intended result.

Our project car is a 1967 Plymouth GTX powered by a 440cid Magnum wedge. Jim Salonisen, the owner of this outstanding classic, explains his motivation for installing a nitrous system; "The GTX is plenty fast, but I only use the car for weekend blasts, so nitrous seemed like a great way to get even more of a good thing."

The engine is completely stock except for an Edelbrock Torker manifold that retains the original Carter AVS (air-valve secondary) carburetor. A high-capacity fuel pump was also installed to ensure ample supply for the enrichment delivery of the nitrous system. Engine output is routed through a Torqueflite automatic transmission with a stock torque converter (2500rpm stall speed). In stock street trim this potent musclecar will run quarter-mile times in the high 13-second range, despite the nearly 3600lb weight.

In stock form the 440 Mopar powerplant produces plenty of torque and because this is strictly a street project, the budget "Power Shot" package from Nitrous Oxide Systems was chosen. This system is designed with engine reliability as a foremost consideration; even so, our dyno tests show a 115-125 horsepower boost and we would expect a full one second drop in elapsed times.

It was evident from the outstanding performance on the very first test that the Nitrous Oxide Systems package is well engineered. No last-

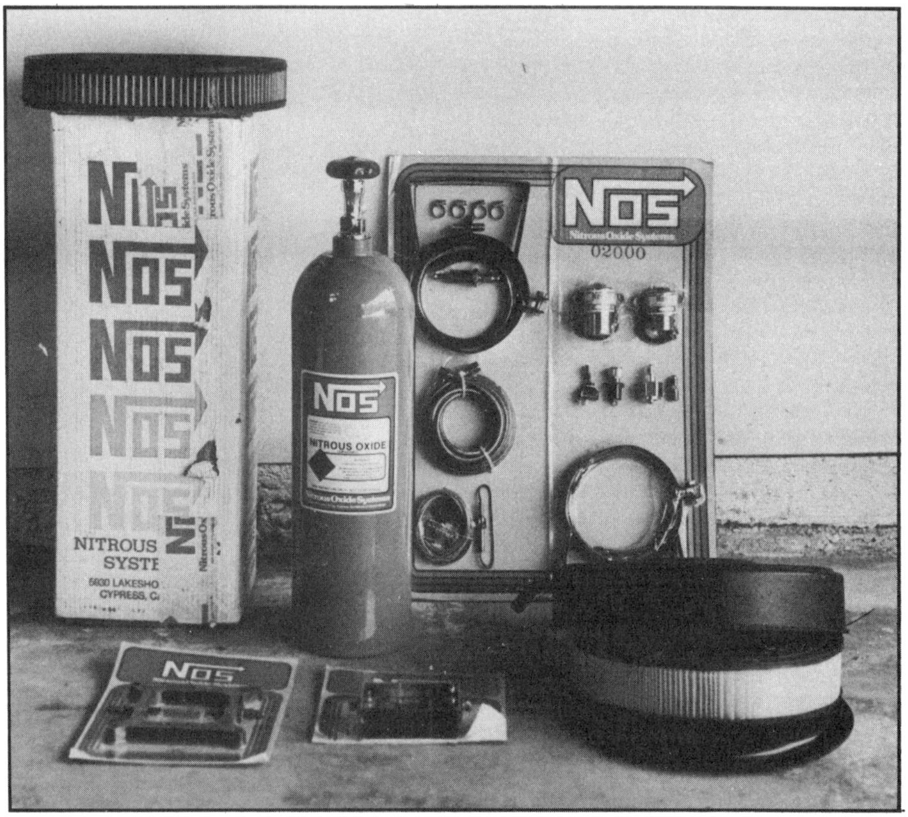

The "Power Shot" kit includes solenoid valves, braided line, electrical connections and tank mounting brackets. (The latest NOS systems have high-flow solenoids mounted on the injector plate.) The injector plate and the digital electronic timer are optional items. The installation adds about 5/8-inch to the height of the carburetor, so to maintain adequate hood clearance a 5/8-inch shorter, but highly efficient, K&N filter was installed.

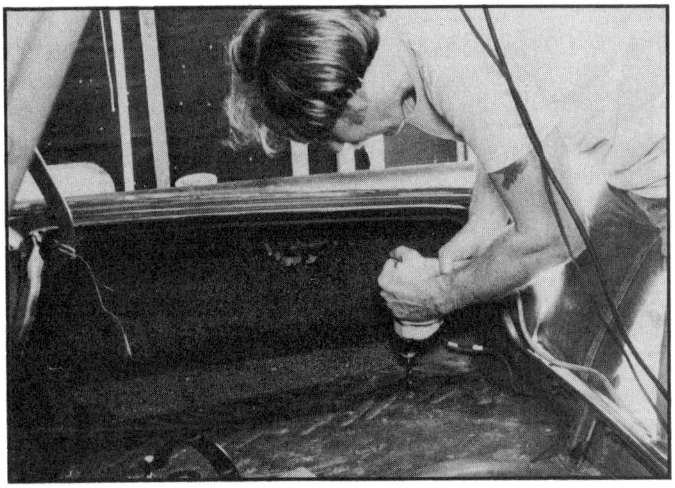

The first step is to locate and drill the holes for the bottle mounting brackets. Care must be taken to ensure that bolt locations are accessible from underneath (avoid drilling into frame sections, fuel tank, etc.). This mounting was chosen as the Mopar has plenty of room in the trunk.

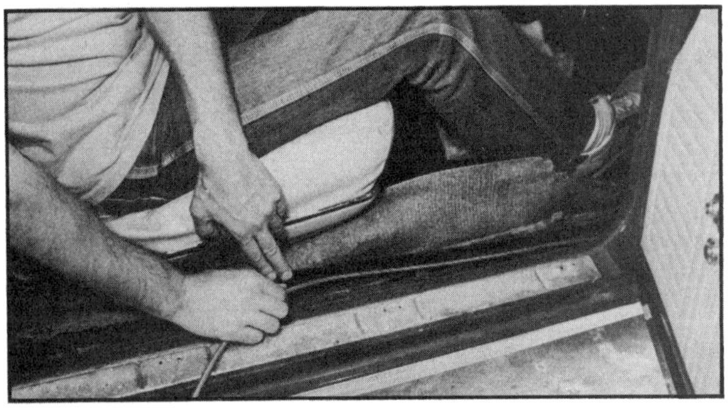

The steel-braid line connecting the bottle to the engine compartment can be located under the car, outside of the frame rails (common in racing applications), or through the driver's compartment. The Mopar has an ideal route alongside the passenger seat. A metal cover plate, which protects the wiring harnesses, provides concealment.

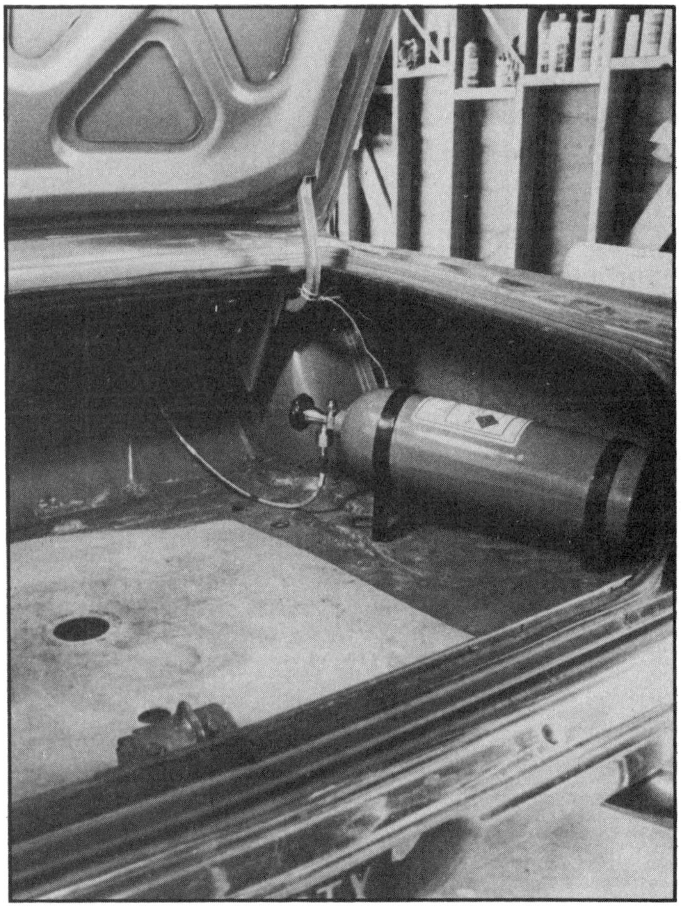

The bottle is located so it can be slipped forward out of the mounts (for refilling). To prevent dirt from entering the system and causing problems with the valves, the open ends of the supply line should be taped closed during the mounting procedures.

The stock engine compartment is spacious. Installation in early musclecars (before the factories added miles of vacuum hose) is usually quite easy; wide open access eliminates a lot of knuckle-busting frustration.

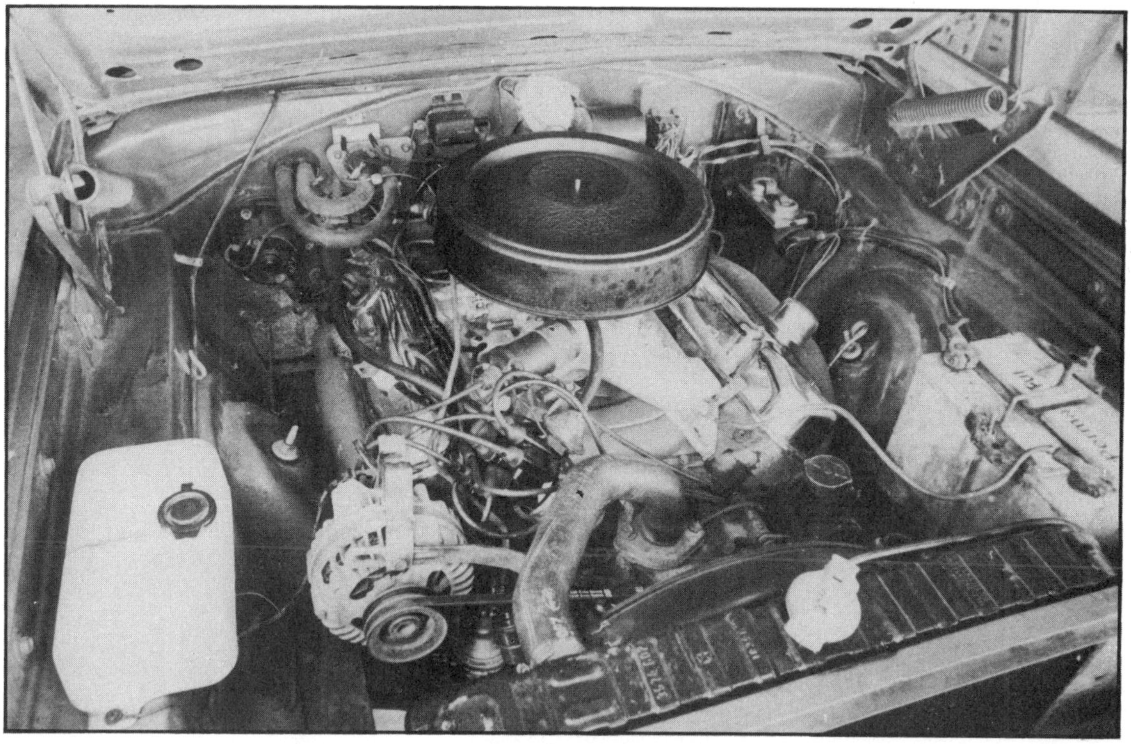

Adapter fittings should be installed in the solenoids before they are mounted inside the engine compartment. To ensure against leaks, NOS recommends Teflon thread tape on both the fuel and nitrous fittings.

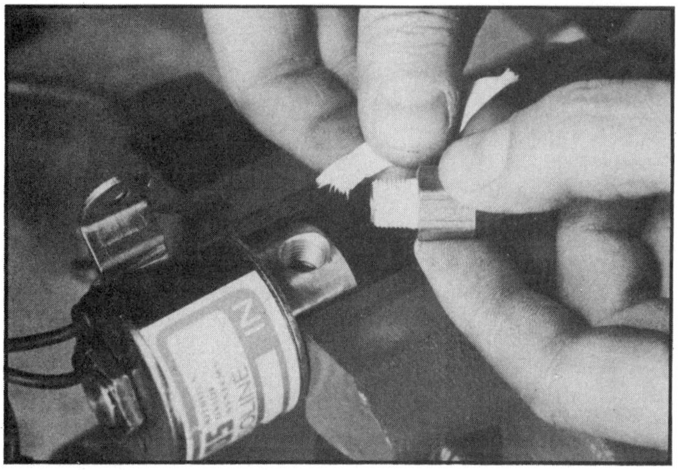

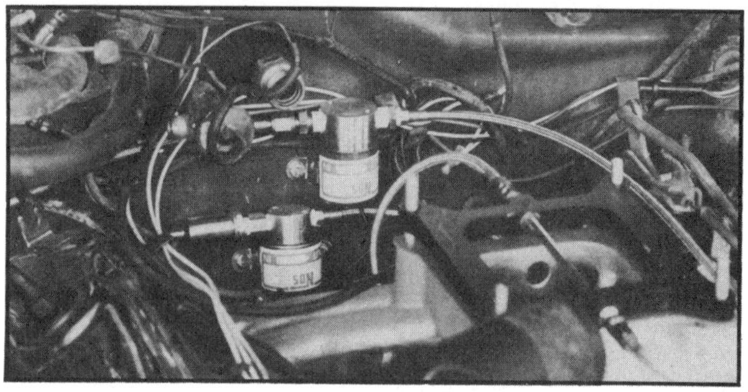

The solenoid valves can now be mounted. In the GTX there is ample room on the firewall. Consider the length of the lines that will connect the valves to the injector plate BEFORE mounting the valves. Also, connect the nitrous line to the bottle and, before you connect it to the solenoid, open the bottle valve briefly to blow out accumulated dirt.

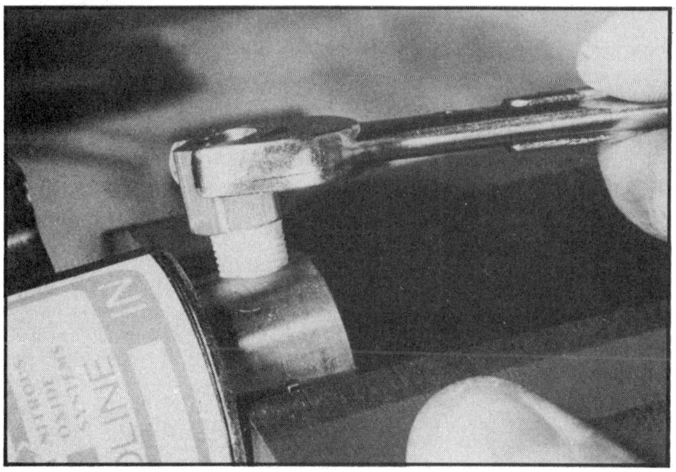

The trick to Teflon tape lies in wrapping it in the proper direction, otherwise the tape will unravel as the fitting is tightened. With the fitting oriented so the threads point toward you, wrap the tape in a clockwise rotation (in other words, opposite to the direction of rotation when the fitting is tightened). You need only wrap 1-1/2 to 2 turns.

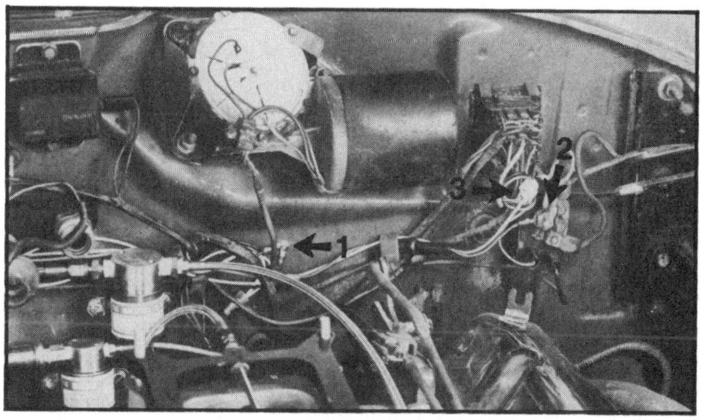

Arrow #1 indicates the electrical ground for the solenoids. Make certain this is a secure connection. If the nitrous valve activates but the fuel valve doesn't (due to an improper ground), you're in for real trouble. Arrow #2 shows the 12-volt electrical source required for the system. Arrow #3 indicates the electrical connection for the backlight of the digital timer (for night driving).

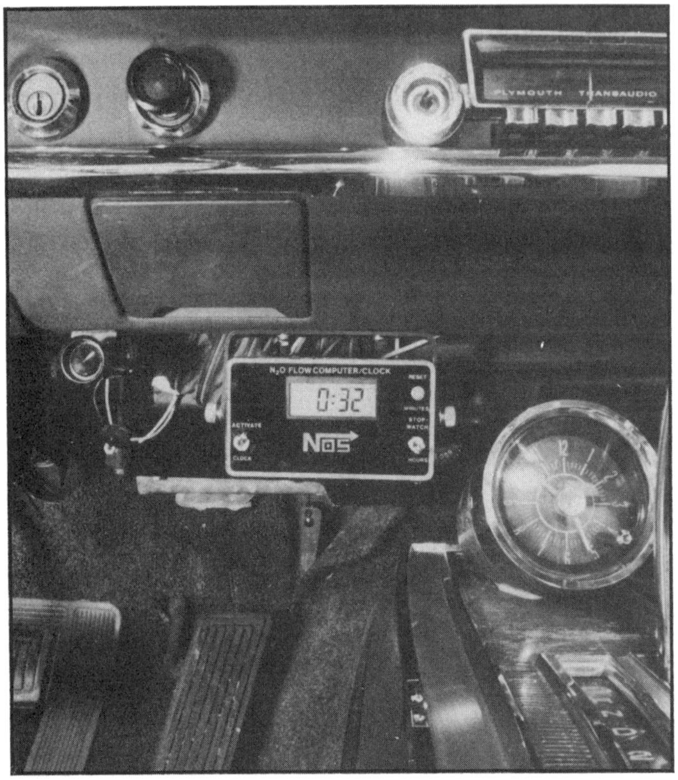

The digital timer/flow meter is actually a stopwatch that counts up the number of seconds that the system is activated. When not in use as a counter, the display can be switched over to a normal clock display. The counter "remembers" the flow display even when the ignition is turned off.

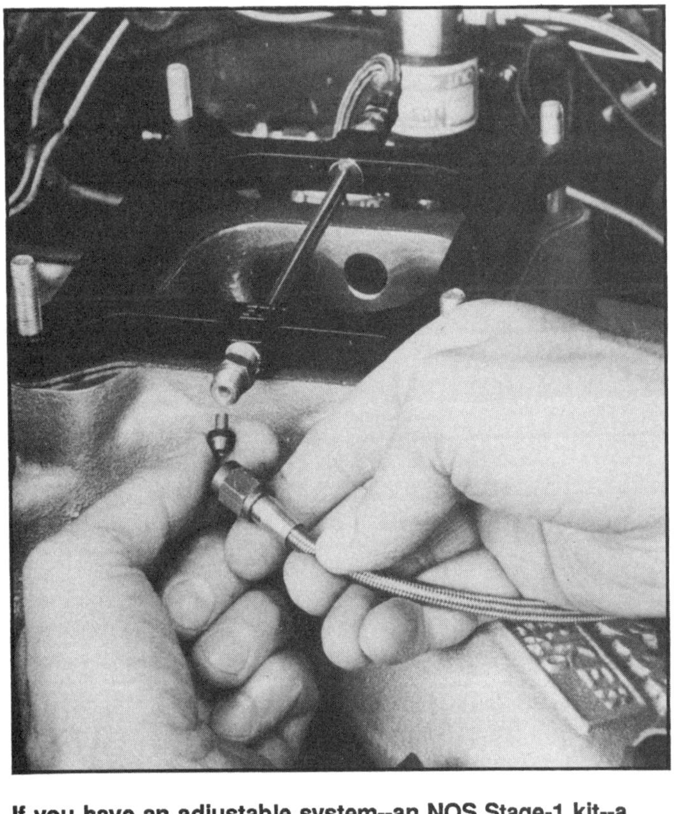

If you have an adjustable system--an NOS Stage-1 kit--a replaceable metering orifice is installed in the fitting on each end of the injector plate. Make certain they are in place and not accidentally left out. Here the injector plate, metering orifice, hoses, and gaskets are installed properly.

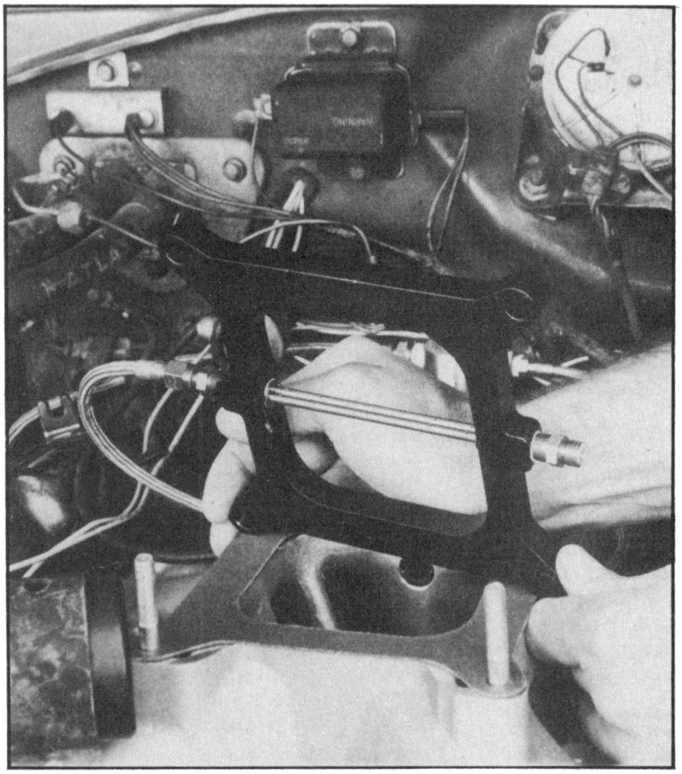

The injector plate meters and injects the fuel and nitrous; fuel enters one side, nitrous on the other. Make sure the plate is installed with the injection orifices aimed into the manifold (down).

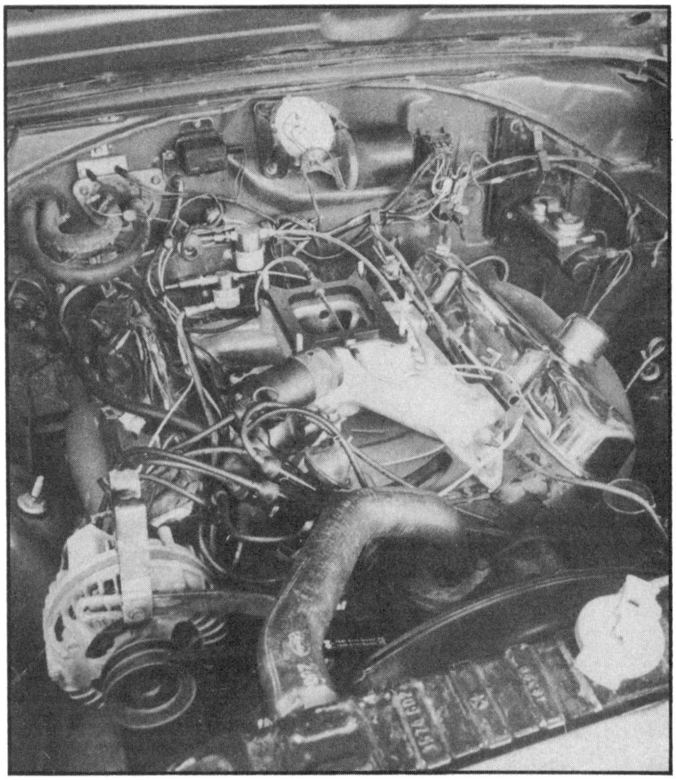

The nitrous can be activated briefly before the carburetor is installed to ensure that the solenoid opens, closes and seals properly. Stand clear and wear eye protection against nitrous or blown dust. The supply line is now charged with pressurized nitrous (the bottle valve is open and the solenoid is closed) and <u>the valves and hose connections should be checked carefully for leaks</u>.

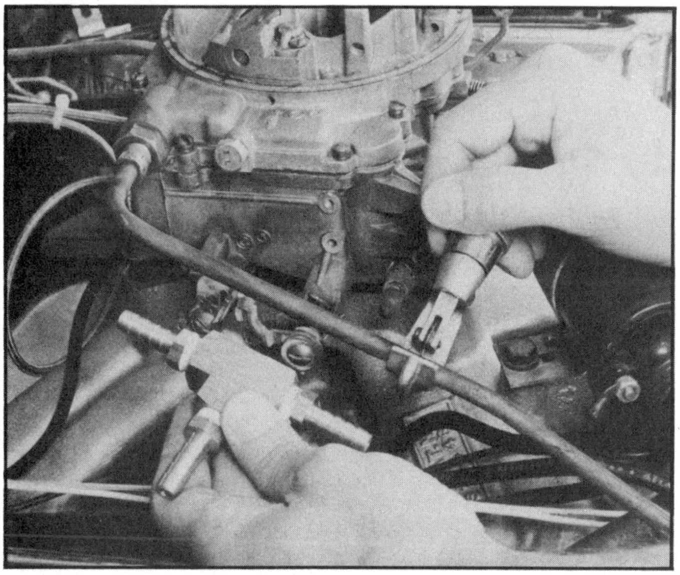

After the carburetor is in place, a T-fitting must be installed in the fuel line to provide a fuel source for the gasoline solenoid. A tubing cutter is used to remove a short section of the factory line.

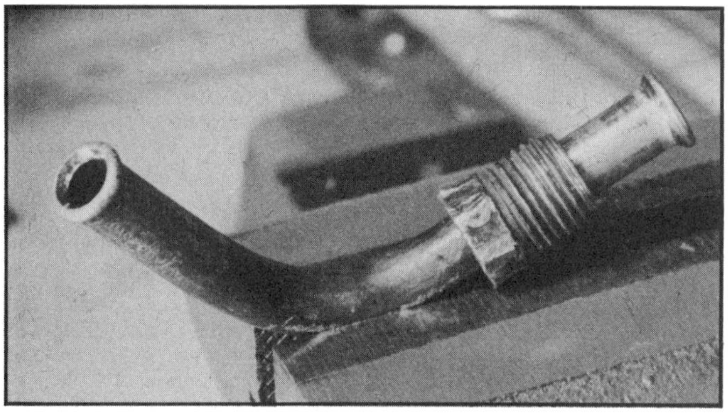

Here is the completed double flare. Note the smooth radius permitting easy hose installation, while the "bulge" helps prevent fuel leaks.

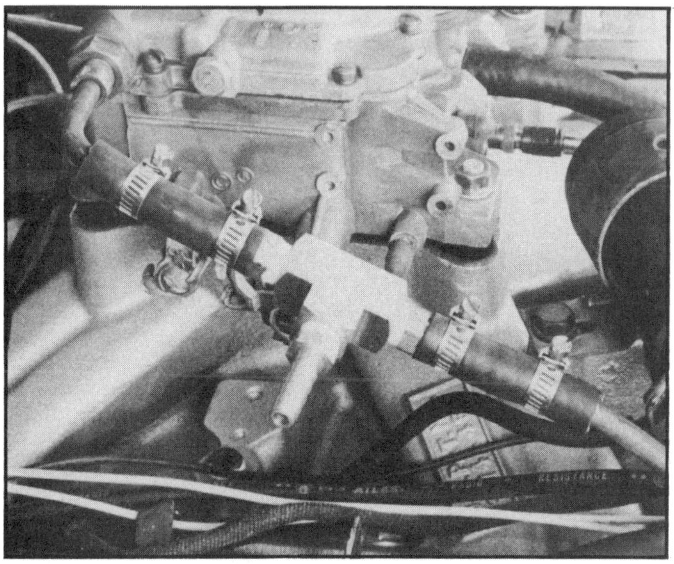

The T-fitting is installed with short pieces of rubber tubing. To ensure reliability use only tubing rated as "fuel-line hose" and stainless steel screw-type clamps.

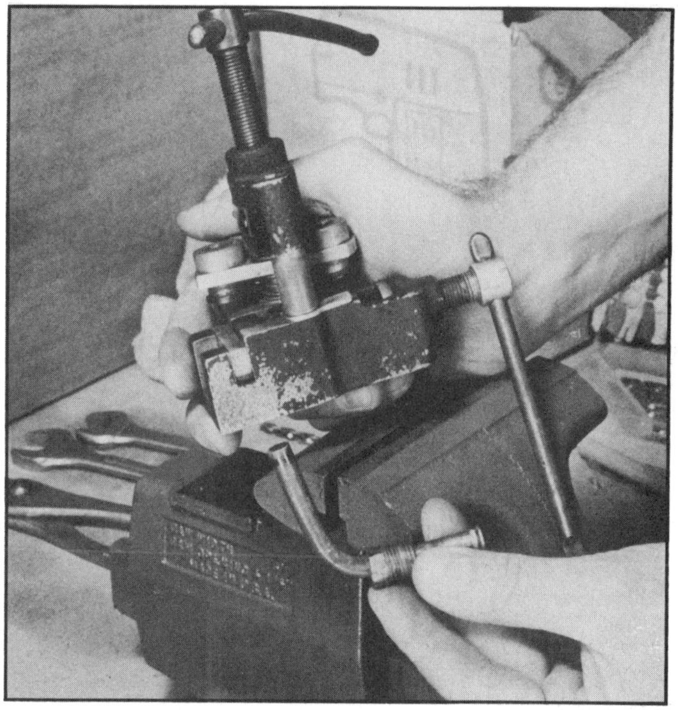

Each end of the steel fuel line should be flared to prevent the rubber hose from sliding off the tube. A shallow double flare is preferred as it has a smooth edge and will not cut the rubber hose as it slides over the tubing. Suitable flaring tools are widely available; this one is a military surplus all-in-one unit.

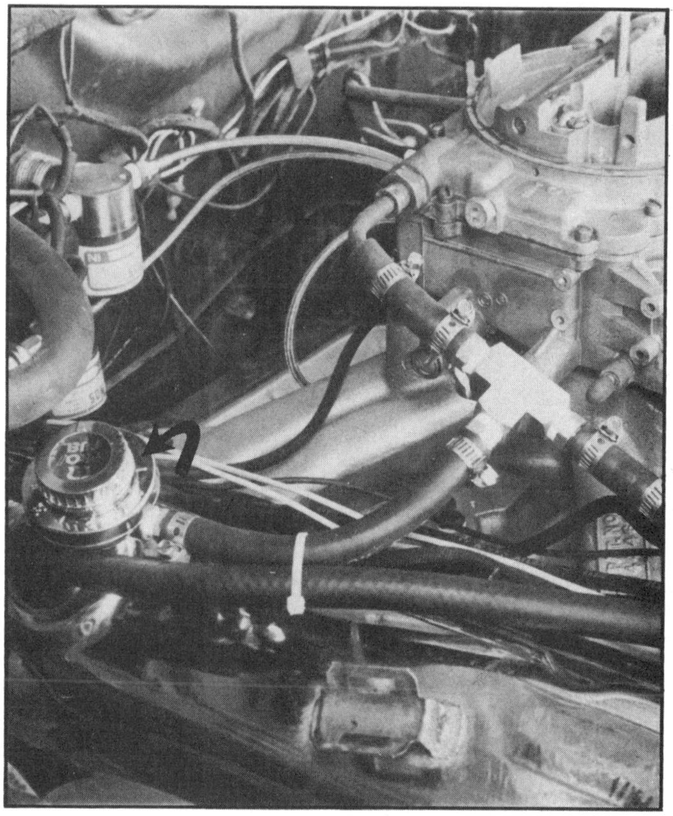

Fuel line is routed from the T-fitting to the fuel solenoid. The high-capacity mechanical pump (installed earlier) is rated at 7psi; and since this is more than recommended by NOS, a fuel pressure regulator was installed to limit the delivery pressure to 5psi.

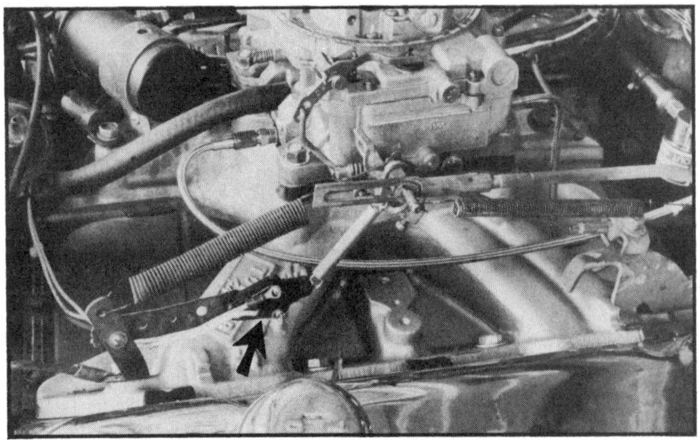

Rather than use a dash-mounted push-button, Jim Salonisen decided that he would prefer a throttle activation switch. The switch is connected to the throttle linkage at the carburetor and is adjusted to "fire" just before the secondaries reach full open.

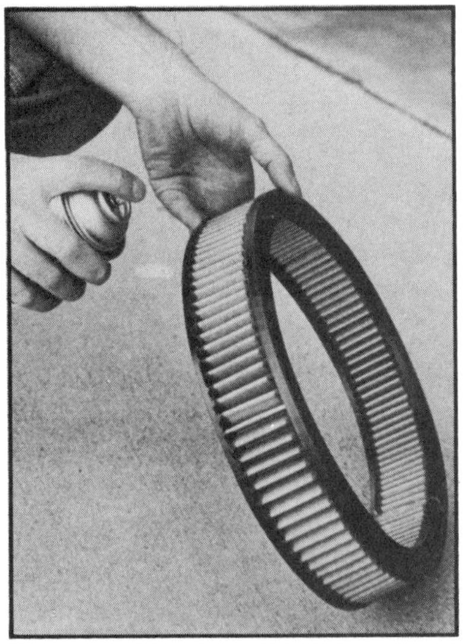

The shorter K&N filter, used to gain hood clearance, is "activated" with an oil applied from an aerosol can. The element can be cleaned with solvent, reoiled and reused. The K&N flows more air than any other high performance filter tested by the author.

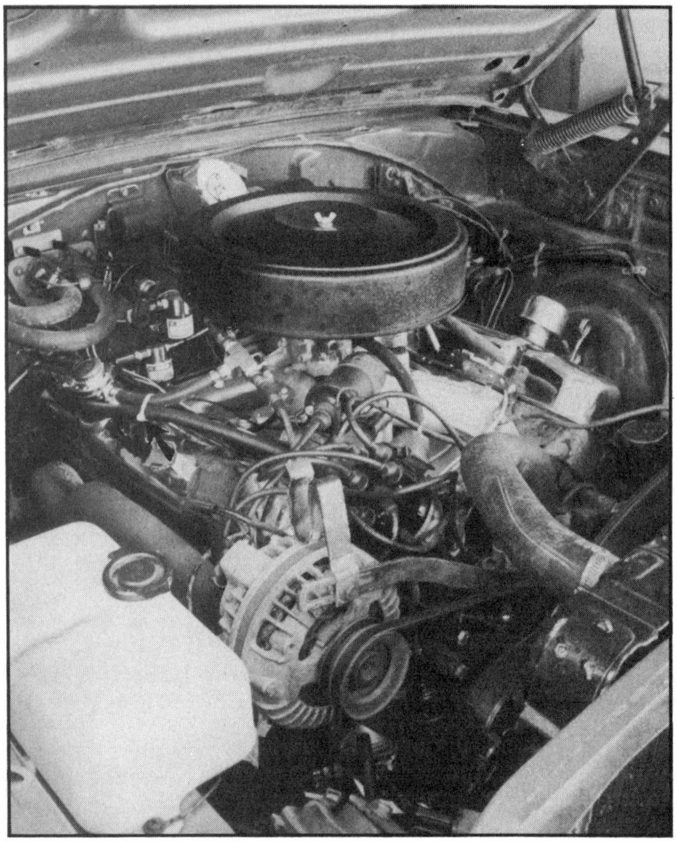

The completed system is neatly hidden behind the engine. Several tie-wraps (locking plastic straps) were used to prevent the braided lines from rubbing the intake manifold and to add a professional touch to the installation. The only thing left is to "try 'er out."

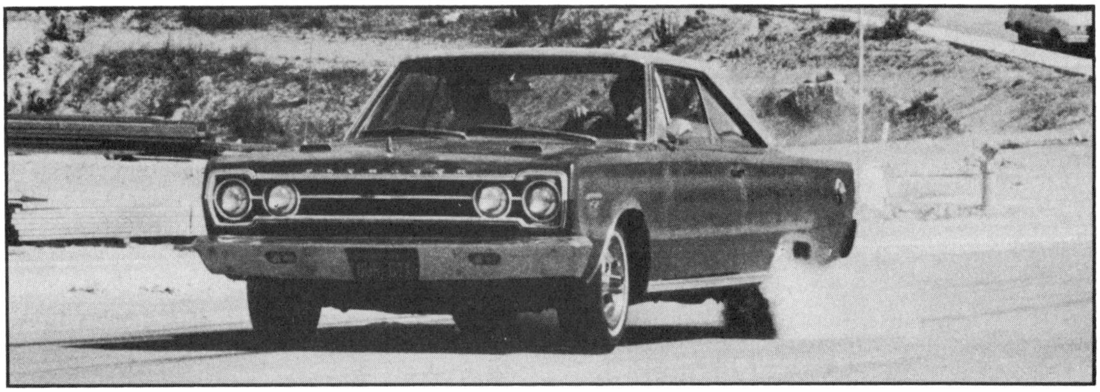

WOW! Stab the throttle at 50mph and the mighty Mopar boils the tires when the nitrous hits full boost and the Torqueflite kicks down a gear.

minute "fiddling" was required, but this kit, like many others, suffers from one drawback--the lack of thorough instructions. The instructions will suffice for someone with a good mechanical background, but the neophyte will feel lost. For example, the braided hose supplied for connecting the nitrous bottle to the engine compartment wasn't long enough for our particular installation. We had to add another section of hose (purchased from a surplus store) and we had to locate and install a #6 AN-to-AN adapter to splice the two lines together. The instruction sheet should discuss this possibility. In addition, no explanation of how to install Teflon tape was provided. The descriptions of the electrical connections were also very terse. The section on the importance of adequate fuel supply--including the possible requirement for a high performance fuel pump--was limited.

However, on the bright side, NOS has informed the author that the instruction sheet has recently been improved. And the only mechanical "problem" of any sort encountered during the installation was the very limited thread depth on the inlet side of the nitrous solenoid. This made tightening the fitting a bit tricky, but did not hold up the project.

The NOS system exceeded our original performance expectations. The 440 Mopar produced incredible low-speed torque and the power output was smooth and strong. When the throttle was pushed wide open at low engine speeds (rpm) the system hesitated for about 1/2- to 1-second before the nitrous reached peak boost. However, the problem was minimized when the system was "burped" to purge hot nitrous from the supply lines. With this technique, full throttle application produced an immediate downshift and a rapid buildup of torque that produced impressive acceleration performance.

REFILLING THE NITROUS BOTTLE

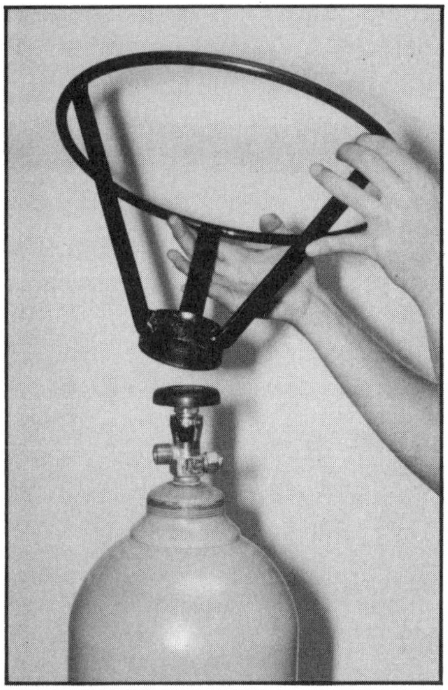

The first piece of equipment needed to make bottle refilling easier is a stand to securely position and hold the large storage bottle.

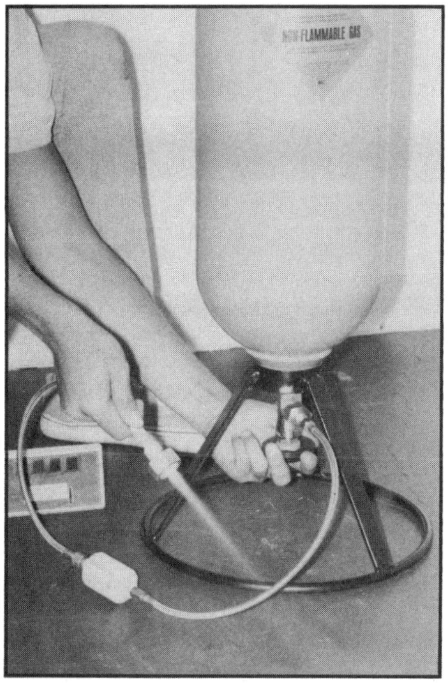

With a supply line attached to the storage bottle, clear the line by momentarily opening the valve and venting some nitrous.

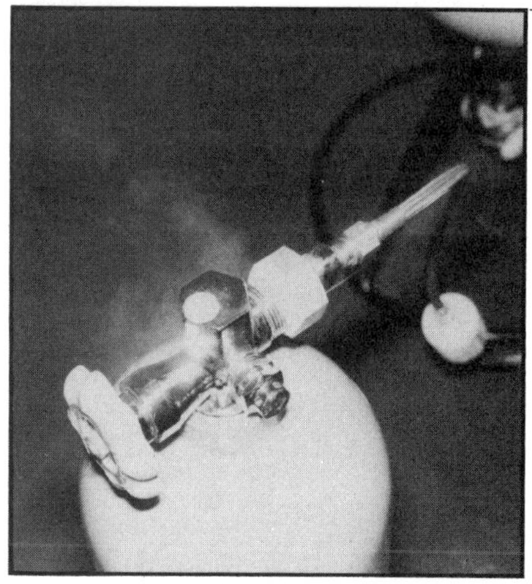

Attach the line to the bottle that is to be filled, but leave the fitting about 1/2 to one full turn short of tight.

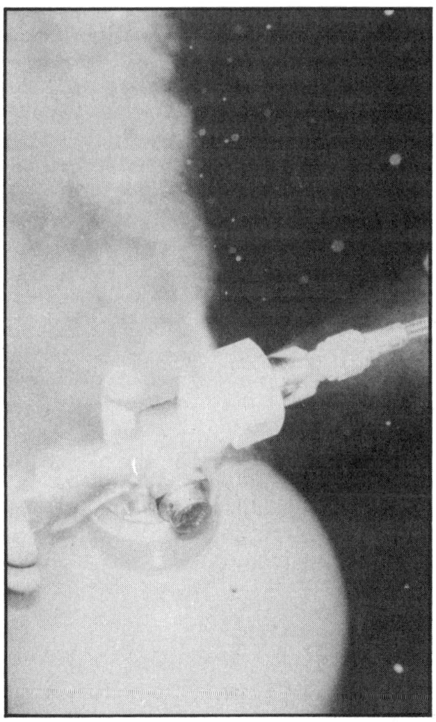

Open the supply line on the storage bottle until liquid nitrous escapes from the still-untightened fitting. (An excessive amount of nitrous is shown here, but this illustrates the effect--to the extreme.) While the nitrous is escaping, tighten the fitting, but do not let the super-cold liquid nitrous come in contact with exposed skin; it can cause freeze burns.

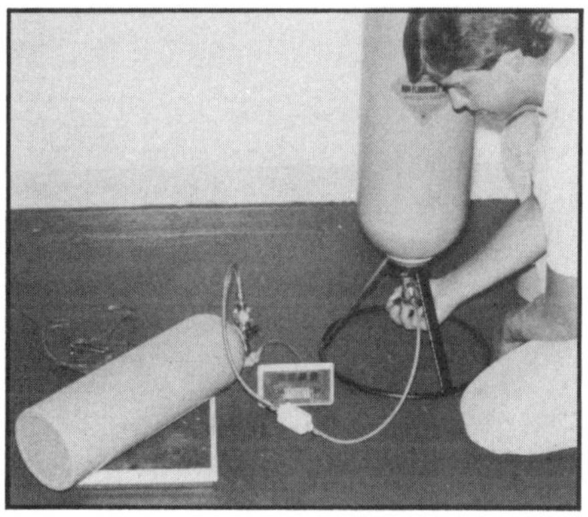

Position the bottle on an accurate weight scale and continue filling. Watch the scale to make certain the amount of nitrous transferred to the bottle does not exceed the rated capacity.

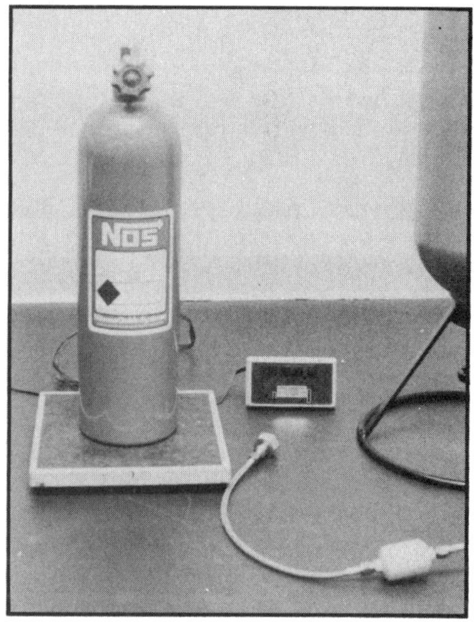

Disconnect the fill line only after the valves on both the storage bottle and the bottle you are filling have been turned off. Remove the fill line carefully, keep your hands clear and allow sufficient time for the nitrous trapped in the hose to bleed off safely.

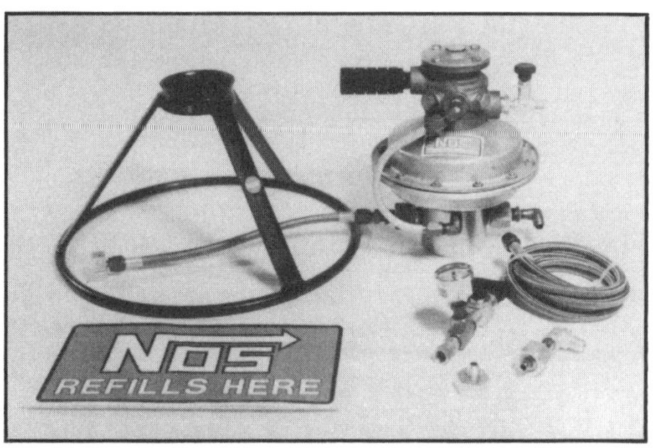

After the bottle has been separated from the fill line, recheck the weight to make certain it does not exceed the maximum fill weight. If you have access to a high pressure air supply (100psi or more), this refilling device makes the job easier. Available from NOS, it is an air-powered pump that transfers nitrous from one bottle to another, no matter what the relative temperatures.

CHAPTER 9

USING THE SYSTEM

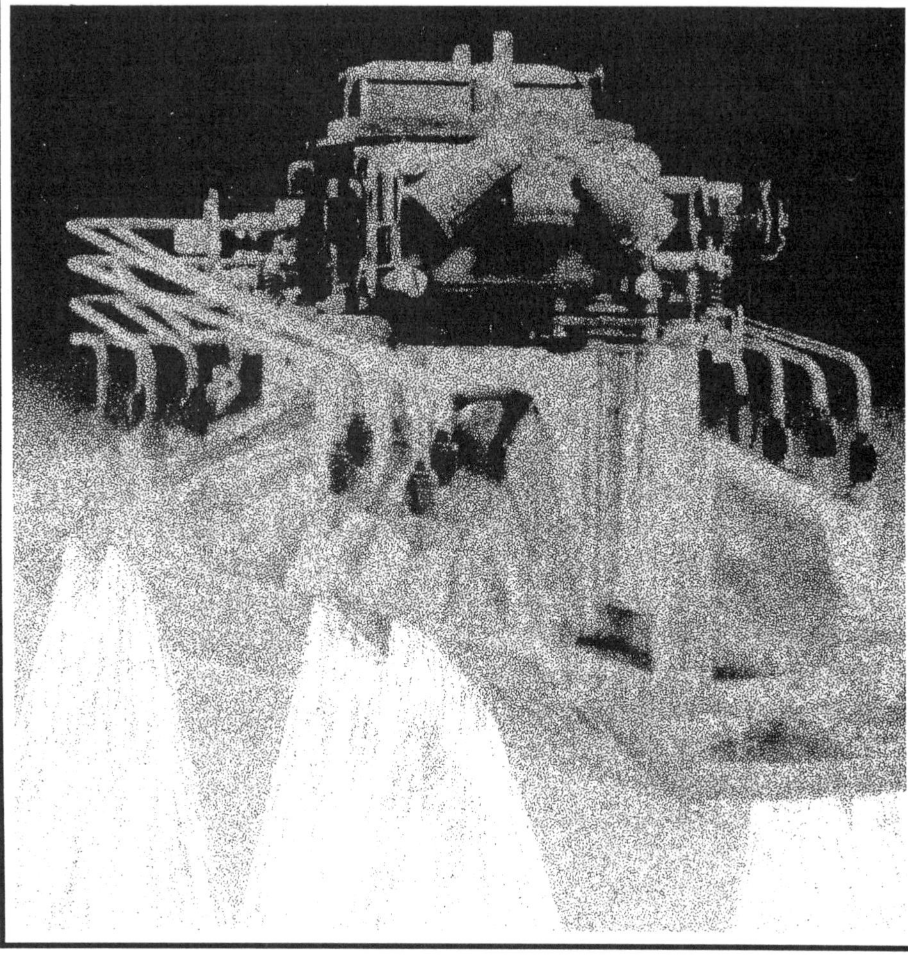

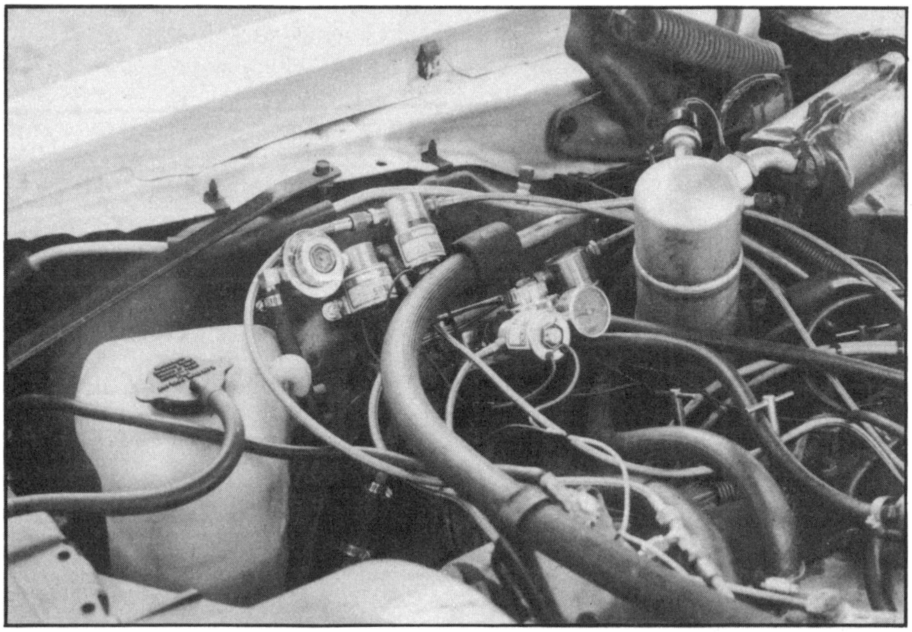

When traction is limited (street suspension and tires), the car will generally respond better if the nitrous system "hits" softly. In this example relatively long lines were used between the solenoids and the point of injection to soften system response.

MAXIMIZING PERFORMANCE

The bottom line with any engine modification is how much quicker or faster it makes the car go, *given the circumstances under which it is expected to perform.* Probably the biggest advantage that nitrous can provide is in drag racing or other forms of motorsport that place a premium on acceleration. This includes competition such as slalom racing, sprinting, and hill climbing. All of these sports greatly depend on how the car performs from a standing start. So, for all practical purposes, we will lump all of them under one heading: drag racing. Let's now look at the ways and means of successfully applying the apparent gains that nitrous-oxide injection will provide.

According to an informal poll among the manufacturers, the majority of nitrous kits currently being sold are designed for street applications. In other words, it is likely that the average nitrous-injected engine will be sitting in a chassis that has a "street-type" suspension and street tires (rather than wide racing tires); and the car will probably have an automatic transmission, since they are commonly used on street vehicles. The addition of nitrous will change the performance requirements imposed on these components, so some "tuning" will inevitably be required to gain maximum advantage from the additional engine power.

SYSTEM INITIATION

In an earlier chapter we briefly discussed system "hit." Due to several variables, each nitrous system reacts a bit differently when initially activated. If the system hits hard, the boost effects develops very rapidly, producing an almost instantaneous increase in engine output. When the system has a soft hit, the boost develops more slowly, and the engine output increases in a more progressive manner. This characteristic will affect the overall performance and driveability of the car.

If the car is regularly driven on the street, a hard-hitting system often causes problems. The sudden increase in low-speed engine torque, combined with the torque multiplication of the transmission and rear-end, produces a shock load that is transferred through the driveline to the tires. This shock generally overpowers most street tires, resulting in a loss of traction. This, of course, means that acceleration performance will drop off. And frankly, the situation can become dangerous if the suspension and driveline are not extensively modified to withstand the increased loading. But there is a suitable alternative, and it hinges on reducing the initial shock load.

If available engine torque is applied progressively to the rear wheels (a front-engine, rear-drive configuration is assumed here), the chassis has more time to "transfer weight" toward the rear wheels, and this increases traction. (We will discuss weight transfer in greater detail in an upcoming section.) When more traction exists, more torque can be applied; this, in turn, creates more weight transfer. There is, quite naturally, a limit to this effect, but substantial amounts of power can be transmitted through a heavy-duty street-type suspension system as long as high shock loadings are avoided. This is possible, even with a nitrous-boosted engine, as long as the activation of the nitrous does not upset the chassis and driveline or severely overpower the tires. In other words, under the conditions described here, the car will accelerate more effectively and quickly if the nitrous gradually boosts power, rather than hitting all at once like a big hammer.

Several variables enter the picture, but one of the easiest ways to "soften" the system hit is to move the nitrous solenoid further from the spray orifices and lengthen the distribution line(s). When the solenoids are positioned further from the point of injection, the initial effects of the nitrous are less pronounced because of the time required to fill and cool these lines. Conversely, if the solenoids are mounted right on the spacer, boost hits harder. As shown in Figure 9-1, the time required to build torque

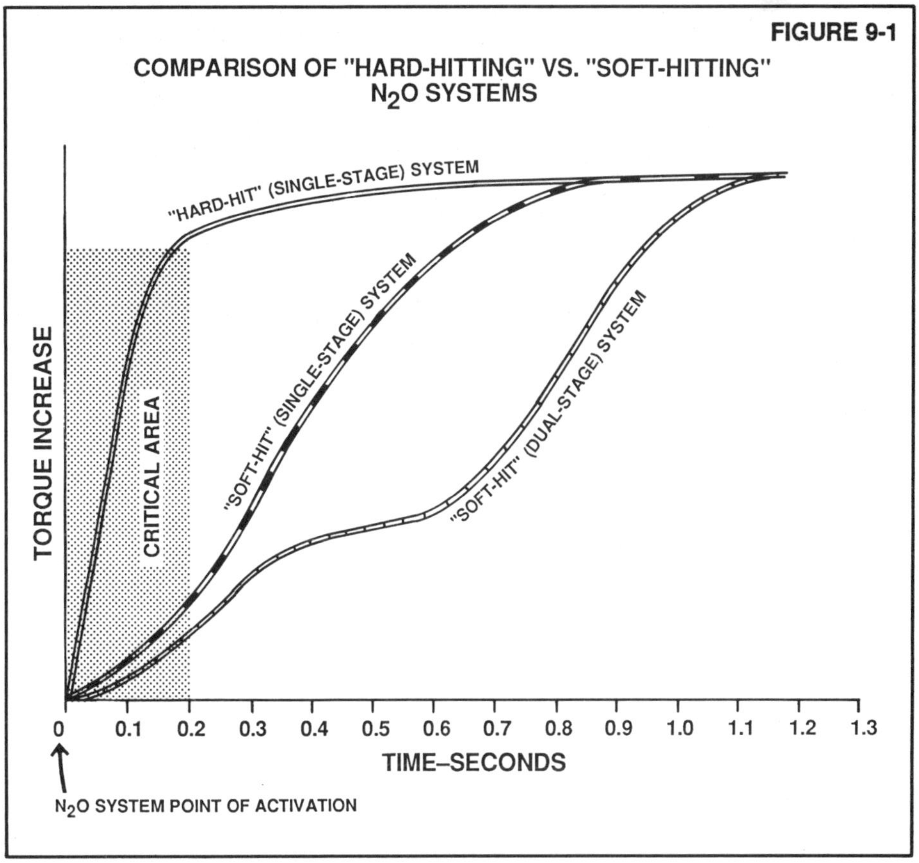

FIGURE 9-1: This is a comparison between soft- and hard-hitting systems. The effect in the first 0.20 second will determine whether the tires lose traction and/or components fail. A hard-hitting system boosts output very quickly, but the transmission and suspension must respond accordingly. A soft-hitting system is better for a street vehicle because typical street tires and suspension can handle the less severe rate of boost increase.

boost dramatically decreases when the system hits hard.

Another solution is to route the nitrous line through an area that will transfer heat to the nitrous. When the temperature of liquid nitrous increases, it converts to gaseous form, and as we have already discussed, this reduces the boost effect. Therefore, when the supply is heated—usually this is accomplished easily with the heat trapped inside the engine compartment—the nitrous is less dense and the system will hit softer. But as more nitrous flows through the line, the line cools, and eventually the nitrous remains liquid all the way to the point of injection. As this happens, the boost will steadily increase to maximum output.

Nonetheless, a high-boost system may not hit soft enough to use all of the available boost in first gear. If the car leaves hard without the nitrous boost, it may only be practical to use the nitrous in the higher gears. In some cases, actuating the nitrous in second gear may provide the same rate of acceleration as in first gear (without the nitrous). If the car is already near the traction limit (unboosted) during the first 50 feet, using nitrous in the first gear may actually cause the ET's to increase because the tires cannot hold traction.

There is another side to this coin. With some systems, the opposite is true: it is difficult to get the nitrous to hit hard. A good example is a system hidden beneath the intake manifold. In this instance the distribution lines absorb so much heat from the hot engine oil that it takes a relatively long time for the tubing to cool down; therefore, the system inevitably hits on the soft side. This may be a disadvantage.

If the car has a good suspension and a lot of tire, it may be able to handle more power than the unboosted engine can develop. Under these circumstances, *a system that hits* *__right now__* *may provide an advantage.* This situation is common with an engine that is designed to produce a lot of horsepower without nitrous boost. Here, the nitrous may only contribute 15 to 20% of the total output, and a

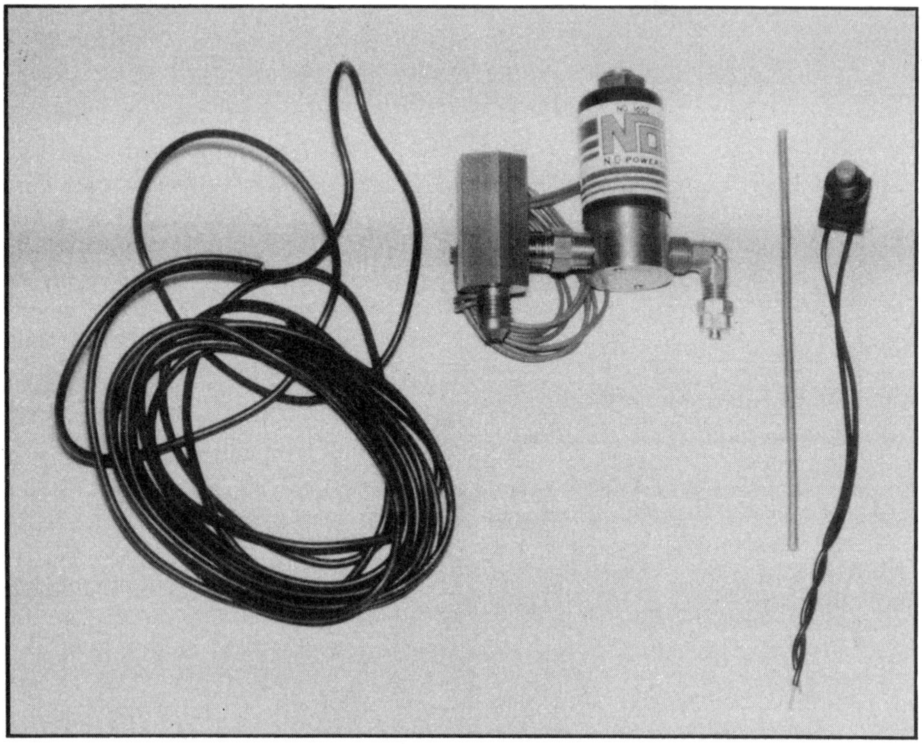

The initial boost effect can be increased by pre-cooling or "burping" the system. A line cooling kit can also be used to "cold soak" the nitrous line. If the suspension responds effectively at launch (drag racing suspension and wide tires), this technique may substantially improve consistency.

hard-hitting system will not greatly upset the traction capabilities. Under these circumstances, the lines from the solenoid to the point of injection should be kept as cool as possible. This is very important. Hit time will also be improved by minimizing the distance from the solenoid to the point of injection. And reducing the temperature of the supply line from the bottle to the solenoid will further improve hit time, but this is really a secondary consideration. .

There are several ways to approach keeping the lines cool. Sometimes a "nitrous bleed" is used to prime the system. This bleed is nothing more than a small secondary solenoid connected upstream of the primary nitrous solenoid. Just before the start of a run, the driver activates the bleed solenoid to purge gaseous nitrous and fills the nitrous line with cold liquid nitrous. It is also possible to vent the nitrous directly onto the fuel and nitrous solenoids. This precools the entire system and reduces the major cause of hesitation.

This system works quite well as long as the nitrous solenoid is placed close to the point of injection. Obviously, if the nitrous solenoid is mounted a long distance from the point of injection, simply cooling the supply line to the solenoid will be a wasted effort because the distribution line—the portion of the line between the main solenoid and the point of injection—may still be warm enough to significantly affect initial performance. Generally speaking, the temperature of the distribution line will affect initial engine performance if it is longer than about 6 to 9 inches.

Another consideration is that when nitrous is injected from an individual nozzle—with an entirely separate nozzle for enrichment fuel—the system tends to hit harder than if a spraybar or a combined nitrous-fuel nozzle is used. This is good if a hard-hitting system is desired. On the other hand, individual nozzles tend to produce less uniform nitrous distribution, and they generally don't mix the nitrous with the fuel as well as spraybars.

If the nitrous system is used for serious bracket racing, it is important to realize that, under certain circumstances, a soft-hit system may produce inconsistent ET's. If the system develops a lot of boost and it hits relatively soft—i.e., it takes more than a full second to reach full boost—ET's can vary because the total engine output may become very sensitive to the temperatures in the engine compartment. On a cool day or when the engine has not reached peak operating temperature, the system can hit much harder. Later in the day, when the air temperature is higher and the temperatures inside the engine compartment are higher, the system may hit with less authority. If this is the case—and consistency is of prime importance—it may be possible to improve consistency by reducing system hit time. Consistency may also improve if the boost developed by the system is reduced somewhat.

AUTOMATIC TRANSMISSION

Like all mechanical devices, an automatic transmission can only withstand so much stress. Steady torque loads applied by the engine do not usually cause a transmission to fail, rather, it's the high stresses created during short-term shock loadings that are the culprit. However, a nitrous-injected engine can produce extraordinary low-speed torque, and if the tires get a good grip, the resultant

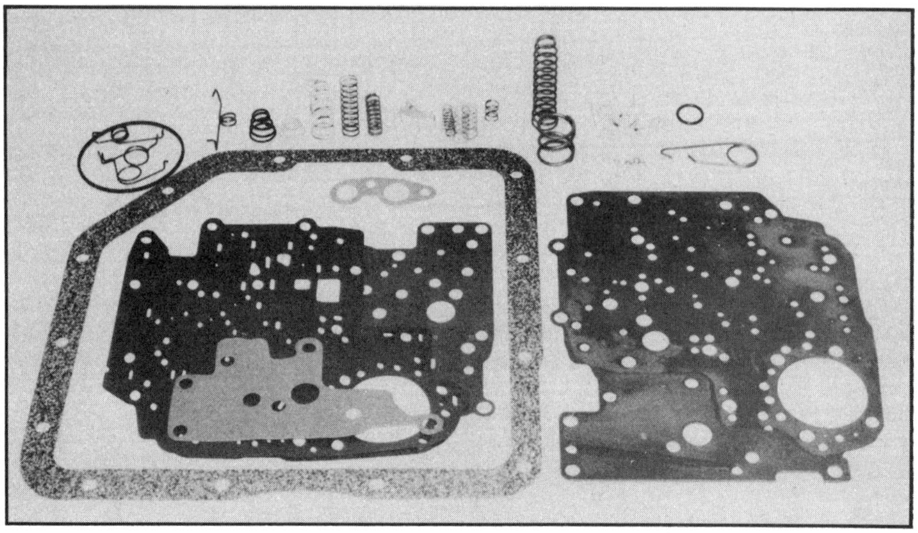

A performance "shift kit" will improve transmission reliability when nitrous is added to a typical street engine. If a high-boost (racing) nitrous system is used, the transmission must be suitably/professionally modified to withstand extreme power levels.

loads can cause transmission components to fail.

The best way to illustrate this point is to cite an example. One of the most popular late-model transmissions is the GM 350 Turbo-Hydramatic. In stock form this trans will handle about 300 horsepower and 375 pounds-feet of torque. This trans will successfully absorb this much power for only short periods of time, however. At higher power levels, the life of a Turbo 350 will generally be very short. As a result, if a 120-horsepower nitrous kit is added to a 300-horsepower engine, one strong pass down the strip at full nitrous boost may terminate the trans with extreme prejudice.

The bottom line here is that this transmission really needs to be beefed up with stronger internal components. It is beyond the scope of this book to go into details, but many transmission shops that specialize in performance or racing work can perform the required modifications; *but be sure to notify the shop that the trans will be used with a nitrous engine.* You should forewarn the shop to take additional precautions to help the trans absorb the extraordinary torque load.

The specific requirements will vary, depending upon the make and model of transmission, but in most cases an auto trans setup for a nitrous engine will live longer if the clutch pack is setup with friction discs that will allow a little slip before full engagement (those surfaced with thin, hard material). Some trans builders will argue with this suggestion. The common line of thought is that some slip will cause the clutch plates to wear prematurely. And to a degree this is true, however the high torque loading—available from nitrous—calls for a small compromise: If the clutch pack locks up very rapidly, other transmission components will probably fail under full nitrous boost (high torque); if the clutch pack locks slowly, the clutch plates will wear more quickly, but the rest of the trans components will live longer. This is a classic case of being forced to live with the lesser of two evils.

There is another device that can emulate a "loose" clutch pack: a high-stall-speed torque converter. Most stock torque converters "lockup" at about 2000rpm—the maximum rpm the engine can obtain at full throttle with the rear wheels standing still—and have very little built in slippage. Although this design permits the highest efficiency and gas mileage, it absorbs little of the shock load generated during shifts. But a higher stall torque converter—2500 to 3000rpm or more—will better absorb shift loads and help prevent loss of traction. Keep in mind, however, that a higher stall speed will also send more torque to the rear wheels and could exaggerate standing-start wheelspin. But if the nitrous system is engaged after the vehicle leaves the staring line, a high-stall converter may *improve low-speed acceleration and prevent tirespin during shifting.* Higher stall converters were sometimes offered as standard equipment on high-performance vehicles and you may be able to locate one in a wrecking yard, or you may have to contact a transmission specialist for a reworked unit.

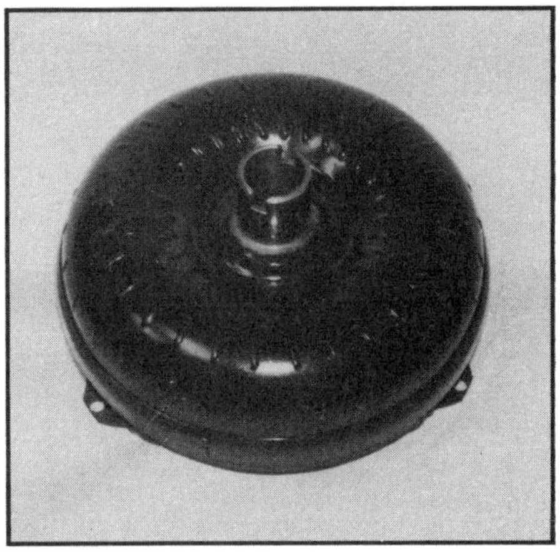

A converter with a 2000rpm stall speed produces hard acceleration at low engine speeds (with nitrous on) and good overall fuel economy in a street machine, but its hard lockup may promote driveline component failure during shifts.

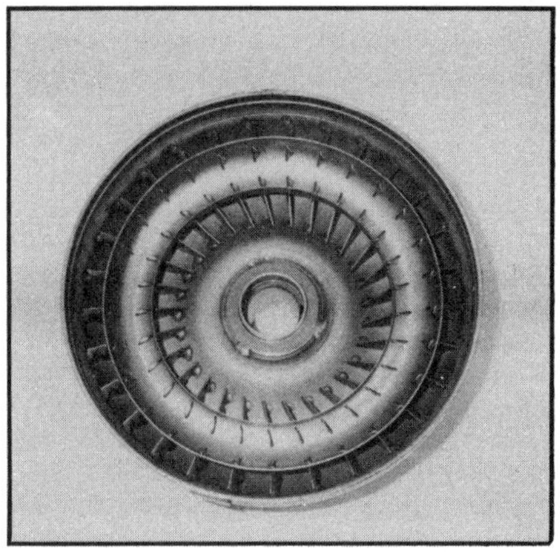

A performance torque converter will improve the response of a nitrous machine, but the stall characteristics must be matched to the torque and power output of the engine and nitrous system.

In most cases, the tires should never lose traction—especially if the chassis is under high side loads (cornering). Poor traction, in these situations, can be dangerous. For example, I once had a 1980 TransAm with a single-stage, 150-horsepower nitrous kit and a 350 Turbo-Hydro modified with a typical street "shift kit." The suspension had also been worked up some and the car could corner pretty well. However, any attempt to change gears while the car was in a corner—even a fairly modest corner—would cause the rear tires to break loose, and the car would try to swap ends in the blink of an eye. Subsequently, the transmission was altered to soften the shift, resulting in a faster and more controllable vehicle.

The situation is about the same during straight-line acceleration. If the tires are on the limit of traction just prior to the shift into second, a hard shift will totally break traction. Eventually the tires will recover, but the race will be lost. The obvious solution is to work with the transmission—whatever make or model it may be—until the shifts become "firm" but not jarringly hard. This will reduce the shock transferred to the tires and will improve overall performance. In some situations—especially when the nitrous system is really potent—this may not be enough. If the engine and nitrous system are really pumping out power, the tires may pop loose no matter how the trans responds. The only solution, then, is to improve the traction capabilities of the chassis.

SUSPENSION

Let's consider what happens when a vehicle accelerates in a straight line. As the car accelerates, weight is "transferred" toward the rear wheels. Since, this is complicated to explain

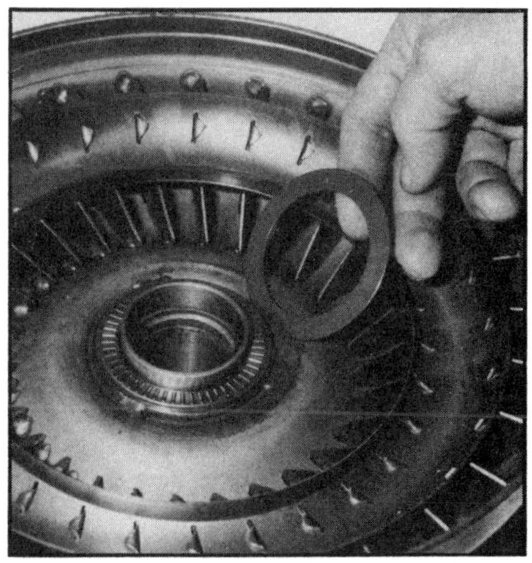

To improve reliability at high torque levels, the flat thrust bearing of this Art Carr torque converter has been replaced with a Torrington needle-roller thrust bearing.

in a pure geometric form, we will assume that when a car is accelerating, the reaction of the suspension will generally shift the weight bias toward the rear wheels. This increases the potential for rear wheel traction, which is just fine because when the car has more power, it can accelerate more quickly and needs more traction.

In actual practice, the suspension of the average street machine or street/strip racer is not able to effectively transform the weight transfer into increased traction. When the driver hits the throttle, 500 horsepower, or more, is transmitted almost instantly through the chassis and driveline to the rear wheels. There is almost no time for the suspension to react to this sudden shock, and the *static weight* on the rear wheels (the actual car weight bearing down on the rear axle) will not be great enough to plant the tires firmly against the asphalt. The net result is, generally, instant wheel spin.

This scenario is common because the suspension systems of production automobiles do not have a high degree of built-in "anti-squat." This is a characteristic—which can be enhanced by proper design—that causes the rear of the car to rise when power is applied to the rear axle. This momentarily presses the axle and wheels harder onto the road surface, improving traction. A suspension with a lot of designed-in anti-squat works very well on the drag strip; but unfortunately, under braking conditions, this same characteristic tends to pull the rear wheels upward, away from the road. This makes the car unstable during hard braking. Quite naturally, the engineers in Detroit do not want their "Custom Cushion Cruisers" to get squirrely during hard braking. So, virtually all production cars have a lot of what can best be described as "reverse anti-squat." Most production chassis react well under braking conditions, but in stock form, they usually react poorly to hard acceleration.

AXLE RATIO

Sometimes the best solution is to alter the chassis setup to accommodate the nitrous effect. If the car has a relatively high axle ratio (compared to normal racing gears) and good tires—soft compound with a wide footprint—the launch should be very effective with a soft-hit system that takes as much as a full second to reach maximum output. This is ideal and would allow the use of injection in first gear. However, most bracket racers have traction difficulties when they use the nitrous system anytime in first gear. These problems may be related to gearing and tires that were originally selected for maximum effect with an unboosted engine. Experimentation with gearing and tires will often improve the situation.

One of the first things to consider is altering the gear ratio. When the gearing is successfully matched to the engine, the nitrous can often be used at launch, through first gear and all subsequent gears. In addition, the system can usually be actuated by a throttle switch. This eliminates the need for a separate activation button and allows the driver to concentrate on steering and shifting.

The object of gearing—either in the transmission or the rear end—is to multiply the torque developed by the engine. Maximum acceleration is achieved when the multiplied torque delivered to the driving wheels is just below, but does not exceed, the limit of traction. Although we are talking about torque at the rear wheel, what actually drives the car forward is the force applied at the point of tire contact on the ground. For example, if 3000 pounds of force is required before a typical street-type tire loses traction, maximum acceleration will be achieved when 2999.99 pounds of force is applied to the contact point. This is simply maximum utilization of the tire. If, on the other hand, 3000.10 pounds is applied to this same tire, the tire will "lose grip," break loose and freewheel (spin). And once this happens, the acceleration capabilities of the car will drop off dramatically!

If the car was geared correctly *without* nitrous, the amount of torque transmitted to the rear wheels, with the addition of nitrous boost, will be too much for the tires to handle. We have already discussed several options to prevent this difficulty—obviously, the simplest solution is to not activate the nitrous until the tire can withstand the extra torque (usually after the shift to second gear)—but *most often the best solution is to alter the final-drive gear so the nitrous boost can be used in first gear.*

The requisite change in rear-end gearing is difficult to predict, but in general, *the gear ratio should be raised approximately the same proportion as the power-output increase produced by the addition of the nitrous boost.* This is a conservative estimate—in many cases the gear ratio can be increased less—but if you have no other experience to draw upon, this will be a good place to begin.

Here's an example. Suppose an engine develops 400 horsepower (unboosted) and the car launches and accelerates well with about a 12:1 overall gear ratio. Then, the output is boosted 200 horsepower—giving a total of 600 horsepower—with the addition of nitrous injection. In this instance, the power has been increased by one-third (33.3 percent), and to maintain maximum acceleration with the nitrous boost activated, the overall gear ratio should then be raised (numerically lowered) by an equal factor: one-third. The 12:1 gearing should be changed for a 8:1 overall ratio (approximately).

Another point to note is that maximum results with nitrous are usually obtained at lower engine speeds. In almost all cases, the optimum shift point will be as much as 500 to 800rpm lower during nitrous activation. Figure 9-2 demonstrates this characteristic. The graph shows tractive effort at the driving wheels produced by an engine in both nonboosted and boosted condition. Note that because torque output is increased at relatively lower engine speed, "short shifting" keeps the engine within the range of highest torque.

FINE TUNING

Returning to starting-line performance for a moment, let's assume the car runs consistently at the local track and the suspension is dialed in so that the car leaves hard without losing traction. But when the car is taken to another track, the grip falls off and the car has a problem with wheelspin. Generally speaking, "detuning" the engine may solve the traction problem, but the car will also record higher elapsed times. A far better solution is to slightly reduce power the instant the car comes off the line, without reducing the power available after the car is moving.

The easiest way to accomplish this is to increase fuel pressure to the gasoline side of the nitrous system. This will reduce low-speed torque without significantly affecting top-end horsepower. For example, increasing fuel pressure by 1.0psi may cause the torque output at 4000rpm to drop by as much as 20 pounds-feet. But power at 6000rpm may only drop by about 5-6 horsepower. This effect is often used to suppress detonation, but in certain circumstances, it can also be a tuning aid. Figure 9-3 demonstrates the effect various nitrous-to-fuel ratios have on engine performance.

Another way to achieve the same goal is to retard ignition timing. The ignition requirements for nitrous have already been discussed in detail, and although adjusting the timing can significantly affect performance, remember that timing alterations will affect power throughout the entire speed range.

Sometimes the best effect is achieved by slightly altering both the timing and the flow of enrichment fuel. Reducing total timing back from optimum will reduce power. Advancing timing can increase power, however, remember a nitrous-boosted engine does not generally require as much timing as a comparable non-boosted engine. And leaning the nitrous-fuel mix will increase power, and enriching the mixture will reduce power. However, *the spark plugs must be inspected carefully for the initial*

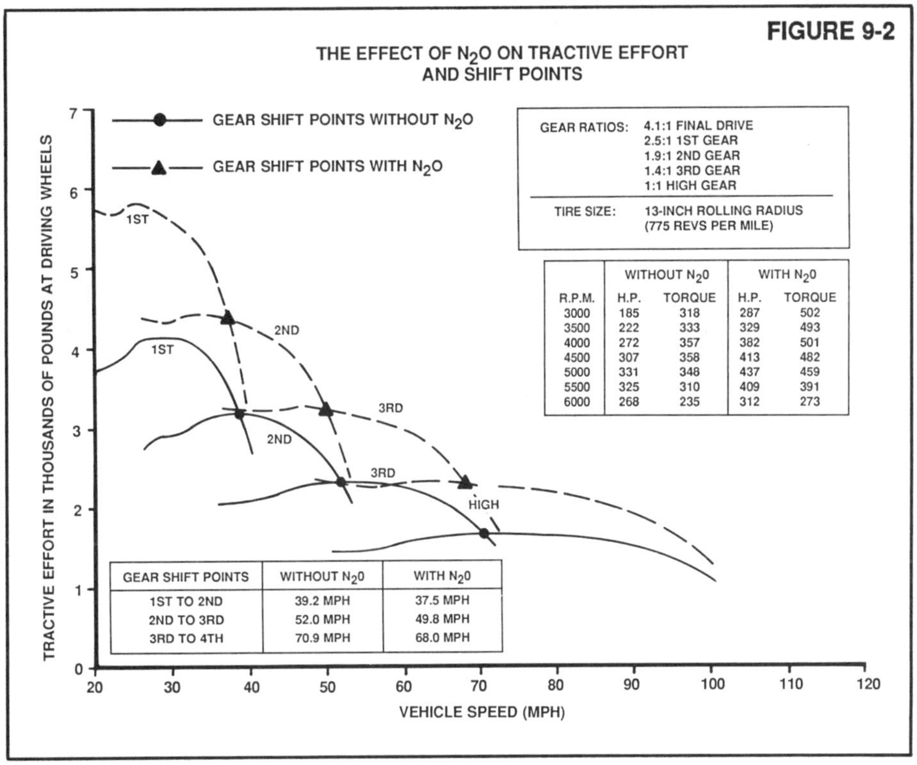

R.P.M.	WITHOUT N_2O H.P.	WITHOUT N_2O TORQUE	WITH N_2O H.P.	WITH N_2O TORQUE
3000	185	318	287	502
3500	222	333	329	493
4000	272	357	382	501
4500	307	358	413	482
5000	331	348	437	459
5500	325	310	409	391
6000	268	235	312	273

GEAR SHIFT POINTS	WITHOUT N_2O	WITH N_2O
1ST TO 2ND	39.2 MPH	37.5 MPH
2ND TO 3RD	52.0 MPH	49.8 MPH
3RD TO 4TH	70.9 MPH	68.0 MPH

FIGURE 9-2: This is a representation of tractive effort with and without nitrous injection. These figures were measured on a Chevrolet smallblock with injection, however, the drivetrain is a calculated simulation. During the 4-speed simulation the optimum shift points dropped 150-200rpm. With a 3-speed automatic the optimum shift points may be as much as 500rpm lower.

FIGURE 9-3: This demonstrates the effect of nitrous-to-fuel mixture ratios. A 40% mixture ratio is the "lean limit" because it produces maximum boost (proportional to the amount of nitrous injected) but if the ratio is leaner, the combustion temperature becomes dangerously high. Enrichening the ratio will generally cause a notable reduction in low-end performance and a modest reduction in top-end power. Curve #2 is a good example of this: a 65% rich mix lost 15hp at 3000rpm, but only 3hp at 5000rpm; a 90% rich mix reduced the power output 25hp at 3000rpm but only 5hp at 5000rpm.

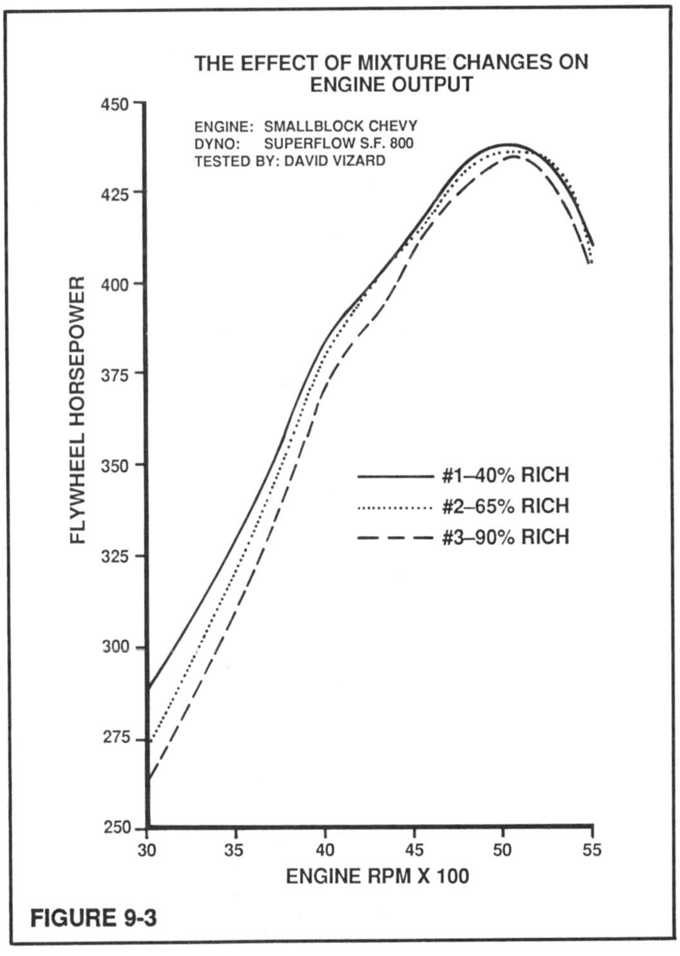

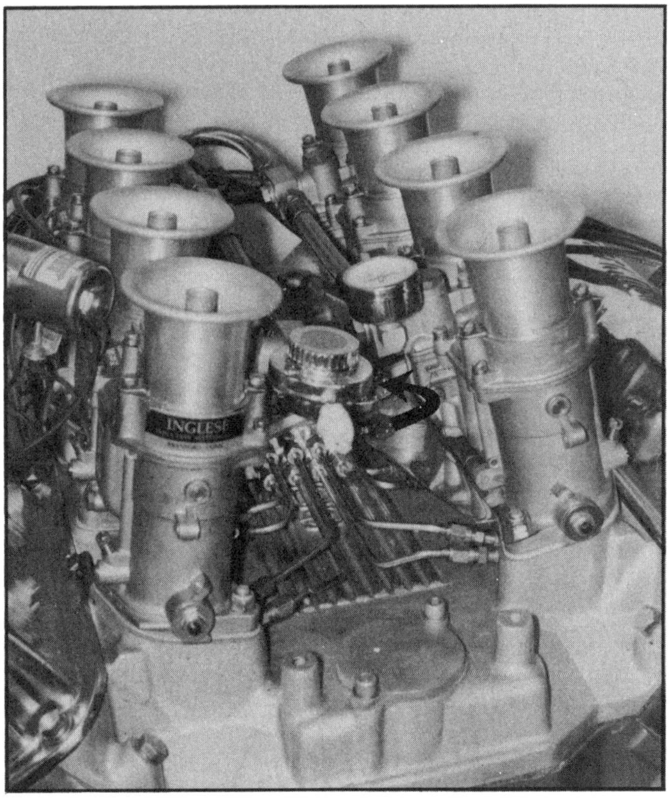

When nitrous is used during the starting-line launch it is often difficult to maintain traction. If a fuel pressure regulator (arrow) is installed in the fuel system, the initial boost response can be moderated by increasing the fuel pressure and, therefore, enrichening the fuel-to-nitrous ratio.

signs of detonation. Remember, an excessively lean mixture will damage the engine.

STAGED SYSTEMS

Even with soft initiation, it is still possible for a 100-horsepower system to break the tires loose in first gear. In this instance, the only solution may be to "sub-divide" the power. Incidentally, this is especially important if a stock torque converter is used. If the vehicle is used for everyday transportation as well as weekend drag races, a stock torque converter is probably the best choice. But the problem is that a 100-plus horsepower boost, when compounded with the torque multiplication present in most torque converters, is simply too much for streetable tires.

In almost all high-boost applications—100 horsepower or more—a two-stage system will improve performance and reliability. In fact, the best all-around setup is a two-stage adjustable system with a low-boost first increment and a high-boost second increment that comes in at higher engine speed. This reduces the low-speed shock transmitted to the transmission and driveline and allows the car sufficient time to take full advantage of weight transfer during acceleration. The bottom line is that a car on street tires will often go faster and break fewer parts when the power is introduced in a more progressive manner.

Once again, my own 1980 Firebird provided some interesting insight. After a 150-horsepower, single-stage system was installed, the ET's immediately dropped 0.90 second. During initial testing, the car had a transmission that shifted like gangbusters and the nitrous hit like the hammers of hell. But, during 20 passes down the strip, the car destroyed three automatic transmissions and two axles! The mechanical problems were eventually worked out, but the biggest improvement came through rebuilding the system into a two-stage setup. After several small modifications, the first stage finally produced a boost of about 35 horsepower and the second stage pumped an additional 75 horsepower into the engine. This gave a total boost of 110 horsepower, as opposed to the original 150 horsepower. But with this setup, the car was 1.2 seconds faster down the strip, and at the time of this writing, had completed over 40 passes without breaking anything.

The lesson to be learned is that *brute horsepower is not always the answer to fast speeds and low elapsed times; the proper utilization of power is more important.* Just for the record, the car weighed 4265 pounds, and on street tires, through the mufflers, with an engine that was built essentially for maximum economy (20 miles/gallon at 60mph) it clocked consistent 12.38 times with a trap speeds of 117.99mph. This was with a suspension system, incidentally, that was set up for cornering, not for drag racing.

ALL-OUT RACING

If the car has wide, sticky tires, rearward weight distribution and a good anti-squat suspension, the chassis will be less susceptible to shock loading introduced by the nitrous system. Under these conditions—when the object is maximum performance, rather than consistency—you might as well use as much nitrous as the engine can stand. If you have enough tire on the car, it will be difficult to break them loose, but if the engine is really cookin', you will probably break some parts. Even when everything in the chassis and driveline is optimized for nitrous, the car will generally react better if the nitrous system hits softer.

Nitrous injection has been used quite extensively in Pro Stock drag racing. This is probably where state-of-the-art nitrous systems are used for maximum effect. And at this time, most engine builders who are using nitrous have opted for engine configurations that produce maximum horsepower with conventional aspiration, and then some extra boost is added with the nitrous system. As a result, most of the current Pro Stock systems only develop about 150 horsepower. And according to some insiders, a few "maximum effort" systems have been used at boost levels around 300 horsepower. Because these systems are used with super-sticky Pro slicks, Lenco transmissions and highly-developed suspensions, the issue of soft- versus hard-hit is moot. These sophisticated cars will handle over 1000 horsepower. Overall tuning seems to be simply a matter of selecting a suitable gear to match maximum engine output.

CALCULATING BOOST

Unless you have a complete dynamometer in the garage, it will be difficult to determine how much boost the nitrous system is actually delivering. However, quarter-mile elapsed times can be used to extrapolate approximate horsepower output. Figure 9-4 shows the mathematical equations for determining horsepower or predicting quarter-mile performance.

In the early days, when extensive dynamometer testing was very rare,

$$HP = \left(\frac{S}{225}\right)^{\frac{1}{.318}} \times W$$

$$S = \left(\frac{HP}{W}\right)^{.318} \times 225$$

HP = Horsepower

W = Weight (Lbs.)

S = Speed (mph)

Figure 9-4: With these equations the nitrous-oxide user can determine the horsepower developed from his system. However, these equations were developed for nonboosted engines, so calculated results must be multiplied by a 0.8 correction factor.

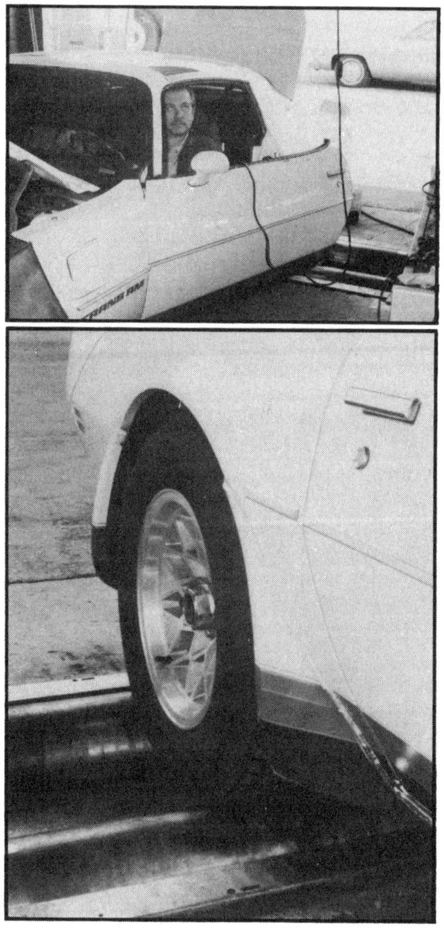

Accurate testing on a chassis dyno is the final proof of any performance modification. The author's Firebird produced about 300 horsepower (at the rear wheels) without nitrous. With the nitrous activated, the measured power should be over 400 horsepower, but the rear wheels would spin wildly and reliable measurements could not be recorded.

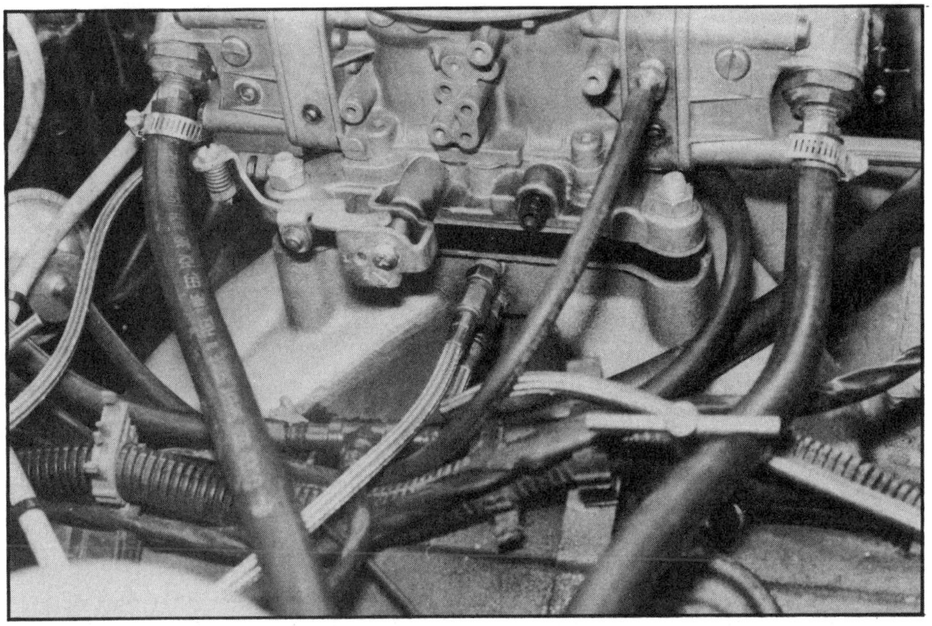

The NOS stage-2 kit on this Pontiac utilizes a spacer plate between the carb and manifold for the first stage, while the second stage is injected directly into the manifold.

these formulas—along with extensive drag-strip testing—were commonly used to verify power output. This method is reasonably accurate, but unfortunately, the formulas cannot be applied directly to determine the power output of a nitrous engine. The reason is not obvious—not unless you understand how these equations were derived. Essentially, they are based on the *average horsepower output* of the engine, although they give—as a final result—the *maximum horsepower.* Within the equations are various constants that can be best described as "fudge" factors. These factors are valid because the power curves of all normally-aspirated engines are roughly the same *shape* (though each individual curve may be displaced higher or lower on the scale, depending on the peak power output of the engine in question). A nitrous-boosted engine, however, does not produce a "typical" curve. A 500-horsepower nitrous-boosted engine has a much higher *average power output* than a 500hp normally-aspirated engine.

Consequently, applying these equations to a nitrous engine will produce a peak power figure that is artificially high. In other words, if drag-strip times "with" and "without" nitrous are used along with these equations to find out how much power the nitrous is adding to the engine, the answer will actually be 10 to 20% too high. For instance, if these equations (along with accurate strip testing) indicate that a nitrous kit is producing a power boost of about 150 horsepower, in all probability, the true boost is more likely to be around 120 horsepower. These equations can provide a reasonably accurate answer, therefore, if the results are multiplied by a 0.8 correction factor.

EFFICIENCY

Nitrous-oxide costs money. No surprise, here. But, it is important to realize that some systems may use nitrous more efficiently. Nitrous is not extremely expensive—it is actually one of the most cost-effective paths to high power—but no one wants to waste money unnecessarily. In the final analysis, system efficiency will have a direct effect on your pocketbook.

Early experiments in the aircraft industry determined that when nitrous was used "to maximum efficiency," it was possible to develop a performance boost of 100 horsepower with a flow rate of around 4.5 pounds of nitrous per minute. In other words, these tests determined that the "best" brake-specific nitrous consumption that could be achieved was about 4.5 pounds per minute per 100hp. However, it is easy to misinterpret this statement. There is no such thing as an "ideal brake-specific nitrous consumption rate" (or brake-specific fuel consumption rate). Obviously, when less nitrous is used to develop more power, the system is more efficient. In other words, if a system only uses 3 pounds of nitrous per minute per 100 horsepower, then so much the better. But, obviously, physical factors limit just how effectively the nitrous can be used.

On the other hand, there are very few factors that limit how *ineffectively* the nitrous can be used. The figure quoted above was the result of extensive, controlled experiments that strived to produce a relatively idealistic situation. But aftermarket nitrous kits for automotive engines rarely perform under "ideal conditions." Real-life variables—such as irregular distribution of the fuel-nitrous mixture through engine manifolding—all tend to reduce efficiency of the typical production nitrous kit. As a result, *most "good" systems actually dispense nitrous at a rate of around 6.0 pounds per minute per 100 horsepower.*

In fact, the real-life numbers for a fairly efficient system usually boil down to something like this: *1.0 pound of nitrous delivered in 10 seconds produces 100 horsepower.* This is an important and valuable yardstick. For instance, if a system delivers 100 horsepower (optimized) and the nitrous bottle contains 10 pounds of nitrous, the bottle will be exhausted after 100 seconds of use. If the output is 150 horsepower, the bottle will last 66 seconds. If the output is 50 horsepower, the bottle will last 200 seconds.

(Of course, you could look at it the other way around and say that if the efficiency is improved, the available bottle time will be greater at a given power output. For instance, if the efficiency of the 100hp kit was improved from 6.0lbs of nitrous per minute to 5.0lbs per minute, the amount of time available from the bottle would increase to 120 seconds.)

However, most systems do not have a provision that allows the nitrous delivery to be adjusted readily. Usually, if the system has a "tuning" provision, it is on the fuel side. If the fuel is adjusted to achieve max power, the nitrous flow remains the same, and the length of time that the bottle will last remains unchanged. In other words, a more efficient system would deliver more power for the same time.

Knowing the rate at which nitrous flows through the system is, of course, the best guide to determine how much nitrous is left in the bottle at any one time. The most common technique is to employ a "counter" that operates whenever the system is activated. This counter totals the cumulative number of seconds that the nitrous is on. Then, if you know the total weight of nitrous in the bottle and the nitrous flow rate, it is possible to calculate the *total bottle activation time.* Subtracting the cumulative time recorded on the counter from the total bottle activation time will determine how much available system time remains.

This sounds complicated, but once

the total bottle activation time is determined, it becomes a virtual constant. It will not change unless the nitrous flow rate is altered. (Although there will be some small variation, depending upon how "full" the bottle is refilled.) Therefore, each time the bottle is filled the total activation time returns to the predetermined constant. To calculate the remaining bottle time, the user need only subtract the cumulative time on the counter from the system constant.

COST

At this point, we've looked at almost every performance angle, except analyzing the costs involved in purchasing and using a nitrous injection kit. So let's first deal with how nitrous affects economy.

A nitrous kit is one of the few performance options that *has no overall effect on engine economy.* Of course, fuel consumption will increase when the nitrous system is activated—this is always the price you pay for horsepower—but when the engine is cruising down the street, the nitrous system does not affect economy or performance in any way. (In contrast, there are many performance-boosting devices that severely reduce mileage, even during normal, day-to-day driving.) Today, this is important as never before. Auto manufacturers have developed engine and transmission packages that produce very good mileage in stock form, and when the vehicle is used for daily transportation, it doesn't make sense to upset this economy potential.

But there is a debit side: When the nitrous system is activated, you are paying for the oxygen that the engine consumes. In most cases, though, the nitrous will be reserved for competition at the local race track. Only rarely will it be used on street. If you view daily traffic as an action scene from The Road Warrior, you can easily go through 20 pounds of nitrous in a day. But with this attitude, it is more likely that your biggest on-going expenses will be replacement tires, traffic citations and hospital bills. Even so, the cost of nitrous-oxide, in relation to the performance potential, is very reasonable.

Let's assume that you're going to spend the day at the drag strip. A typical street system in a late-model vehicle will probably consume about 1.5 to 2.0 pounds of nitrous per pass. At current prices, that will amount to approximately three dollars per pass. In a full day of racing, that could be about 15 or 20 dollars of nitrous; not an unreasonable sum.

There are many modifications that give very good performance for the dollar spent. Some of them approach or exceed nitrous in terms of "cheap horsepower." But usually, modifications that produce horsepower less expensively are not capable of producing as much peak horsepower as nitrous. For instance, it is sometimes possible to gain 15 or 20 horsepower by merely changing the air filter and recalibrating the carburetor. This may cost no more than 40 dollars. Two dollars per horsepower is pretty good, but the maximum limit is only 20 horsepower, and this kind of increase is not always possible because some vehicles already have efficient induction systems. Sometimes this kind of "low-buck hop-up" works, and sometimes it doesn't.

With nitrous, the power increase is guaranteed (as long as a good system is used). A typical budget kit may cost about 300 dollars and often less. If the system produces 120 horsepower (a conservative figure because many budget kits will produce 150 horsepower), the cost is only 2.5 dollars per horsepower. But to this, we must add yet another factor: a nitrous kit is quick and easy to install. Also, it is just as quick and easy to remove. This may be important. If you limit engine modifications to a nitrous kit, you can remove the kit when you sell the vehicle. (A "stocker" is usually easier to sell than a modified vehicle.) And in most cases, it's very easy to transplant the nitrous system to your new ride. This means that each dollar you spend on a nitrous system will go a long way!

Very few performance modifications can produce this much horsepower and still be as cost-effective as nitrous. Turbocharging is a suitable example. Some bolt-on turbo kits produce excellent performance. A typical turbocharger installation will cost at least 2500 dollars—and often a lot more—but 2500 dollars is a reasonable estimate for comparison. We will assume that this is an effective turbo kit and produces 150 horsepower. Now, suppose you keep the car for two years, and during that time you take it to the drag strip 40 times and make 8 passes each time. The only additional cost, beyond the purchase of the system, will be about 50 dollars for the gasoline used at the strip.

Let's see how this compares to nitrous injection. A typical nitrous kit that produces 150 horsepower will cost about 300 dollars, but you may want to add some extras, such as a nitrous counter, throttle switches, etc. So the total cost, installed, should be about 450 dollars. The approximate cost of fuel will again be 50 dollars (I am assuming that the turbo engine and the nitrous engine will provide about equal fuel efficiency). But there will be the additional cost of nitrous. In this amount of time, with average use, the total nitrous consumption should be about 720 pounds, with a total cost, at current prices, of about 1,080 dollars.

When it is time to sell the turbocharged vehicle, it will probably be easier to leave the turbo system in place because it is elaborate job to remove the turbocharger and all of its special components. But we can assume that if you find the right buyer, the turbo kit will add about 500 dollars to the resale price. So the net price of the turbo kit, minus the resale price, will be about 1,750 dollars. This makes the total cost for using the turbo system for two years about 1,800 dollars.

Removing a nitrous system is pretty easy, so we can assume, given the same circumstances, that you will remove the system and use it on another vehicle. It will, therefore, not affect the resale price. So, the total cost of running the nitrous for two years is 1,580 dollars, plus you still have a 450-dollar nitrous kit.

In this simplistic scenario, you will be 670 dollars ahead if you use nitrous instead of a turbocharging system. Real life does not often follow predictable pathways, but experienced performance enthusiasts recognize the economic value of nitrous. And no matter what modifications are considered, it is very tough to beat the overall horsepower-per-dollar value of nitrous.

Things can be even more attractive if you have an all-out race car. Let's assume you are running a smallblock Chevy that produces about 580 horsepower (this is fairly common for 10-second machines). A nitrous engine that pumps out 580 horses is not likely to cost more than 6,000 dollars (including shortblock, heads, induction and nitrous kit), and it should be dead reliable. Yearly operating costs will look something like this (assuming no major engine trouble): If you attend 20 events a year and make 8 passes at each event, the total gasoline, spark plug and oil bill will be about 100 dollars. If the engine is equipped with a 200-horsepower nitrous kit (a common setup), it will consume approximately 320 pounds of nitrous, which comes to about 450 dollars. The total engine and fuel cost for the year will be 6,550 dollars.

In comparison, a non-nitrous engine that produces 580 horsepower is going to be more than a little "high-strung." It will require top-grade racing hardware and will cost about 12,000 dollars! Annual costs will again include about 100 dollars of consumables (though actual fuel costs may be higher when you consider driving around the pits, tuning time, long burnouts, etc.). Total costs for the year will be 12,100 dollars.

Again, this is a simplistic view, but the difference in total operating cost of the non-nitrous racing engine is 5,500 dollars *more* than the nitrous engine. This cost difference means that a racer could almost buy a spare nitrous engine (he certainly could buy a spare short block), and this doesn't even consider the reliability problem that plagues high-rpm, naturally-aspirated engines.

SAFETY

Using nitrous in automotive applications is not intrinsically dangerous in any way, so long as the user is familiar with system functioning and has an unwavering respect for the inherent volatility of high-pressure gases and liquids. Without question, nitrous-oxide must be handled carefully. The procedures are simple and relatively convenient, but just as every mechanic must learn not to bring an open flame near gasoline fumes, the nitrous user must learn to handle nitrous-oxide properly.

Nitrous-oxide has been used clandestinely by some racers for many years, but when aftermarket street-oriented kits became widely available, some users failed to understand the potential hazards, I even know of a few people who have had some rather hair-raising experiences. One that springs to mind is a guy who had just bought a new '79 Corvette. This is a handsome car, but the stock engine is choked with makeshift factory smog controls (compared to the sophisticated smog equipment on current factory engines). So the owner decided to revamp the engine. It was torn down and equipped with all the usual "go-fast" parts: intake manifold, big carb, high-lift cam, headers, etc. The list of specialized parts included, of course, a nitrous kit. And a pretty healthy one at that. For the first few days, the engine functioned perfectly and he was very impressed with the performance, especially when the nitrous was operating. However, one day the owner tried to start the engine and it literally blew up, sending the carburetor and chunks of intake manifold through the hood of the car. The hood was splintered into little pieces and the top half of the engine was totally destroyed. This proved a bit unexpected for the driver, who for a moment, thought The End was very near. And the passenger, needless to say, was impressed by the demonstration.

But what caused the explosion? The answer is simple and a useful object lesson. While the engine was *not running*, the driver had pressed the nitrous firing button a couple of times to demonstrate how easy it was to operate the system. However, the nitrous shut-off valve was open and each time he pressed the button, nitrous was released into the intake manifold. As he started the engine, he pumped the throttle a few times, and this, of course, dumped a large amount of raw fuel (from the accelerator pumps) into the manifold. Then, unfortunately, the engine "kicked back" into the manifold—the engine was fitted with the type of long-duration, high-overlap cam that tends to promote backfire into the manifold during low-speed cranking—and the highly concentrated mixture of gasoline and nitrous trapped inside the manifold exploded.

To avoid problems of this type, *there are some safety rules that must be rigidly observed.* If you handle nitrous regularly, these precautions will become a matter of second nature. Nitrous is safe, as long as you are alert to the potential hazards.

The best place to begin is right at the source—the nitrous bottle. The first rule is: *Do not expose any nitrous bottles to direct sunlight for an extended period.* Accumulated heat from the exposure will cause the temperature of the bottle to rise precariously, to the point where the blow-off valve might actuate. The blow-off valve is nothing more than a pressure-sensitive plug in the shut-off valve. This plug is preset to rupture at a certain pressure and release the gases in the cylinder in a controlled manner.

There is enough margin of safety to allow normal handling, and a few minutes of exposure to direct sunlight will not normally cause difficulties, but do not leave the bottle sitting in direct sunlight for long periods. Remember this when looking for a suitable place to mount the bottle inside the car. The very *worst* place to mount a bottle is under a large, sloping rear window. It will be exposed to direct sunlight and the effect will be magnified by the "greenhouse effect" of the glass. In most cases, an enclosed trunk space will become warm enough to maximize the working pressure inside the bottle, but as long as the car is not parked for long periods in intense summer heat, the trunk

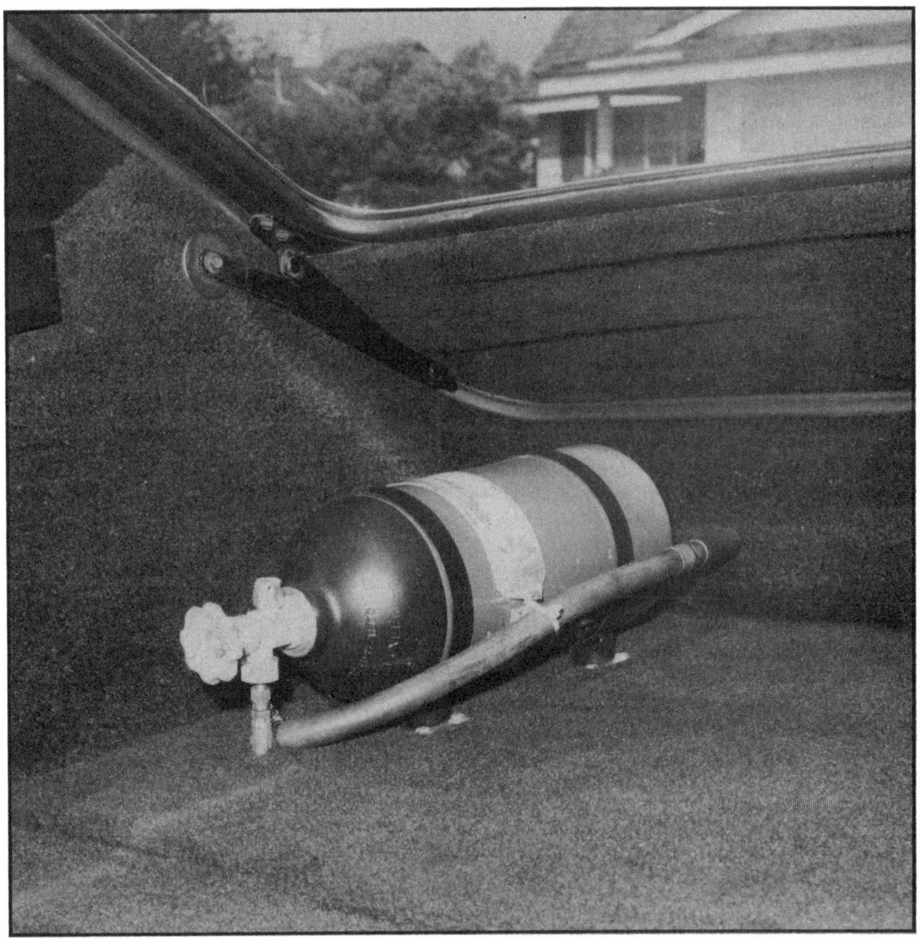

To improve safety and performance the bottle must be kept as cool as possible. Do not mount the bottle under a hatchback glass window (a reflective film on the window will not solve the problem). The bottle must be protected from direct sunlight.

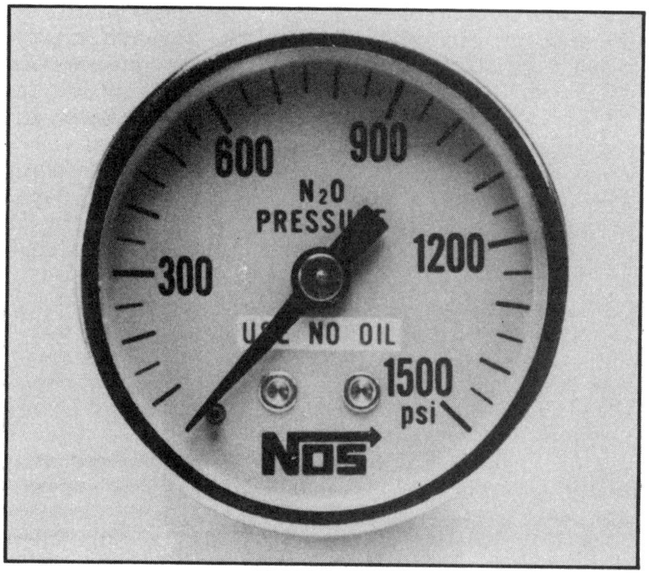
600
900
N2O
PRESSU
300
1200
NO OIL
1500
psi
NOS

The gauge says "USE NO OIL" for a good reason. If oil or grease is used on the threads, the nitrous may combine with combustible byproducts to form an explosive mixture.

space should not become too warm for safety.

Do not ever tamper with the blow-off valve. I have seen bottles that have had the blow-off valve drilled through and replaced with a threaded plug. This is patently stupid. If this safety feature is defeated and, for some reason the bottle is overpressurized, it may rupture. Violently! There is enough energy in a pressurized nitrous bottle to reasonably simulate a hand grenade. And though the motion picture version is quite colorful, a real hand-grenade explosion is deadly.

"Overfilling" the bottle can also activate the blow-off. In some instances the blow-off valve has been plugged so the bottle could be intentionally overfilled. This is Russian roulette with a hand grenade. *There must be a minimum of 32% free space above the nitrous in the bottle.* Otherwise, pressures can rise to dangerously high levels.

Never permit oil, grease, or any other readily combustible substance to accumulate in areas that nitrous might also contact, such as valves, regulators, gauges, hoses, threads, etc. This could, in some instances, produce an explosive mixture. In the same vein, if the exterior becomes greasy or oily, the nitrous bottle will be difficult to grasp and handle safely. If you drop a 25-pound bottle on your foot, you will have good cause to remember the incident for quite some time.

A top-grade nitrous storage bottle is actually very tough; but it must not be abused. The weakest spot of the bottle is, in fact, the shut-off valve assembly. *The bottle, and especially the valve assembly, should always be protected from mishandling or sharp impacts.* Remember, if the bottle were to be ruptured and a gasoline or fuel spill occurred at the same time, the slightest spark would set off an intense fire. And even if the mixture did not catch fire, the super-cooled nitrous could potentially "burn" the driver or rescue personnel. This can be minimized if the bottle is mounted securely inside the car and located as far away from the sides of the vehicle as possible. The supply hose should be armored—this type of hose is commonly known as "Aero-Quip" or "braided-steel" hose—and *must be routed in such a way that it will be protected during an accident or component failure.* For example, the line should be routed through a steel tube as it passes the general area of the flywheel. This provides additional protection in case of a flywheel failure.

Never use a bottle that is not specifically designed and intended for storing pressurized nitrous-oxide. A nitrous bottle should always be painted blue to alert safety officials of the contents. Do not fill a carbon-dioxide bottle with nitrous-oxide. In the past, it was common for "cheaters" to camouflage a nitrous bottle as a carbon-dioxide, fire-retardant bottle. In case of an accident, this could be hazardous. In fact, you should never do anything that may cause confusion about the contents of any pressurized bottle or storage cylinder. Also, if you suspect, for any reason, that a foreign substance or contaminant has entered the bottle, notify the gas supplier when the bottle is returned for refilling.

Another problem, incidentally, is the possibility of nitrous leaking past the solenoid into the engine when the vehicle is not in use. During startup this could cause a manifold explosion like the one described earlier. To avoid this kind of leak it is a good idea to turn off the nitrous supply either with a remote valve or at the bottle valve when the vehicle is parked or when you are certain that the system will not be used.

There may be, for one reason or another, occasions when it is necessary to dump nitrous-oxide into the atmosphere. Never do this in an enclosed space; always jettison unwanted nitrous in a well-ventilated area—or better yet, outdoors. When doing so, *never point the nitrous outlet at anyone because the super-cooled nitrous will cause freeze burns if it contacts bare skin.*

As explained in Chapter One, nitrous-oxide is not hazardous, per se, but if it is present around a fire, it will greatly intensify the flame. Precautions must be taken whenever it is transferred from one container to another to prevent accidental leaks. To help identify the presence of gaseous nitrous—and, consequently, the possibility of an accidental leak somewhere in the system—Puritan Bennet

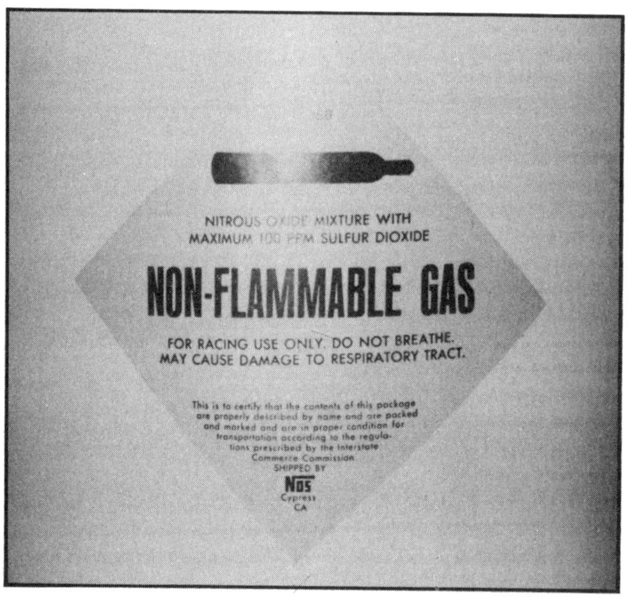
NITROUS OXIDE MIXTURE WITH
MAXIMUM 100 PPM SULFUR DIOXIDE
NON-FLAMMABLE GAS
FOR RACING USE ONLY. DO NOT BREATHE.
MAY CAUSE DAMAGE TO RESPIRATORY TRACT.
This is to certify that the contents of this package are properly described by name and are packed and marked and are in proper condition for transportation according to the regulations prescribed by the Interstate Commerce Commission
SHIPPED BY
NOS
Cypress
CA

Nitrous Plus has been developed specifically for racing and automotive applications. Effects of the sulphur-dioxide additive eliminate abusive behavior and allow this nitrous derivative to be dispensed by commercial suppliers.

(one of the major manufacturers of nitrous) and the performance industry have collaborated to produce a unique product called Nitrous-Plus. This is simply nitrous-oxide with sulphur-dioxide added in minute concentrations (100 parts per million). Sulphur-dioxide has a nasty smell—it reminds me of rotten duck eggs—and it adds enough odor to the nitrous to make it readily detectable if it leaks from the system. Nitrous-Plus is considered safer than ordinary nitrous and can generally be obtained more easily.

Of course, this evolution has not been without criticism. Some nitrous proponents claim that the sulphur-dioxide will be detrimental because it may increase corrosion in the engine, particularly inside the cylinder bores. During combustion, the sulphur-dioxide can combine with other elements—mainly byproducts released from the fuel—to produce sulphuric acid. However, gasoline-fueled engines already produce sulphuric acid in small amounts. (The residue usually collects in the pan and is removed during oil changes.) So the likelihood of increased corrosion linked to the presence of sulphur-dioxide is small.

As far as performance is concerned, the addition of sulphur-dioxide should, in theory, slightly improve power. Sulphur-dioxide contains more oxygen than nitrous-oxide, and when it decomposes, slightly more oxygen is liberated. However, since the amounts are so small, the effect is virtually inconsequential.

As a side issue, Nitrous-Plus may improve performance but in an unexpected way. At the same time Nitrous-Plus was developed, a new family of valves and fittings was also designed specifically for use with the new gas. This was intended to prevent confusing Nitrous-Plus bottles with ordinary nitrous bottles. But this new hardware has larger ports and orifices and can flow larger quantities of nitrous. Using a bottle with this larger valve will almost always improve engine performance a little bit. A regular street system may pick up two or three, maybe five, horsepower, and a high-output racing system may gain as much as 10 to 15 horsepower.

RACE SAFETY RULES

Although the same common-sense safety procedures apply at the race track, there are a few other points to consider.

Most reputable manufacturers can supply nitrous equipment and suitable installation instructions that conform to the regulations imposed by major racing organizations. However, local regulations may be a little different. When nitrous-oxide first appeared on the racing scene many unusual safety restrictions were established to protect the racer. The intent was legitimate, but most of these restrictions have subsequently lapsed because they have proven to be inappropriate. It would be wise, nonetheless, to check with track officials or tech inspectors for any local requirements.

Some regulations require a dump tube that will vent the pressurized nitrous outside the vehicle if the blow-off valve is activated. This is really not a bad idea in any nitrous installation, but it is especially important if the bottle is mounted inside the driver's compartment. Most rule books call for the bottle to be installed outside of the driver's compartment. The trunk is, of course, the best and most logical location, but some racing vehicles based on hatchback designs do not have a separate trunk. In such a case, some track officials allow the bottle to be mounted in the driver's compartment, but this may be hazardous in a somewhat unexpected way.

The blow-off valve on a completely full 60-pound bottle of nitrous-oxide accidentally activated in the back of a full-size Dodge van that I was driving. It was, to say the least, a memorable experience. It sounded like a pistol shot when the safety disk ruptured. The entire contents of the bottle flooded the interior of the van and though I was not close enough to suffer freeze burns, the immediate danger seemed to be asphyxiation. The gaseous nitrous displaced all of the air inside the van, but fortunately, the average person does not suffer asphyxiation, loss of consciousness or death unless oxygen is withheld for several seconds (usually more than one minute). It was not difficult for me to roll the window down, bring the vehicle to a stop and beat a hasty retreat. (A driver strapped inside the rollcage of a race car might have a dicey time, though.) The biggest danger, as it turned out, was the dense fog that the nitrous created inside the vehicle. This obscured my vision for a moment, but as soon as I rolled the window down, the fog cleared away, removing the immediate hazard.

This is an interesting story, but the point is this: Even if a vent tube is not required, it is good insurance. If the bottle is inside the driver's compartment, a safety-minded driver should consider a vent tube mandatory. And if the bottle is mounted inside the trunk, a vent tube is still a good idea.

Throughout this book I have discussed important safety measures that apply primarily to the engine. These guidelines may not relate directly to the safety of the driver, but they are, nonetheless, important. If this information is viewed in a serious light and used in conjunction with the safety considerations outlined in this section, the reader can enjoy the tremendous performance advantages of nitrous-oxide without hazard to life or limb.

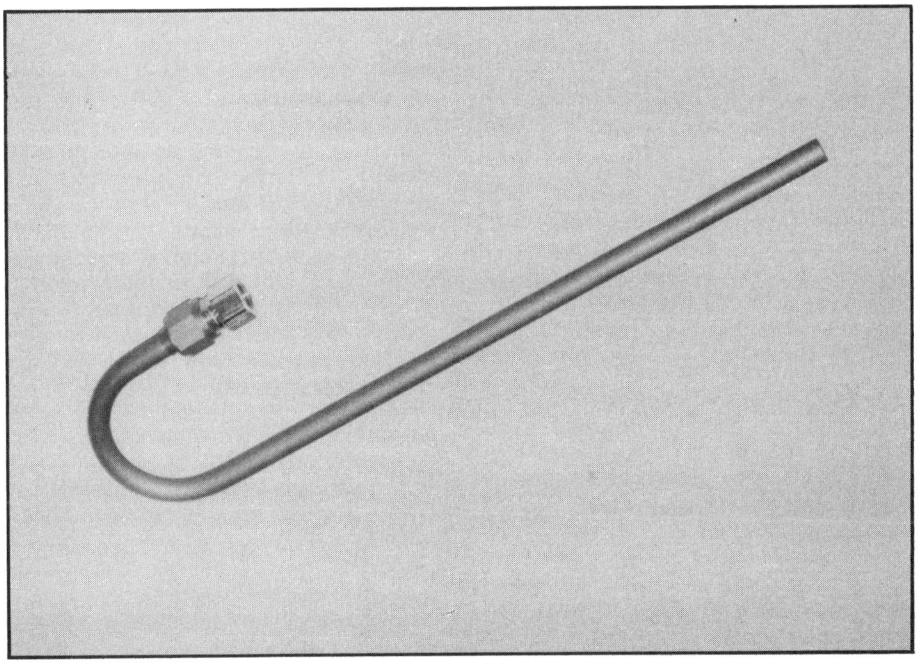

Racing regulations often require a dump tube that will discharge nitrous outside of the vehicle if the safety valve on the nitrous bottle ruptures. Many race tracks do not enforce the rule, but this is a good safety precaution for any nitrous system.

CHAPTER 10

BUILDING A NITROUS ENGINE

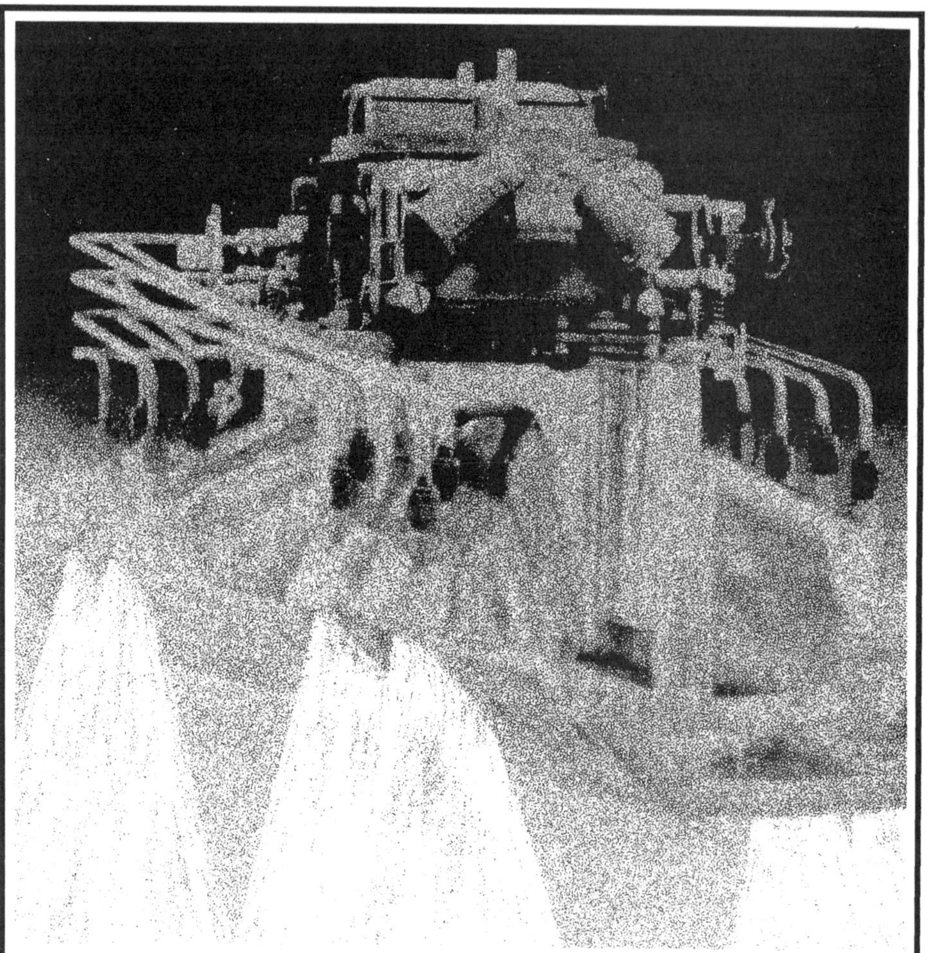

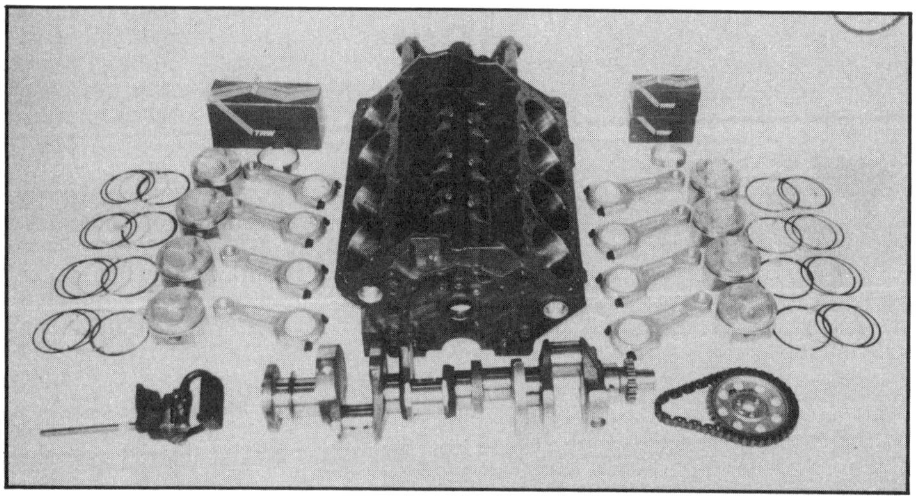

Power and reliability can be improved if engine components are selected and the engine is assembled with an eye toward optimum compatibility with nitrous-oxide injection.

ENGINE COMPONENTS

Nitrous injection can produce spectacular performance from an engine that is almost totally stock; however, the effect of nitrous-oxide can be heightened if the engine components are selected and/or altered to complement the nitrous system. This chapter looks at various procedures that can be used to enhance the performance from nitrous-oxide injection.

CYLINDER BLOCK

When the engine is designed and assembled specifically with nitrous in mind, the basic strength of the cylinder block should be considered. Unfortunately, the all-time most popular performance engine—the venerable smallblock Chevrolet—does not have the all-time strongest block. It is common for the little Chevy block to fatigue rather quickly at the 600-horsepower level achieved by Grand National stock-car racers. On the other hand, it will withstand considerable stress and develop a lot of horsepower in drag-race trim. (In this type of racing, though, the engine develops max power for a relatively short time.) In the final analysis, the little Chevy's main advantage—light weight—is often offset by the flexing it exhibits during high-stress operation. This is not a problem in average street or racing trim, but when the peak power is boosted to very high levels by nitrous injection, block flex can become a serious limitation.

If you are free to choose any available block (engine type) and are not restricted by brand loyalties, financial limitations and/or sponsorship commitments, it will pay dividends to consider a larger, heavier and stiffer block. For instance, the beefy 350cid and 455cid Oldsmobile blocks or any one of the various big-block Chevrolets can withstand a lot of nitrous boost without any serious difficulties. There are other considerations, but the main thing to look for is strong, thick cylinderwalls and reinforced main-bearing webs that utilize heavy-

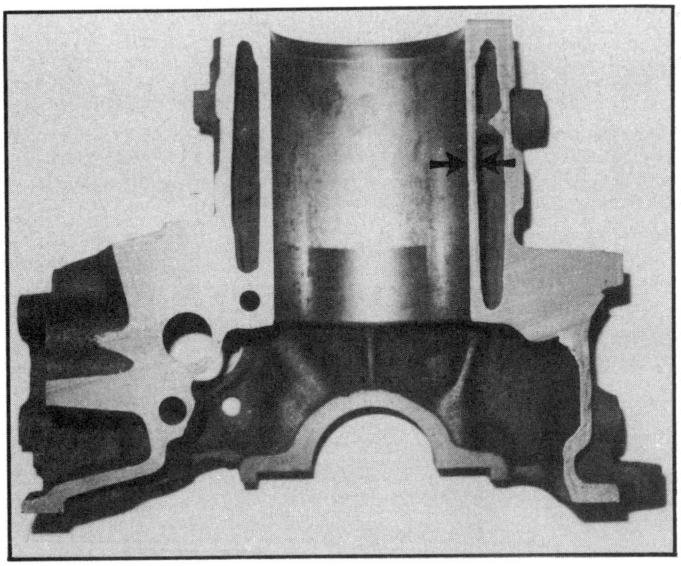

Modern lightweight cylinder blocks have relatively thin cylinderwalls. Overboring will reduce wall strength; so when the engine is boosted with nitrous, keep the bore stock or limit enlargement to the smallest practical overbore.

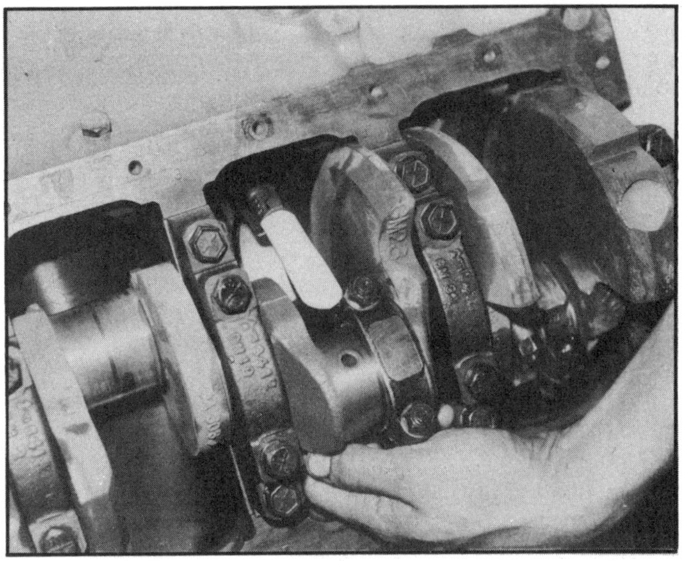

A 4-bolt block is desirable in an all-out engine, but not absolutely essential. As long as detonation is avoided, a 2-bolt block is suitable for a street engine boosted with a typical street nitrous system.

duty, four-bolt main caps.

CRANKSHAFT

Just as with the cylinder block, the crankshaft selected for a nitrous engine should be as strong as practicable. A production cast crank will withstand a lot—at the time of this writing a lot of cast cranks are being successfully used in drag-race engines—but no engine builder would use anything but a premium forged crank in a serious circle-track engine. Most street engines will live practically forever with a cast crank, but if you are planning a strong dose of nitrous for your asphalt rocket, consider a good forged crank (provided a suitable one is available for something less than a hostage ransom).

Accumulated fatigue can cause a crank to fail. This is not as important in a drag-race engine as it is in any sort of an endurance engine. To give you an idea of how quickly fatigue can sideline a crank, consider this: At high-horsepower loads, it is estimated that at 6000rpm the typical crank may have a life-span of 400 hours; at 6500rpm the life will be decreased to 100 hours; and at 7000rpm the life may only be one-half hour!

Crankshaft fatigue is caused by two factors: (1) flexing of the crank due to cyclic loads applied to it by each power stroke and (2) the resultant vibrations transmitted through the crank by engine operation. These forces are considerable, and without a suitable "vibration dampener" a crank will fatigue very quickly. However, a stock-type crankshaft dampener is "tuned" for a limited engine-speed range (hopefully the speed range in which the greatest vibrational excitation occurs). Make certain that whatever crankshaft you select, the dampener is properly matched to the expected engine-speed range.

A typical stock dampener (i.e., a crankshaft-mounted center piece surrounded by a rubber insulation ring and an outer cast-iron or steel flywheel section) is not really very effective. It can only dampen vibrations over a limited speed range. However, there are viscous dampeners available, in which the flywheel is contained in a chamber filled with a silicon-based fluid. Such dampeners are not frequency sensitive. They absorb vibrations effectively over a wide range of engine speeds. If the price is within your budget, such a dampener is definitely an advantage. Hydraulics Houdaille is a good source for this type of dampener. Also capable of doing a good job are the friction-type dampeners produced by Fisher Dynamics and Innovations West.

As far as pre-assembly preparation of the crankshaft is concerned, standard racing techniques apply—depending upon the size of your pocketbook. Indexing the crank, sizing the journals, checking that the crankshaft is straight, radiusing oil holes, etc., are all part of a full-on crank job. Also, to increase the fatigue life, it is a good idea to consider shot-peening and/or Tuftriding.

PISTON SHAPE

The piston is the primary compo-

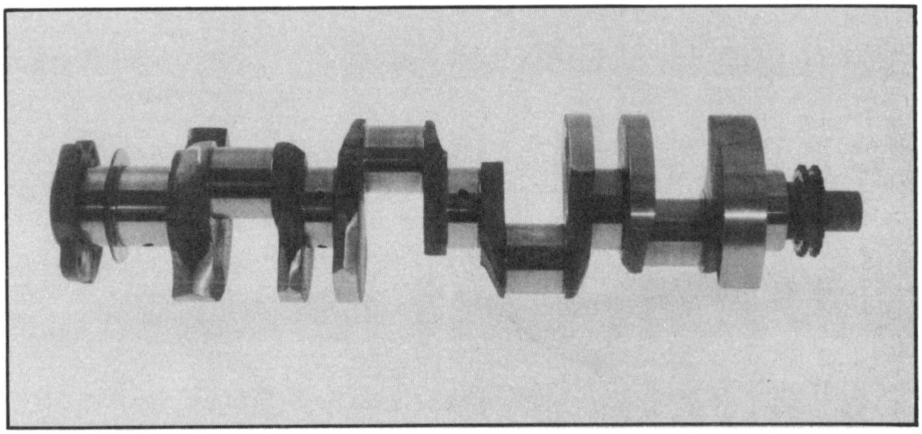

If the power output is significantly higher than 300 horsepower, a properly prepared forged crank will improve the reliability of a compact engine (most small-blocks). However, large engines (big blocks) operate successfully at relatively high outputs with cast cranks (if the basic crank design is fairly stout).

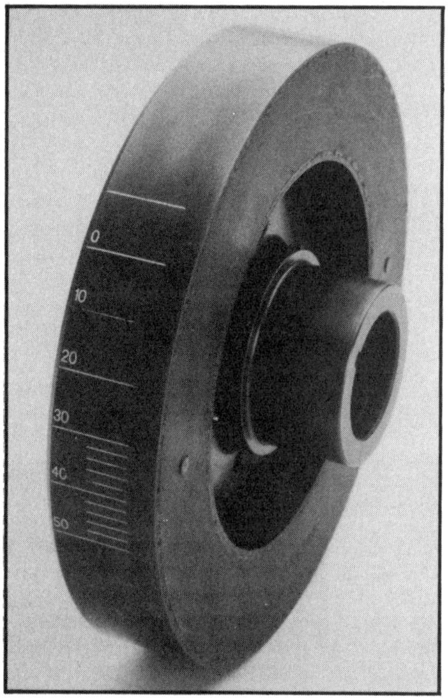

High cylinder pressures increase the torsional vibrations generated by a high-speed engine, and internal modifications may alter the resonating frequencies. As a result, a conventional dampener may not be effective. However, the unique Houdaille hydraulic dampener will cancel a wide range of torsional anomalies.

nent that takes the brunt of transmitting power developed in the cylinders to the flywheel. It exists in a very hostile environment. It is driven up and down the bore at tremendous speeds, and it must effectively seal gases that are at very high temperatures and violently varying pressures. All things considered, it is amazing that the piston can survive at all.

We've already discussed what happens if the mixture is too lean: the pistons simply melt. But it is also possible to damage the pistons even when the mixture is not at fault. Usually this happens when the amount of nitrous going into the cylinders produces pressures that are too high. This problem is, of course, more severe when the compression ratio is relatively high. Under certain conditions, heavy doses of nitrous and too much compression can hammer a piston to death in a matter of seconds.

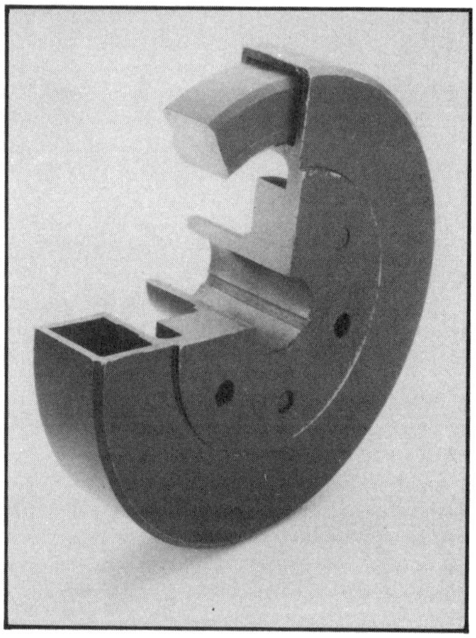

The Houdaille dampener has an internal flywheel that rides in a bath of high-viscosity oil. It is virtually indestructible and is accepted by almost all racing sanctions. The bottom line is that it lengthens engine life.

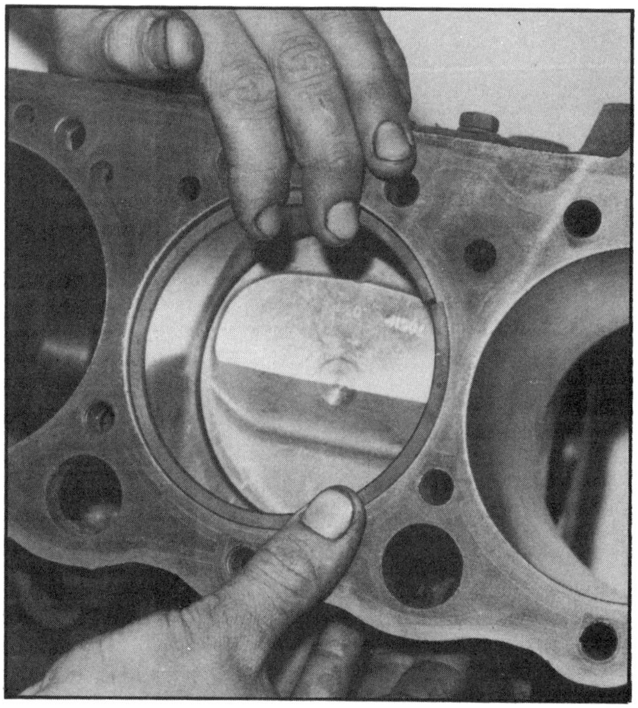

The ring gaps are vital because of high cylinder pressures and operating temperatures when the nitrous system is functioning. The cold gaps should be about 0.001- to 0.0015-inch wider than the manufacturer's recommended minimum limit.

For maximum performance and reliability the crown of the piston should be as nearly flat as possible, consistent with achieving the desired compression ratio. Fortunately, with most engines, an 8.5 or 9:1 compression ratio is possible with a relatively flat piston crown. Indeed, some engines will require a dished piston to lower the compression to this range. In this case, the dished portion should not have any sharp ledges or crevices. Shallow dishes—preferably offset toward the spark plug—are, theoretically at least, the best.

CAST PISTONS

As long as the piston crown is thick enough to withstand the temperatures and pressures of combustion, a piston will be durable under most circumstances, However, the life expectancy in a nitrous engine will depend on several other variables.

First, let's consider the question of a cast or forged piston design. Most cast pistons are produced primarily to be inexpensive; therefore, they are not inherently suitable for high-performance use. However, the word *most* does not mean *all*. There are some cast pistons that have been designed with performance in mind.

In 1986 the APT Corporation of Riverside, California, introduced a nitrous piston for the smallblock Chevy that has the requisite features for long life on the highway. It should also withstand a typical high-powered street nitrous kit. This piston is made from a special alloy that is much harder than even forged pistons, yet it has the toughness of a forged piston. The crown of this piston is slightly thicker than most cast pistons. Also, a special cooling fin design on the underside of the piston not only stiffens the critical crown area, but also reduces crown temperature by increasing the surface area for crankcase oil splashing on the piston underside to take heat from the crown.

It is not commonly understood that the strength of aluminum decreases very rapidly with temperature. If the operating temperature of the piston crown can be reduced by 20 or 30 degrees, the strength of the

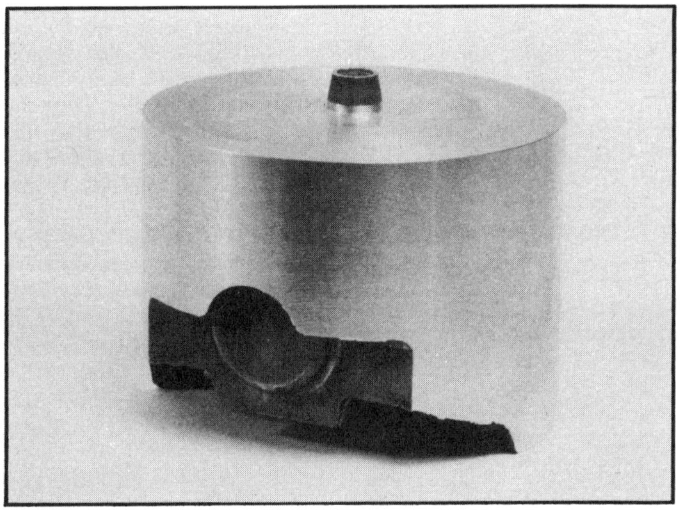

Pistons are available in unfinished form from TRW and Speed-Pro to accommodate special applications. For ultra-high output nitrous engines, "starting from scratch" with one of these forgings may be required.

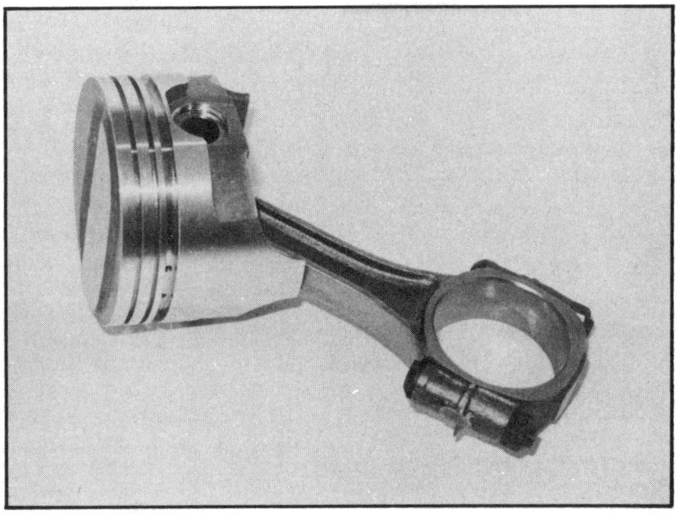

High quality forged pistons are available from local TRW and Sealed Power dealers. These pistons have been designed for most popular engine families and are a good selection for any street-strip nitrous engine.

crown will be improved by as much as 10%. And one of the advantages of making a cast piston is that deeper cooling fins can be manufactured with the casting process than in the forging process. As a result, the underside of some cast pistons (the APT piston is a good example), may have as much as 40% more cooling area. Incidentally, this drop in the operating temperature can add an extra measure of safety by keeping the engine below the detonation limit.

There is also good reason to believe that a hard cast piston—like the APT piston—will maintain skirt and ring groove shape better than a typical forged piston. The APT piston is a very good selection for a high-powered street Chevy because it also has a full-skirt design that gives superior ring support. This effectively keeps the rings squarely in contact with the bore, even during the extreme pressures generated by nitrous injection. According to APT, this particular piston was designed for nitrous motors producing up to about 450 horsepower. Unfortunatly, this piston is somewhat difficult to obtain, however, a piston designed for similar usage was just released by Speed-Pro (see buyers guide, pgs 126-127).

FORGED PISTONS

When we use the term "forged piston," we need to qualify it somewhat. Many forged pistons currently available are simply "stamped" or "impacted" cast pistons. In other words, just before the material solidifies in the mold, it is hit with a large punch that compresses the contents into something akin to the micro structure of a true forging. Such pistons, though designated as "forged," qualify for the title in a very general way.

True forged pistons are stronger than the average production cast pistons, but some "impact forged" pistons may not prove reliable when the peak output of a nitrous-boosted engine exceeds about 450 to 500 total horsepower. With everything just right, these pistons will stand 500 horsepower for *maybe* a total of about 500 miles of competitive endurance racing; and they will, of course, be fine for limited drag-strip use. However, many of the "impact-forged" and "true-forged" pistons require wider skirt clearances than a cast piston and this often leads to reduced ring stability against the bore wall, increasing blow-by and reducing power out-

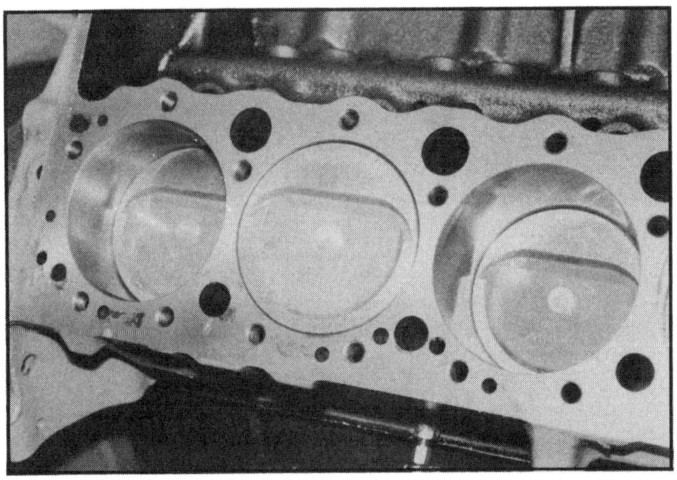

This dished-deck TRW piston is an outstanding choice for a street-bound smallblock. With closed-chamber heads the compression ratio is typically about 9.0:1—yielding good all-around performance, both unboosted and with nitrous boost up to about 150 horsepower.

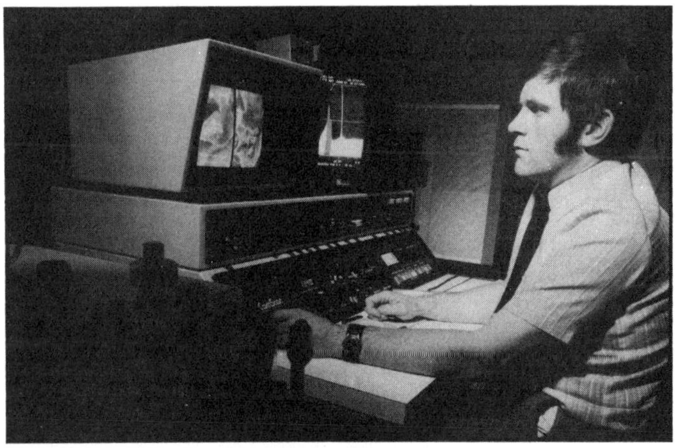

The metallurgic makeup of the piston greatly affects reliability. A scanning electron-beam microscope and an X-ray fluorescent analyzer are used at Cosworth to inspect racing pistons during the manufacturing process. Although expensive, Cosworth pistons are noted for their exceptional durability.

put.

If you are building a "sky-is-the-limit" nitrous engine, there is little option but to use forged pistons or expensive custom-machined specialty pistons. When selecting a piston for this type of engine, choose one that has thick, sturdy ribs abutting the pin boss. Many piston manufacturers have only a few forging dies, and several different piston models are "finish machined" from the same rough forgings. And since most racing or performance pistons must be capable of relatively high compression ratios, the rough forgings usually have large domes. However, in an effort to reduce weight, the underside of the dome is often machined at the factory. As a consequence, if—during engine pre-assembly—the engine builder decides to machine the crown to reduce compression, some areas of the crown dome/deck can become dangerously thin. If an unsupported area of the crown is reduced to a thickness less than 0.300-inch, there is a high likelihood of failure under extreme conditions (racing or heavy nitrous use).

To avoid crown collapse, it is desirable to select a piston that has a relatively thick crown with a flat or slightly dished top surface (depending upon compression requirements, of course). *Pistons that have been designed for turbocharged application are good choices.* Two specialty sources come to mind: Cosworth Engineering and Gale Banks Engineering. Of course, there are also several other piston manufacturers that produce suitable performance pistons for most domestic V8 engines.

Apart from having the right material and a suitable crown design, there are other important factors to consider. First, when nitrous is used it is necessary to position the ring pack lower on the piston. If the piston material above the top ring land is too narrow, it may collapse onto the top ring as a result of the high heat and cylinder pressures involved. This will trap the ring and destroy ring seal. It is also possible to trap the top ring in such a way that it presses hard against the bore, causing a very high friction level. Of course this leads to severe bore scoring and possibly total seizure. And, even if the top ring land holds up, the band between the top and second grooves may collapse if it is too thin. The wide land widths found on most street pistons—as opposed to the narrow spacing used on some race pistons—will prove more reliable on the average nitrous engine.

Basically, the top ring width should be at least 1/16-inch, and preferably 1/8-inch, positioned further down the piston than is normally the case. It is a good idea to use a slightly thicker ring than would otherwise be the case. If the engine is normally fitted with an 0.043-inch compression ring, step up to a 1/16-

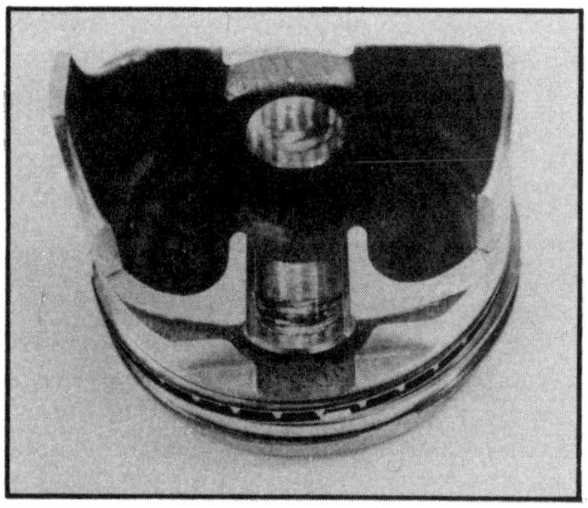

The pin clearance should be increased by at least 0.0002- to 0.0003-inch in a nitrous engine. If total output is in the 600 horsepower range the pin clearances should be about 0.0007- and 0.0009-inch. Positive pin oiling from the ring lands should be provided at power levels above 400 horsepower.

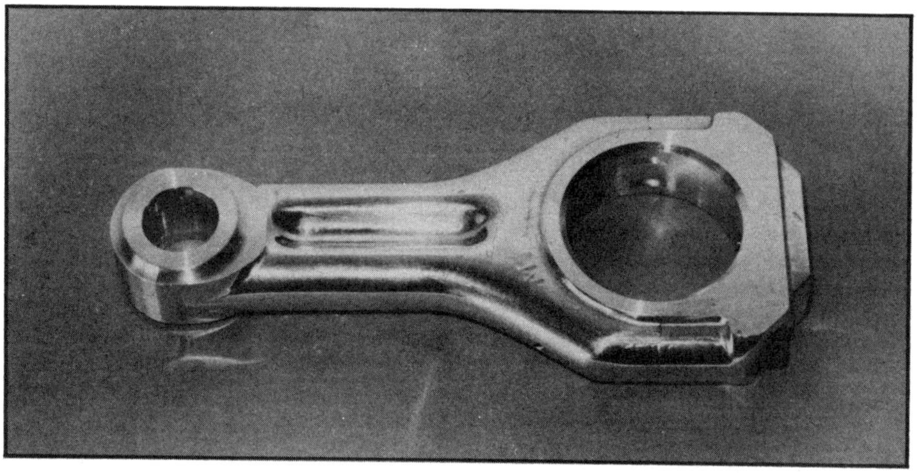

Because of the lower operating speeds, aluminum rods can be used successfully in a nitrous engine. In most cases the aluminum rods will last about twice as long (compared to aluminum rods in a high-rpm racing engine).

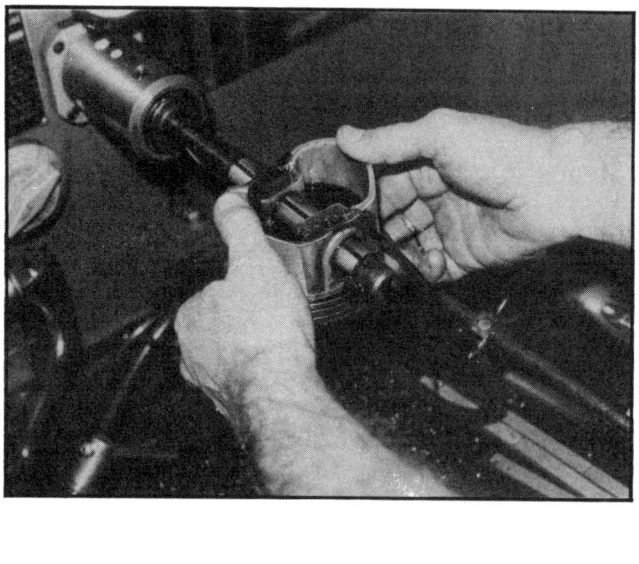

A local machine shop can hone the pin bores to increase the pin clearance.

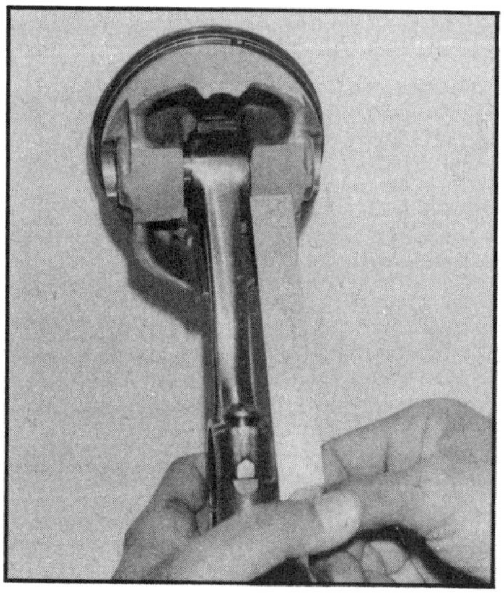

When heavy doses of nitrous are used at low engine speeds the compression loads on the connecting rod are quite large. About 1000 lbs/ft of engine torque at 5000rpm caused this Chevrolet steel rod to bow.

inch top ring. Remember, the two justifications for a narrow ring are: (1) that it seats quickly and (2) that at high engine speeds, it won't "flutter" in the groove. When nitrous (and the consequent high cylinder pressures) is used in the engine, there will be plenty of pressure behind the ring to hold it in place and ensure a good seal.

Because of the very high heat resistance, the new (as of 1984) ceramic rings produced by TRW are well worth trying. These rings have more heat resistance than a regular stainless or moly-filled ring. (But they require special bore preparation, so follow the manufacturer's instructions to the letter.) Another combination worth considering is the Sealed Power Head Land ring and piston. The high placement of this unique ring is contrary to all that has been said so far about nitrous ring placement, but the size and excellent heat conductivity of this ring saves the day. This piston/ring combination is worth a close look if the max engine speed is below 6000rpm and the nitrous horsepower boost is restricted to about 150hp. Under these conditions, this combination gives excellent bore life and good performance.

Moly-filled or stainless rings can also be used effectively in a nitrous engine. Some engine builders have reported success using a Total-Seal second ring. This unique ring has, as far as the gases are concerned, no visible end gap. A similar ring is manufactured by Childs and Albert, a company that produces various components for race engines, and I have had good results with their products.

It is important to have a very rigid piston pin and, as noted earlier, solid well-anchored pin bosses in the piston. Unless the pin is very rigid, it will bend; and in bending, it will cause piston distortion. And *piston distortion at the pin bosses is one of the major contributing factors of piston failure.* Don't even consider a "super-lightweight" pin for a nitrous engine. A good starting point is a typical Pro Stock pin and adding at least 0.030-inch more wall thickness—as a minimum! In most cases, stock pins are among the stiffest pins available. Although they may be a bit heavy, at least you will know for certain they won't bend and cause premature failure.

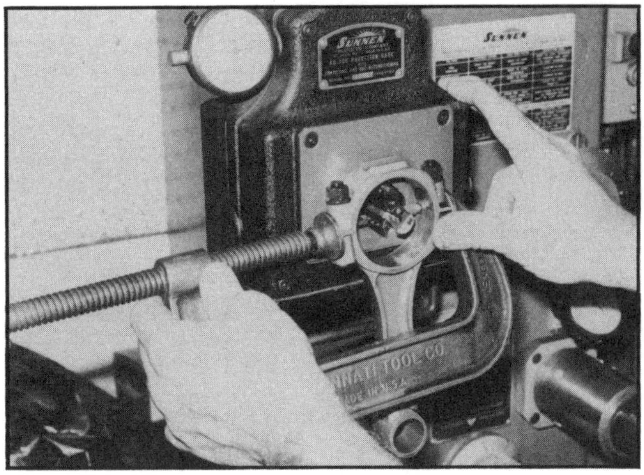

To give maximum bearing crush, rod big ends should be finished to the minimum recommended diameter. The clamp across the rod slightly deforms the rod, so the journal becomes more nearly round during operation.

CONNECTING RODS

Connecting rods almost always fail due to tensile loads, and a nitrous engine increases compressive loads but *reduces* tensile loads. Tensile loads are a by-product of high engine speeds, but because of the high torque developed by nitrous-oxide, a nitrous engine produces peak power at relatively modest crank speeds. As a result, the prime cause of rod failure—excessive engine rpm—is substantially reduced.

Indeed, aluminum rods—which are highly resistant to tensile loads for short periods of time (compared to steel rods)—can be operated reliably for relatively long periods at the low crank speeds typical of most nitrous engines. However, in most instances, it is not really necessary to go to the expense of aluminum rods, unless you are building an all-out racing engine. Very often a properly prepared set of stock rods will do the job adequately. For instance, a big-block Chevy nitrous engine that develops about 700-800 horsepower can function adequately with stock rods. Likewise, a 600-horsepower smallblock Chevy (with nitrous) will usually get by with stock rods. If the peak power level is pushed above these limits, a premium rod may be necessary. Or, if the engine is used for circle-track or some form of endurance racing, where high engine speeds are required (and the amount of nitrous is considerably less), a premium steel connecting rod will be required to withstand the long-term tensile loadings generated during unboosted operation.

ROD BEARINGS

As with any high-performance assembly, a nitrous engine should be fitted with the best premium bearings available. Bearings are relatively inexpensive, and there is no legitimate reason to use anything less than the best. Select top-quality bearings—such as Federal Mogul, Clevite, Sealed Power, TRW or Childs & Albert—and fit them properly.

When nitrous is used, the face pressure on the rod bearings will be considerably higher during a longer portion of the power cycle. Under these circumstances a greater oil "cushion" on the bearings will significantly reduce the possibility of bearing failure; consequently, the big-end bearing clearances can be increased slightly. But the maximum clearance *need not be significantly greater than that used for normal race preparation.* In all cases, however, remember to add wide chamfers to crank journal oil holes, as this will improve oiling and eliminate fracture-starting sharp edges.

CYLINDER HEADS

Although it is possible to achieve good horsepower with a nitrous engine that does not have expensive,

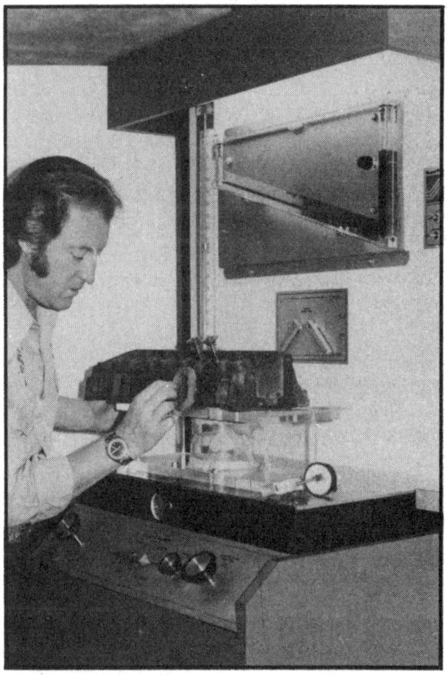

Cylinder head preparation is important in an all-out racing engine. The author modifies and tests heads on a Super Flow SF-300 flowbench. Air mass-flow energy, velocity, velocity distribution and swirl are some of the factors that affect overall performance.

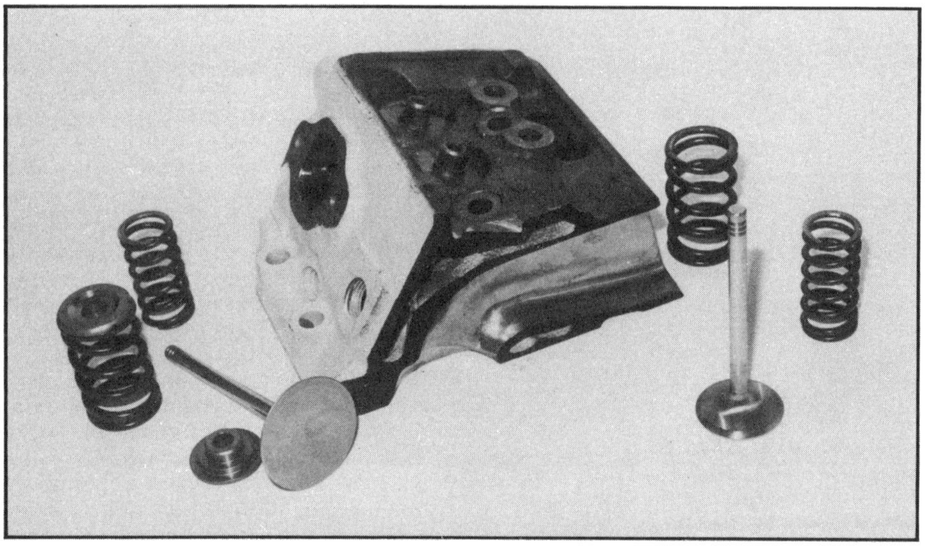

Shape is the most critical aspect of port performance; but with nitrous, a polished surface finish can be beneficial. This does not aid flow, but it reduces the heat transferred from the port wall to the liquid nitrous, allowing a denser charge to enter the cylinder.

highly-developed cylinder heads, modifying the cylinder heads on a nitrous-injected engine is worthwhile if you are after every last drop of horsepower. Modified heads can also improve, although to a far lesser degree, the effect of the nitrous injection.

Enlarging the intake ports of most production cylinder heads will generally aid top-end power. However, the price of improving high-rpm power is often a drop in low- and mid-range performance. Fortunately, a well-designed nitrous system can be used to bolster the performance in these areas. As a result, when nitrous is employed, the manifold and head ports can be designed or modified with a specific eye toward top-end horsepower. This does not mean that the ports can be "hogged out" indiscriminately. If you are going for all-out max performance, it is a good idea to talk to the best available cylinder head expert to find out what can be done to enhance top-end power.

At this point it is important to mention that the optimum valve sizes for a nitrous engine may not meet classical standards. A substantial proportion of the oxygen entering the cylinder of a nitrous-injected engine is in liquid form. This means that the ratio between the intake volume and the exhaust volume is not going to be the same as it is for a normally-aspirated engine. The total induced *intake volume* will not change; but due to the fact that the nitrous is mostly liquid, the *charge weight* will increase dramatically. After combustion, therefore, the exhaust volume will increase substantially. As a result, it is important to re-evaluate the ratio between exhaust and intake flow.

Several variables affect the flow of a specific port and valve combination, but most cylinder head experts believe that, with a normally-aspirated engine, maximum performance is achieved when the intake flows about one-third more than the exhaust. In other words, the exhaust flow should equal about 75% of the intake flow.

If possible, this balance should be altered slightly in a nitrous engine, but just how much altering it needs depends on how much nitrous is used. It is difficult to be specific here because very little research has been done in this area. But an educated guess is that when max power is increased by 20% due to nitrous injection, the flow balance of the exhaust side should be increased by about 5%. For example, if an engine is developing approximately 40% of the total horsepower from nitrous-oxide, the exhaust valve should flow about 85% of the intake valve. Likewise, if 60% of the power is developed with nitrous, the exhaust flow should be about 95% of the intake.

However, this formula may not apply to all cylinder heads. The popular Chevrolet "Turbo" smallblock head is a good example. Since these cylinder heads already have valve sizes that occupy most of the combustion chamber, it would be very difficult to reduce the intake valve by much more than 0.050-inch and increase the exhaust valve by a like amount. Under these circumstances, it's not practical to raise the exhaust flow to more than about 80% of the intake flow. This means that a reasonable compromise may be required. Flow balance is important, but it is not wise to unnecessarily restrict the intake just to attain the desired balance. This will hurt power more than it will help.

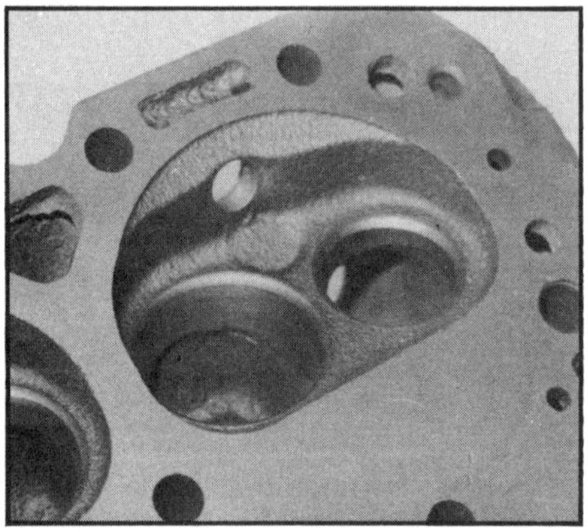

Cylinder heads with closed chambers are usually less susceptible to detonation. The term "closed chamber" generally refers to a combustion chamber that is relatively small with one or more quench areas.

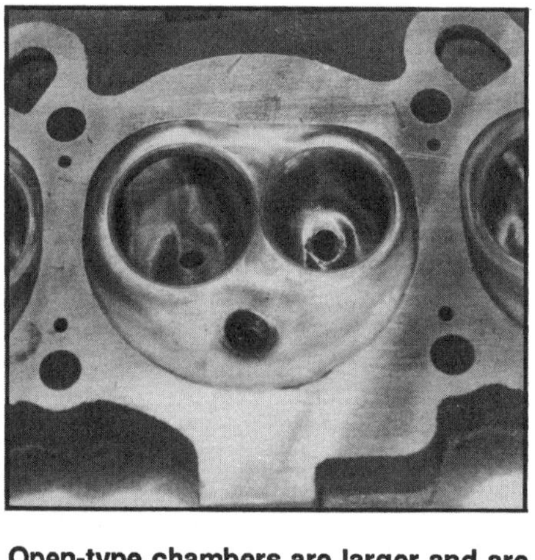

Open-type chambers are larger and are sometimes fully dome-shaped. It is more difficult to achieve high compression with open chambers and they are more prone to detonation.

HEAD MODIFICATIONS

Whenever possible, it is best to determine port flow balance requirements, and then select a bare cylinder head that will best fit these requirements. For example, the conventional Chevy smallblock street heads that are equipped with 1.5-inch exhaust valves and 1.94-inch intake valves are a good choice. For use with nitrous, it is a good idea to stay with the 1.94 intake size and, consequently, there is enough room in the chamber of most of these heads to fit a larger exhaust valve. This general head design is available with several different chamber and port sizes, but by using oversize replacement valves it is usually possible to increase the diameter of the exhaust valve to 1.6 or even 1.650 inches.

In most cases, *it will pay to improve on the exhaust flow at least as much as the intake.* On a conventional engine, some head experts estimate that increasing the max airflow of the intake is about 10 or 20 times more effective than a comparable increase in exhaust flow. However, this same effect does not apply to a nitrous engine. Keep in mind that exhaust flow is much more critical on a nitrous engine, and make certain that whoever is prepping the heads understands the difference.

If you intend to modify your own heads in a limited time and get the best return for the effort, work around the valve seats and polish the intake port. Spend the rest of your effort reworking the exhaust port and installing larger exhaust valves. (If the combustion chamber has limited space to accommodate larger exhaust valves, the flow balance can be improved somewhat with the camshaft selection. However, we will deal with this later).

Most V8 cylinder heads have limited potential for modifications in the combustion chambers because of the adverse effect this has on compression. If too much metal is removed from the chambers—especially around the valves—a large piston dome will be required to achieve a relatively high compression ratio. Large domes will inevitably hurt max horsepower, and as such represent a compromise.

A large piston dome protrudes prominently into the chamber at top dead-center, and this segments the chamber into little pockets. As a result, the combustion in some areas of the chamber will be less effective. This varies with the specific design of the chamber and dome, but in most cases the dome doesn't have to be too high before it will cause a substantial power decrease—and here, substantial means SUBSTANTIAL. There have been instances when peak power has dropped by 200 horsepower because the piston dome was 1/8-inch too high!

However, with a nitrous engine, the compression ratio need not be extremely high. It is possible, therefore, to modify the chamber in the area around the valves to achieve greater airflow—as long as the modification does not weaken the chamber. Remember, a well-modified pushrod engine has a brake-mean-effective pressure of around 180psi in the combustion space. A nitrous-injected motor in the lower speed ranges can have a brake-mean-effective pressure in excess of 400psi. With this much cylinder pressure, many V8 heads—in modified form—may suffer from cracking problems. So proceed cautiously.

HEAD MOUNTING

Head gaskets can be a problem on any high-rpm, high-compression engine. The same is true of nitrous-injected engines, only worse. In many instances, a good competition head gasket will get the job done. I have had good results with Felpro Blue head gaskets. If these head gaskets fail, then I believe it will be necessary to backup the fire ring of the head gasket with a copper ring. Once the block is machined for O-rings and copper O-rings are properly fitted, the problem will probably disappear (a tool that allows the home mechanic to cut the required grooves can be obtained from numerous tool suppliers).

For engines that are likely to produce up to three or four horsepower per cubic inch, regular head bolts may not be adequate for the job. It is wise to change to high-tensile studs to hold the heads in place. With the right assembly techniques, they can achieve a higher clamping pressure from the same torque setting.

INTAKE MANIFOLD

The design of the intake manifold will, of course, affect fuel-air distribution. A good single 4-barrel intake manifold—such as an Edelbrock Victor or Victor Junior—generally produces acceptable fuel distribution in a normally-aspirated engine. If the nitrous injection adversely affects overall fuel distribution, the problem can generally be traced to a mixing problem at the point of injection (in most cases the streams of nitrous-oxide are not thoroughly mixing with the enrichment fuel).

Despite the best efforts, it is not always possible to get equal amounts of nitrous to enter each manifold runner. The consequences of this have been discussed in earlier chapters, however, it may be necessary to accept the fact that achieving precise distribution within a single-plane, open plenum, high-performance manifold is, or can be, quite difficult with some nitrous kits. But to make the point clear, if good mixing is ensured at the point of injection, distribution variations will be minimized.

A *divider plate* may improve the distribution in some intake manifolds. If it does, the problem may lie in carburetor or manifold port characteristics and the general specification of the rest of the engine. If an open-plenum manifold is used and a distribution problem exists, try adding a divider plate before you make any other changes. Usually the divider doesn't need to reach to the bottom of the manifold. It will be effective if it extends about three-quarters of the way to the floor of the manifold plenum. When some sort of spacer is used in the nitrous system, the easiest way to add a divider is to simply weld it to the spacer, so the divider will be positioned properly when the spacer is installed to the manifold.

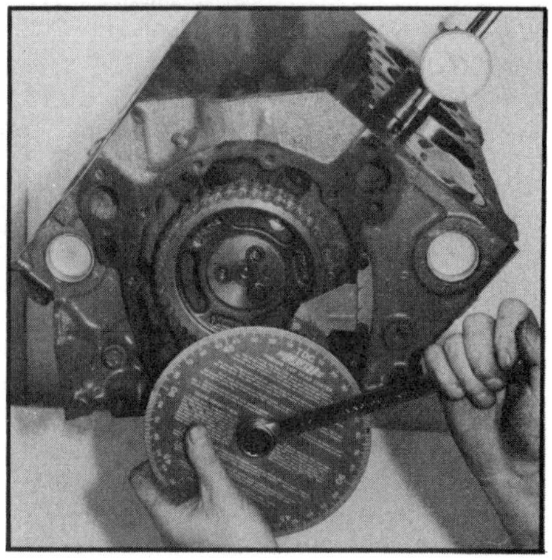

Camshaft timing is critical with a nitrous engine. Some of the author's tests indicate that a typical smallblock Chevy responds well with an additional four to six degrees of lobe displacement angle and the cam about eight degrees advanced.

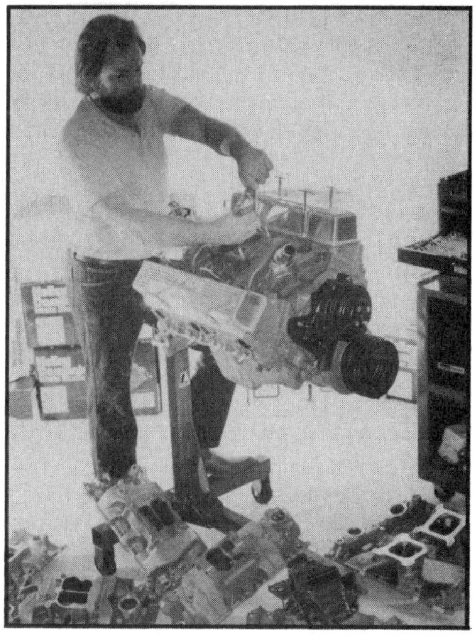

Numerous aftermarket manifolds are available for most domestic engines. A manifold that provides good performance during unboosted operation will also work well with nitrous. The most critical factor is uniform delivery of nitrous and enrichment fuel through all of the manifold runners.

MANIFOLD SPACER

Many performance engines re-

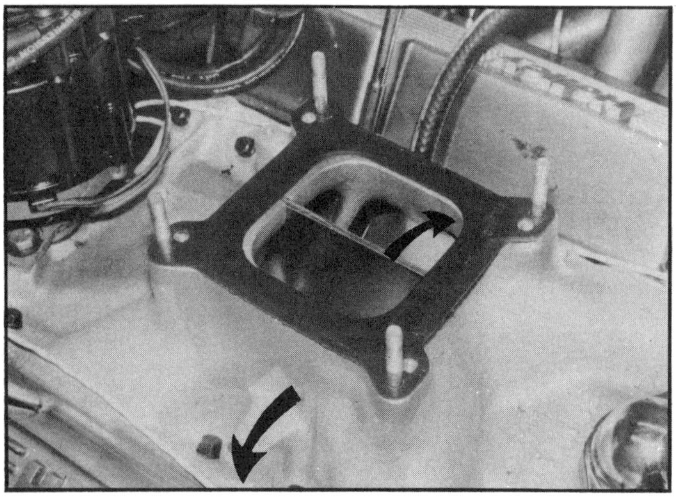

If cold-start performance is not critical (warmer climes), blocking the heat riser in the manifold may be worth about as much as seven horsepower during nonboosted operation and about 15 horsepower with nitrous (riser passage runs between cylinder-head mounting flanges across center of manifold--arrows indicate approximate location).

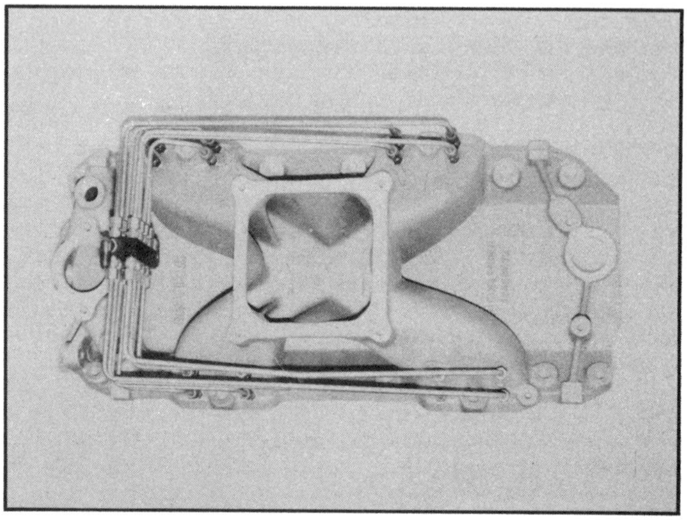

This Weiand big-port manifold works well on big Chevys—especially engines displacing 454 inches or more. The plenum flange is for a Holley Dominator; but on smaller engines (427cid or less) an 850cfm Holley, with an adapter, will improve low-speed response.

spond very well to an undivided spacer—about two inches thick—placed between the carburetor and manifold. Some engines seem to prefer a 4-hole spacer. The best setup depends on the specific intake manifold, carburetor, and camshaft combination.

The effects of a spacer are largely a matter of flow dynamics within the induction tract. These dynamics are complex, but in simplest terms large, open-type spacers increase the overall volume within the manifold plenum, and this generally results in improved high-rpm performance. Also, a spacer allows the fuel and air more time to mix before entering the manifold runner. Either effect may help performance, depending upon the engine and induction combination.

The effects of a 4-hole spacer are somewhat different. In this case some of the benefits are related to improved airflow in the area immediately beneath the throttle bores. The 4-hole spacer will also increase the plenum volume—but not as much as an open spacer—and give more time for the fuel and air to mix, though these effects are not as pronounced as with an open spacer. Nonetheless, some engines distinctly prefer a 4-hole spacer.

The spray orifices of some nitrous kits are already installed in relatively sophisticated spacers. For example, the 10,000 RPM system utilizes a 4-hole spacer to mount spray bars between the carb and manifold, and Rom Hammel attributes the improved performance—sometimes as much as 10 to 12 pounds-feet of extra torque throughout the rev range—to the spacer design.

If you are considering a nitrous kit that utilizes a smaller 0.50- or 0.75-inch thick spacer to locate the spray orifices, it might be interesting—assuming there is sufficient hood clearance—to try adding a 2-inch spacer beneath the nitrous spacer. If you do this, remember to put the nitrous spacer above the open spacer, because this will give the nitrous and fuel more time to mix before entering the port runners.

SINGLE CARBURETOR

The selection of the carburetor will affect overall performance. The type or brand will not be important (whatever you prefer will probably work fine), but for maximum performance the *airflow ratings* of the carburetor should be selected with an eye to the overall engine performance and the

If there's no vertical space constraints, the Edelbrock Victor Junior is a strong performer. A spacer with a plenum divider often improves low-speed power without sacrificing top-end performance.

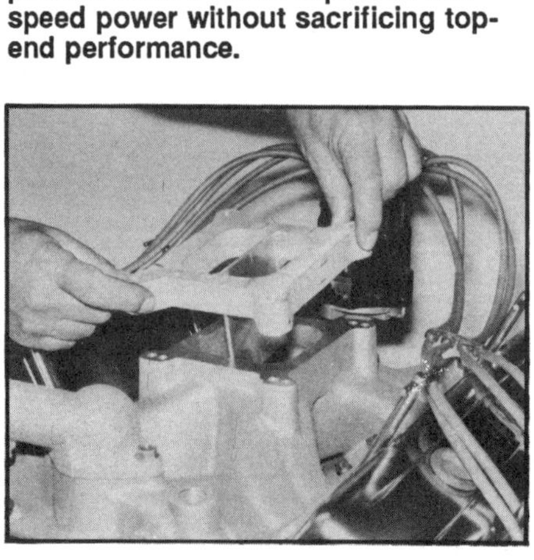

specific effect of the nitrous system.

In most cases the engine will be fitted with a single four-barrel carb. In situations where low- and mid-range performance is important—particularly street-type engines—it is helpful to use a carburetor with relatively small throttle bores. The small bores promote high air velocities through the venturis at low engine speeds (rpm), which provides rapid fuel-flow response and, as a result, excellent low-speed torque. On the other hand, a small carburetor will restrict top-end power because of the restricted maximum airflow capabilities.

However, carburetor response at low engine speeds is less important when the nitrous system is designed to boost low-rpm performance. And as is typical with this type of nitrous system—especially a single-stage system—the high-rpm nitrous boost will be less effective. As a result, a larger carb should enhance high-speed power without detracting from low-speed response (which is now boosted by the nitrous). In this case, selecting an 850cfm carburetor, instead of a 750cfm carburetor, could increase maximum power by 15, 20 or maybe as much as 30 horsepower on a large-displacement race-type engine.

Now consider a nitrous system designed to boost top-end power. In this instance the engine must be tuned for peak power, but with nitrous boost, it is practical, within certain limits, to reduce the carburetor rating in order to improve low-speed response. This approach can significantly improve the starting-line performance of a drag car. The smaller carburetor

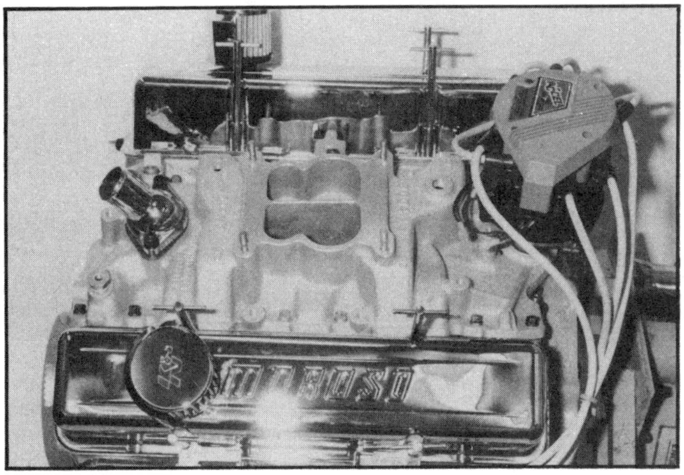

Manifold height is a limiting factor with most street machines, and the low-profile Weiand 8004 manifold works well with a typical spacer-plate spraybar system.

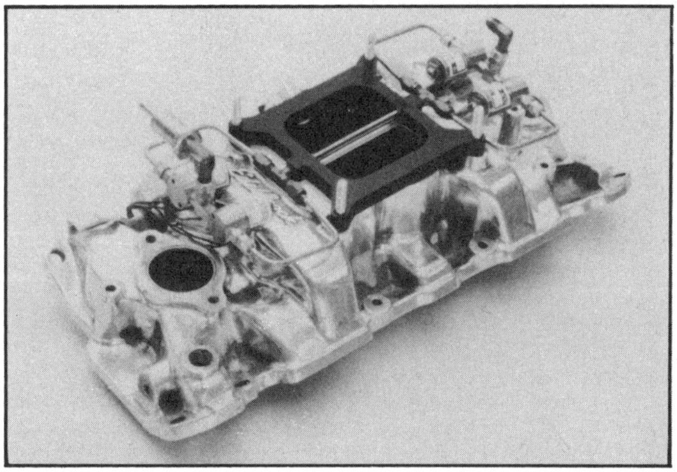

The Edelbrock Performer manifold works well on most street engines. It is shown here with an NOS Stage-2 kit.

should improve the launch characteristics of the engine and the nitrous will boost top-end performance. In effect, the nitrous and enrichment fuel will overcome the relatively restrictive airflow of the carb.

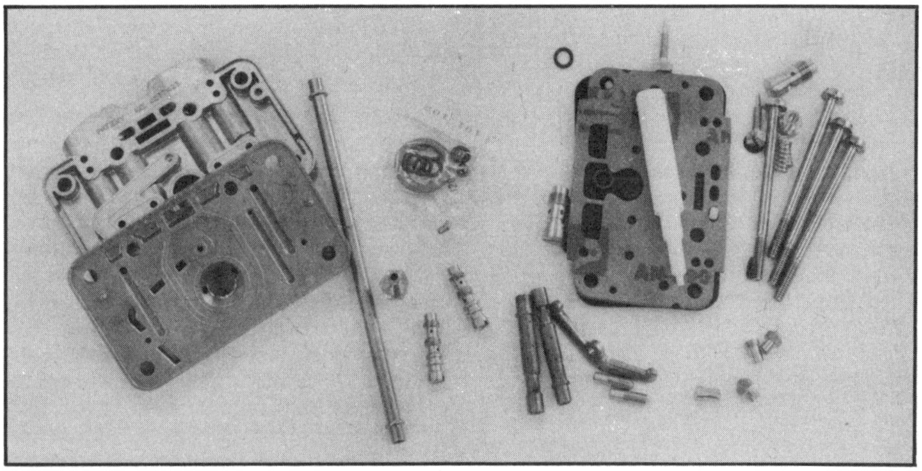

If the "unboosted" air-fuel ratio is not proper, the amounts of nitrous and fuel injected by the system may upset the overall fuel and air balance. This conversion adapts Weber calibration jets to Holley metering circuits. The modification allows the main metering jets to be changed without removing the float bowl.

DUAL 4-BARRELS

Many high-echelon race vehicles—such as Pro Stock drag machines—employ two 4-barrel carburetors and a racing-type manifold. These inductions systems almost always work well with nitrous injection. Carburetion capacity is rarely, if ever, a problem with this setup. The plenums on modern tunnel-ram manifolds intended for high-rpm racing are quite shallow, and it is important to ensure that the nitrous and enrichment fuel are thoroughly mixed at the point of injection.

There is also an important benefit when a 2x4 induction is used. With some attention to the placement of the nitrous and fuel orifices, the distribution can be calibrated to the specific needs of the engine. The best systems use multiple points of injection at both ends of the manifold and a stream of nitrous and fuel injected directly into each manifold runner. Under these conditions, the potential for near-perfect distribution exists.

The air-fuel ratio is critical—without and with nitrous injection. Virtually all of the dyno tests in this book were completed with a Holley electronic carburetor because it provides fast and accurate calibration.

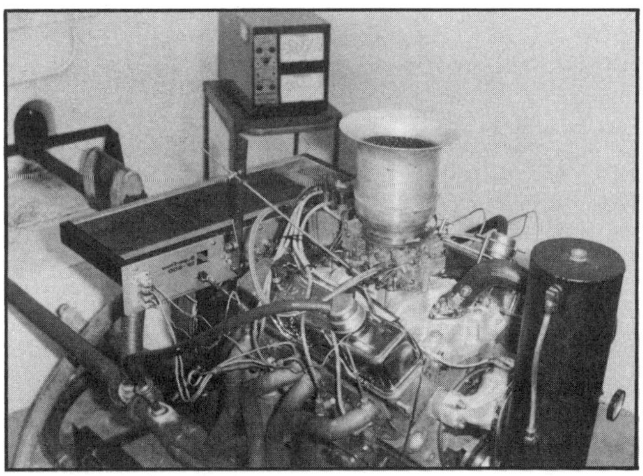

CAMSHAFT

Any cam that works in a non-injected performance engine will work *better* when used with nitrous, however the engine will generally produce more torque at a relatively lower engine speed. In other words, assuming that the cam reaches max torque around 4000rpm in a non-nitrous engine, when the nitrous is in operation, the "fat part" of the torque curve may begin as low as 2500rpm (depending on the amount of nitrous used).

Most performance cams are not designed for low-speed operation. These cams have a lot of valve-open duration and, consequently, excessive overlap. As a result, during the overlap sequence, the intake and exhaust can actually flow in reverse directions within the engine. These unusual conditions are well known to racing mechanics, and for our pur-

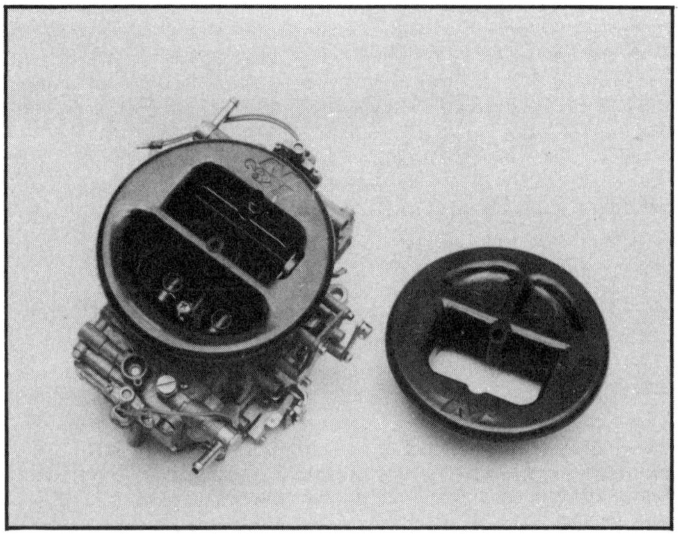

A simple velocity stack will significantly improve airflow into the carb and, hence, increase horsepower. Gains of 10 horsepower are common on a high-output smallblock Chevy, and increases as high as 22 horsepower have been recorded.

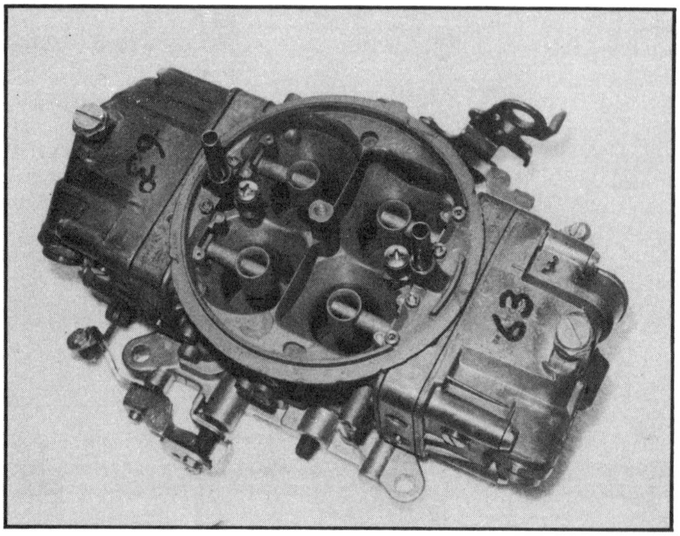

A professionally modified carburetor is expensive, but it may be worth more power on an all-out racing engine. This Braswell-modified Holley features improved flow, increased booster signal, four-corner idling, calibratable air bleeds and other racing-oriented refinements.

poses we will just assume the primary problem is reverse flow of spent exhaust gases past the intake valve as it raises off the seat in the so-called "blowdown" phase during crossover from the exhaust stroke to the intake stroke. Much of this "intake dilution" is due to the relatively slow exhaust velocity at the end of the exhaust stroke.

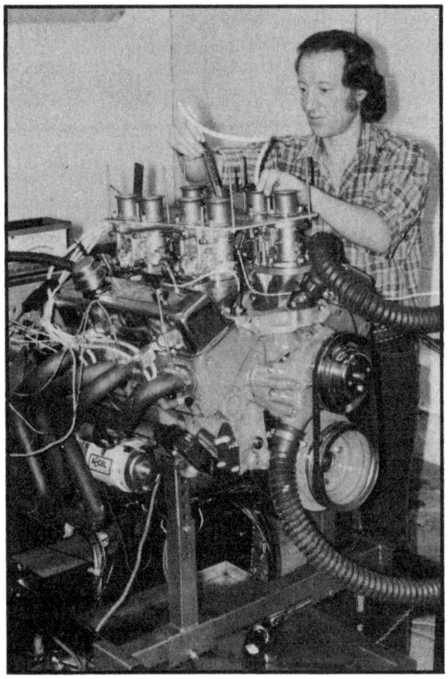

Since the nitrous system provides boost oxygen and fuel, the carburetor is not crucial—as long as it provides suitable performance during nonboosted operation. This innocuous 350cid truck engine produces 620 lbs/ft of torque and 520 horsepower—on nitrous, naturally.

However when the nitrous injection is activated, the substantial amount of exhaust created by the nitrous system causes the exhaust gases to flow out of the cylinder at considerable velocity. With a properly designed exhaust system this flow will cause an increased "extraction effect," which will continue throughout the complete exhaust cycle. When the overlap period is reached, the exhaust is still traveling fast enough and in the proper direction to resist any change of direction. This greatly reduces the possibility of reverse flow into the intake port. Indeed, the exhaust may have enough velocity to actually induce the intake charge to start moving into the cylinder even before the piston has reached top dead-center.

All of this boils down to one thing: the bad side effects of an extended overlap period are substantially reduced and the engine will generally run very strongly at lower engine speeds (with the nitrous in operation). And any cam that "works" without nitrous will generally be satisfactory with nitrous-oxide. However, it may not be the ultimate. Often, changes to the cam timing will improve power.

The first thing to consider is the exhaust. If we could use a larger exhaust valve and improve the flow through the exhaust port to cope with the extra exhaust, we might find that there is no need for additional exhaust timing. Unfortunately, this is impractical with most production cylinder heads. But a viable alternative is to open the exhaust valve a little earlier. It is difficult, however, to say exactly how much earlier, be-

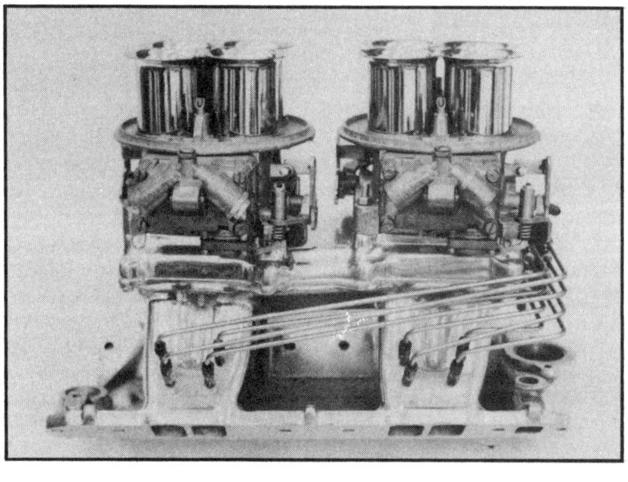

Performance intake manifolds are generally very efficient in stock form, but some builders love to fiddle with the port runners. This effort to find a few "extra" horsepower requires specialized equipment, including a completely instrumented flow bench and years of experience.

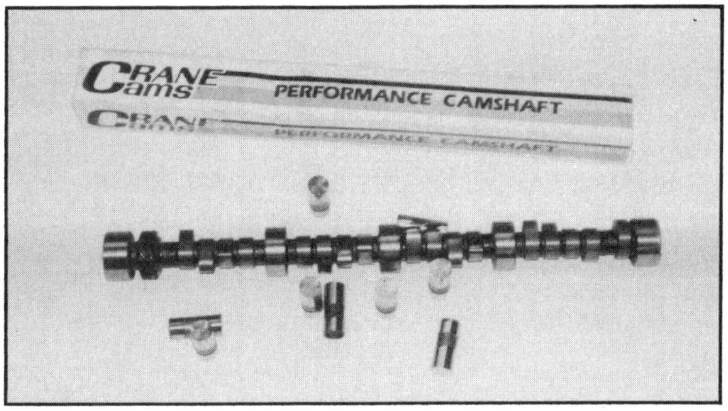

Many of the street hydraulic cams produced by Crane Cams have relatively large lobe displacement angles (112 degrees). Consequently, these cams perform very well in nitrous-injected engines.

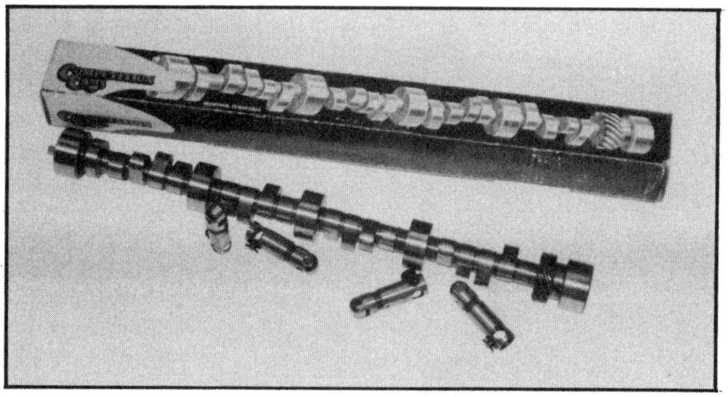

Even though roller cams are not generally suitable for street-type engines, they are common in competition engines. This roller cam produced 30 additional horsepower compared to a similar flat-tappet cam of identical duration and timing.

cause the ultimate exhaust opening point depends upon several engine variables. It is possible, though, to alter the cam phasing to see if any improvements can be found. (Typically, opening the exhaust 5 degrees earlier will show some improvement in most low-speed engines and 10-15 degrees earlier may help some very high-rpm engines.)

In addition, closing the exhaust 5 or maybe even 10 degrees sooner can also improve low-speed power. In this discussion "low-speed" refers to about 4000rpm or so. This will certainly improve the engine idle and responsiveness (while it is not being boosted with nitrous). In other words, what we've done here is to move the entire exhaust cycle into the power stroke by 5 to 10 degrees.

As far as the intake is concerned, with nitrous boost we find that it is not necessary to have the intake valve open quite as long. Remember, a nitrous engine produces max power at relatively lower engine speeds (compared to a normally-aspirated engine). Consequently, the engine can benefit from slightly shorter intake timing and the peak power point will usually occur about 1000rpm lower in the speed band. At the bottom line, this means that the total intake duration can be reduced by 10 to 15 degrees. (A typical race cam may have around 305 to 320 degrees of intake duration, and the nitrous equivalent should have about 290 to 305 degrees).

Some protagonists of nitrous injection claim that it is better to use more intake timing and, to a degree, there is justification for this. Longer intake timing will curb low-end power and reduce the likelihood of detonation. However, I believe if low-end power is a problem—in that there may be too much torque for the traction capabilities of the chassis—it would be much better to "trim" the nitrous system or ignition advance at low speeds to produce less power. If *unboosted performance* (without nitrous) is important, the longer timing on the intake valve will increase top-end power, but remember, because of the torque characteristics of nitrous, in general it is more effective to use the nitrous to develop low-speed torque rather than twist the engine tighter to make high-rpm power.

VALVETRAIN

A super-lift valvetrain is not necessary or desirable on a nitrous engine. Many drag-race smallblock Chevys are equipped with cams that produce as much as 0.750-inch lift at the valve. This places tremendous stress on the valvetrain, and the valve gear tends to break down under this kind of loading. With nitrous injection, the power output can readily be increased (within limits) by simply supplying more nitrous-fuel to the engine. It is not necessary, therefore, to "overlift" the valves in an effort to force more intake charge into the engine.

With nitrous augmentation, it is usually possible to achieve very high power levels from a smallblock Chevy with net valve lifts of about 0.650-inch. Indeed, lift numbers in the range of 0.580- to 0.600-inch will produce very respectable and reliable results from nitrous boost. Nevertheless, the best camshaft for any given situation will depend on the design and specific configuration of the engine and the required relationship between unboosted and boosted modes of operation. If nitrous is being used for an occasional punch of power, the camshaft should be selected to obtain maximum effect during unboosted operation. This may require more lift than absolutely necessary for optimum nitrous operation.

One area that is worth exploring is the advantage provided by roller-tipped valve lifters. As most performance enthusiasts know, a roller lifter can follow a more "severe" lobe profile, which results in "faster" valve-opening rates. Even with identical nominal lift and timing figures (but faster valve rates), a typical roller cam can produce as much as a 20 to 30 horsepower output increase over a flat-lifter cam. This can be especially helpful on the exhaust side of a nitrous engine. Pushing the exhaust open more quickly allows the exhaust to achieve higher flow rates during the early portion of the flow cycle. In a general sense, this improves exhaust

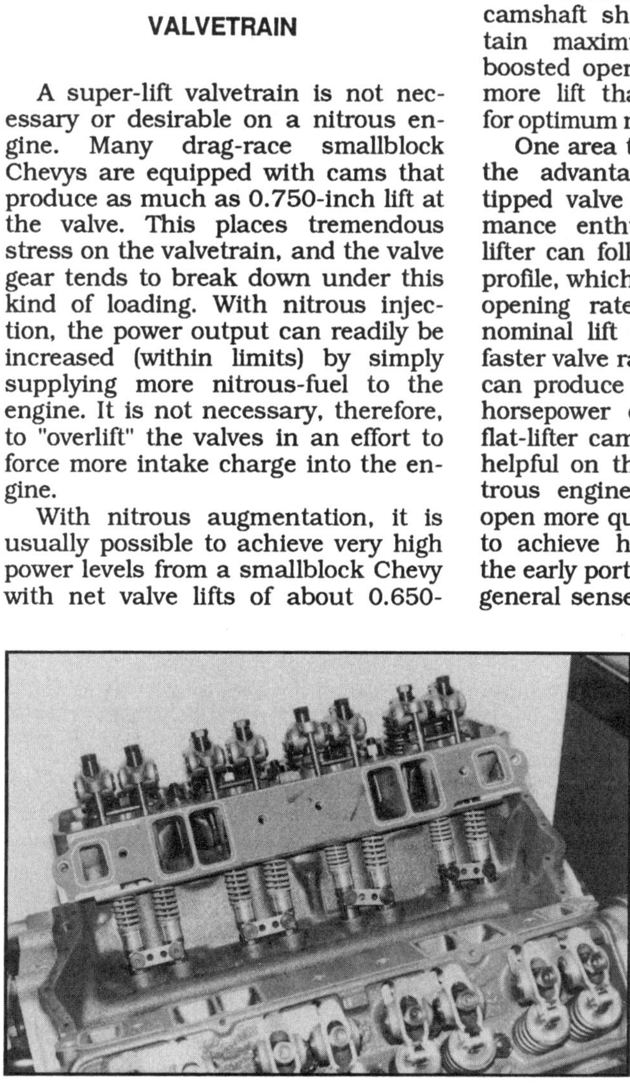

Because nitrous engines develop peak torque and power at relatively lower engine speeds, it is usually not necessary to use rev kits and fancy high-rpm valve gear.

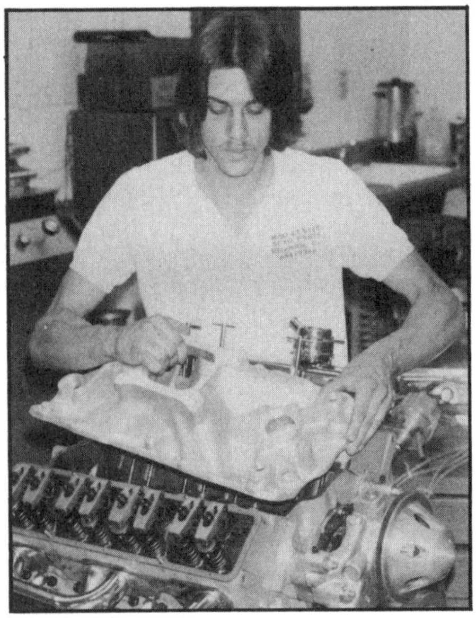

Although nitrous injection makes it a lot simpler for the performance enthusiast, the combination of intake manifold, valvetrain, cylinder heads, and exhaust system is still crucial for maximum power.

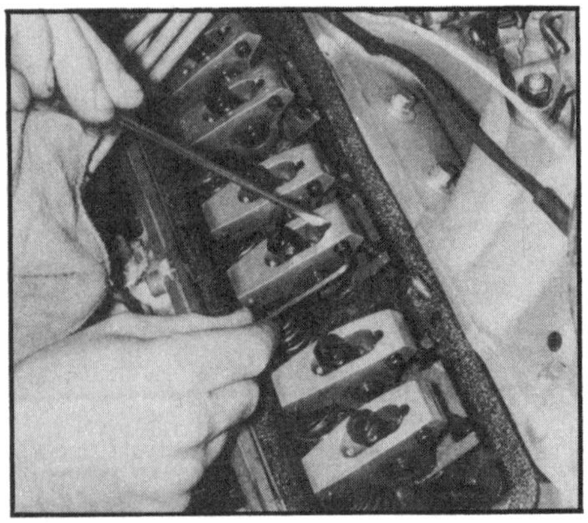

Dyno tests with various cam and rockerarm combinations showed that lift and duration was an important factor on the intake side of the smallblock Chevy; but on the exhaust side, duration affected power far more than the amount of lift.

"breathing," an important consideration during periods of nitrous operation.

In all candor, a flat-lifter cam (with either solid or hydraulic followers) that is well-matched to the load requirements will work adequately for most situations. For an all-out engine, though, a well-matched roller cam will probably be a little bit better.

IGNITION CHARACTERISTICS

It is easy to believe that nitrous-oxide places extra demands on the ignition system. Quite to the contrary, nitrous acts as both an ignition accelerator and ignition enhancer. Some portion of the nitrous inevitably converts to a gaseous form before it enters the combustion chamber, and the available "extra" oxygen content from the nitrous enhances the ignitability of whatever fuel may be present.

This can be an advantage. For instance, in the recent past a system was developed to inject *gaseous* nitrous-oxide into supercharged Top-Fuel drag engines during idle. This technique effectively "cleans up" the very rough idle characteristics associated with these engines. Primarily as a result of more effective and reliable ignition operation, when the throttle is punched open, the engine reacts instantly, without the hesitation or stumbling that is typical of a "loaded up" engine.

The problems with nitrous arise primarily when the nitrous injection *isn't* being used. To understand this, we need to look at the general spark-plug requirements of a nitrous-injected engine.

SPARK PLUGS

The major limitation of any engine—including a nitrous-injected engine—is detonation; and one of the primary sources of detonation is overheated spark-plug electrodes. *If detonation from this source is to be avoided, careful attention must be paid to the selection of spark-plug heat range.*

The increased combustion temperatures created during nitrous injection will almost always require spark plugs that are two or three heat ranges colder than normal. This is an expected and reasonable response to the effects of nitrous; however there are always exceptions and, in all instances, a careful examination of the spark-plug conditions will be required to ensure that detonating does not occur during nitrous operation.

After a few exploratory activations of the nitrous system, the spark-plug conditions must be checked. If there are any signs of spark-plug overheating, *do not use the nitrous system!* Exchange the spark plugs for replacements that have a colder heat rating. If the engine is operated with overheated spark plugs, there is a high likelihood that detonation will chew up a piston or two.

If plugs are overheating but it is absolutely necessary to use the nitrous, a *temporary* fix is to reduce the combustion temperature by increasing the amount of enrichment fuel. This will usually help cool the spark plugs, but remember, this is no more than a crude band-aid fix. To maintain safe combustion temperatures, the enrichment fuel of most out-of-the-box nitrous systems is already calibrated on the rich side. Adding more enrichment fuel will inevitably reduce the peak horsepower.

SPARK PLUG SELECTION

In the final analysis, just how "fussy" an engine is to spark-plug temperatures depends on the type and specific configuration of the engine. The recommendations given here are intended as useful general guidelines, however, the only sure cure for detonation is a methodical and careful monitoring of spark-plug conditions.

In general, it is wise *not* to use resistor-type spark plugs in a nitrous engine. Of course, resistor plugs are used in production engines when suppression of radio interference is important, but some brands are far less forgiving to variations in combustion temperatures.

Spark plugs that use a copper alloy in the electrodes are far more forgiving—in terms of operating temperatures—and they will generally tolerate relatively high temperatures without the central electrode overheating. Virtually all major brands now produce a copper-core plug (i.e., a plug with a central electrode made from a copper alloy), and this type of plug is highly recommended for a nitrous engine.

Sometimes the central electrode of the plug runs cool enough, but the side electrode doesn't. When this occurs, a colder plug is of no help whatsoever. Indeed, the side electrode can be a common source of detonation. If the side electrode becomes too hot, it will melt and cause the onset of detonation. In extreme cases the electrode may completely disappear. *And on the way to its demise, it will induce detonation, causing the piston to melt and, possibly, damaging the exhaust valve seats.*

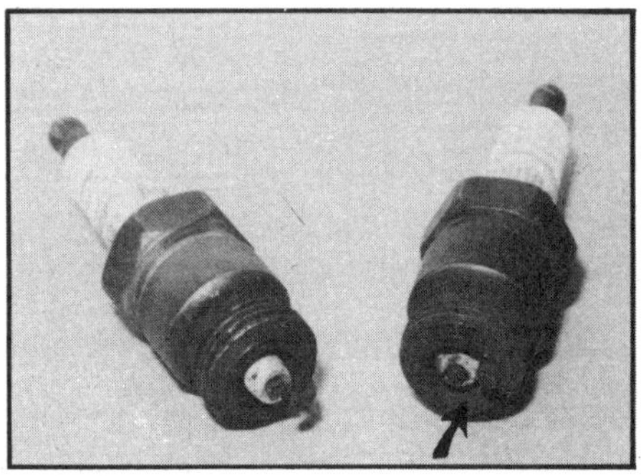

These spark plugs were perfectly adequate for a naturally-aspirated engine producing 1.2 hp/inch. However, when the nitrous system was activated, boosting the power to about 1.8 hp/inch, the tip melted in a period of 10 to 15 seconds.

Under these circumstances it is necessary to use a plug with *shorter* side electrodes. (Here, "shorter" refers to the total length of the electrode, measured from the tip to the point where it joins the shell of the plug.) Usually, extended-nose plugs have a relatively short side electrode. Some models have a short, straight electrode that is welded to the face of the outer shell and projects across to the central electrode. In other words, this design is much like a retracted-nose plug. If overheating of the side electrode appears to be a problem, this type of plug will generally withstand high heat loading better than a conventional plug. (If one of these plugs melts, the engine is probably already beyond saving!)

In extreme cases it may be necessary to use "retracted-nose" spark plugs. This type of plug is commonly used in racing engines, but very few street engines require them. However, with high-horsepower nitrous systems—those that are more suited to competitive racing—a retracted plug may be required to solve overheating problems. Whenever heavy loads of nitrous are used, it is a good idea to try retracted-nose plugs. In some cases the engine will gain horsepower, *even though there may not be signs of overheating with conventional spark plugs.*

There are also some spark plugs that have "side-wire" electrodes. These plugs do not fair very well in a nitrous engine because the thin electrode cannot conduct heat fast enough to prevent overheating. This type of plug often works very well in a normally-aspirated engine, but they should not be used in a nitrous engine.

In general, a nitrous engine is less sensitive to plug gap than an engine running on straight gasoline. Very often wide plug gaps will improve power slightly in a conventional engine, but when gasoline and nitrous are used, most engines seem to lose sensitivity to the size of the plug gap.

For best results during unboosted operation, the typical smallblock Chevy nitrous engine requires plug gaps no wider than 0.030- to 0.035-inch. It is generally acknowledged, however, that the relatively small Chevrolet combustion chamber is very efficient—provided the piston dome does not block-up the chamber and prevent even flame propagation—and even a minimal spark usually works fine. On the other hand, many other engines demonstrate a greater sensitivity to gap widths. Engines that have hemispherical or large open-type combustion chamber configurations and engines that have relatively large cylinder bores may respond to wider gaps. Quite often, experiments with the plug gap will produce interesting results, but the upper limit is generally about 0.055-inch. (Remember, of course, that very wide spark-plug gaps are only practical when the entire ignition system is capable of producing and reliably transmitting very high voltages.)

The situation also changes when alcohol is used. Often the fuel "droplets" entering the chamber are quite large and the mixture becomes difficult to ignite, even in the presence of nitrous. Under these conditions, opening the gap to 0.050-inch may produce better results; but this is really just another band-aid fix. If a wide plug gap produces positive results, there is always the possibility that another problem is present—often one of carburetion, fuel injection or manifold distribution shortcomings.

AFTERMARKET IGNITION SYSTEMS

Most manufacturers of nitrous kits recommend using a good electronic ignition system. Even though nitrous assists the initiation of ignition in the chamber, a good ignition will keep the engine running in top shape in both boosted and unboosted modes. As noted above, the proper spark plug (heat range) for nitrous operation will probably be colder than the plug that would be optimum for non-nitrous running. It is, however, essential to use a cold plug to prevent problems when the nitrous is activated, and a high-voltage electronic ignition will keep these "cool" plugs from fouling during normal, everyday operation.

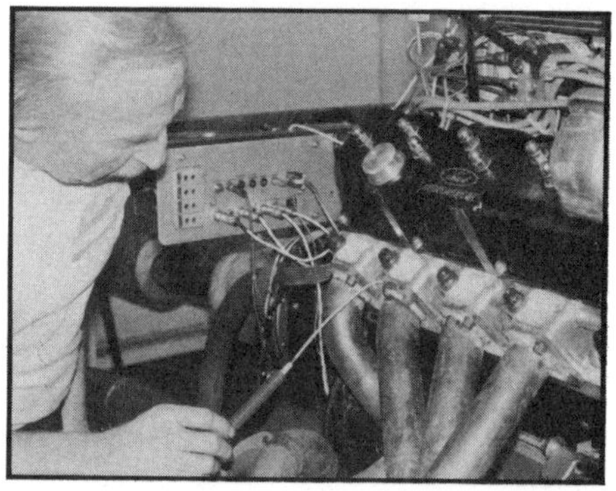

While "dialing in" a high-output engine it is a good idea to periodically check the piston deck for signs of detonation. When a small light is inserted though the spark-plug hole, a substantial area of the piston dome can be viewed.

A conventional Kettering-type (breaker-point) ignition with some sort of "souped-up" coil would probably provide sufficient secondary voltage to fire the plugs in all but the most radical nitrous engine. However, Kettering ignitions have never been noted for their long-term reliability. And considering the number and common availability of high-quality, breakerless electronic ignitions currently available on the aftermarket, there is no reasonable or defensible argument for using a Kettering ignition on a modern performance engine.

Some electronic ignitions will work with conventional breaker-point distributors, but a breakerless distributor, or a conventional distributor that has been changed over to breakerless operation with some sort of conversion kit, will virtually eliminate the need for any periodic maintenance. Most of the currently available factory or specialty breakerless distributors are absolutely reliable, and there are a variety of models to fit virtually any engine.

For example, the General Motors HEI production system (High Energy Ignition) is a good choice for a nitrous engine with a rev limit of about 5500rpm. The HEI delivers a high-quality spark—especially at low engine speeds—even when plugs are

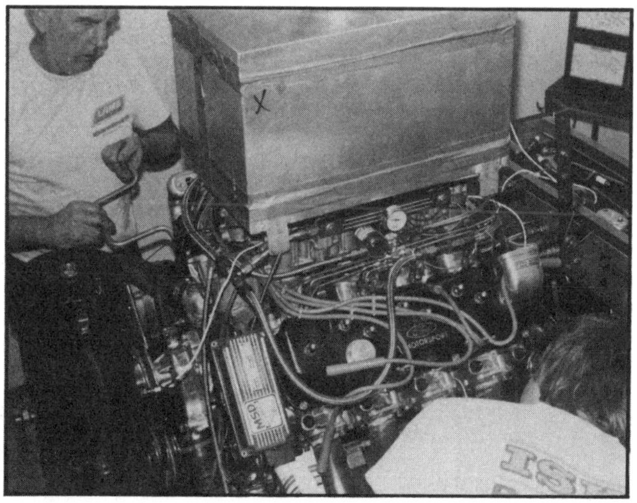

This smallblock Ford engine pumps out almost 800 horsepower. The highly efficient MSD (Multiple Spark Discharge) ignition system, including the breakerless distributor, is from Autotronic Controls.

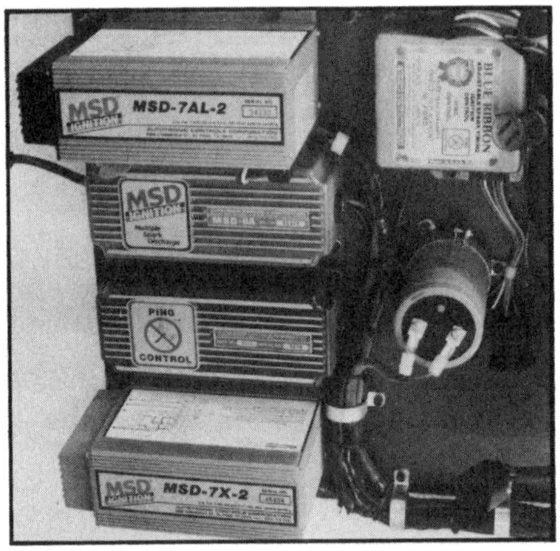

The system on the author's dyno allows various ignition modules and coils to be selected during engine operation. This permits easy and accurate back-to-back evaluation of ignition systems.

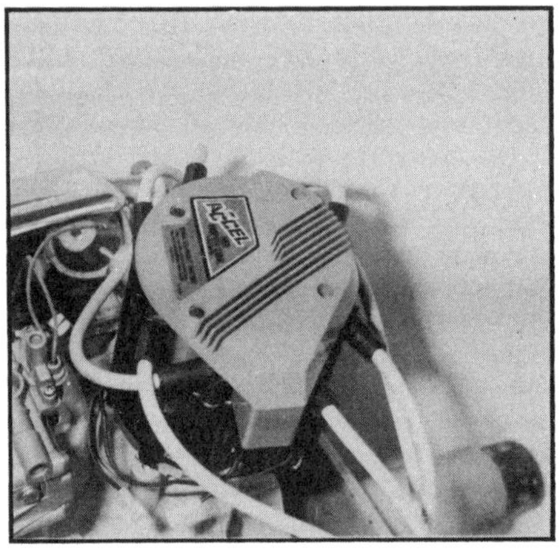

The stock GM HEI ignition system is adequate for most street applications; but at high rpm, the coil does not produce enough secondary voltage. This can be remedied by installing a high-energy coil.

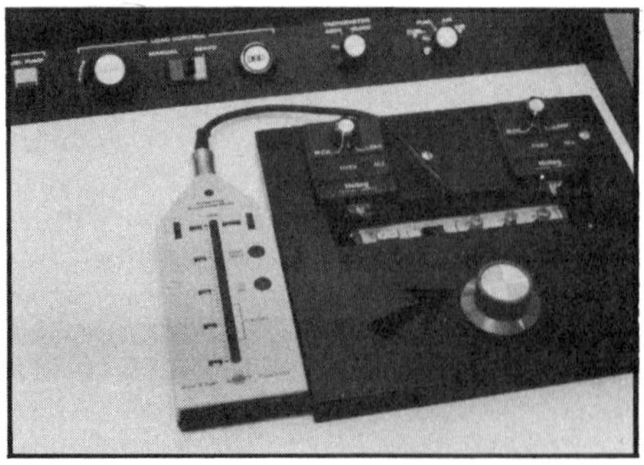

During testing on the author's dyno the ignition advance can be remotely advanced or retarded in increments as small as one-half degree (note control knob on the console). This allows precise exploration of ignition characteristics. The vertical scale to the left is a noise meter; a high-boost nitrous system will raise the noise level about 5db.

fouled and/or have wide gaps. Unless the situation has deteriorated to extreme limits, a stock HEI will deliver enough voltage to fire the plugs during boosted or unboosted operation.

However, it is important to realize that the HEI is strongest at the low end of the rpm range. In other words, it delivers a very intense spark at cranking speeds (this ensures that the stock GM engine will start quickly), but at higher speeds the spark quality drops off. This is due to the relatively weak coil used with the system, and the fact that the "saturation time" of the coil is insufficient above 5000rpm to deliver an optimum spark. This can be a problem with a racing engine, but the HEI should be adequate for most street engines.

If the situation requires it, the HEI system can easily be reinforced by using a high-output coil (both Accel and Autotronic Controls make high-voltage coils for the stock HEI). It is also possible to use an electronic add-on system—like the Autotronic Controls MSD6 and matching coil—to give the ignition a real jolt.

IGNITION TIMING

Nitrous injection changes the ignition timing requirements of the engine. The ignition timing can be optimized when the nitrous is not in use, but *as soon as the nitrous is introduced, the optimum timing for max power will change.* Because the nitrous creates better combustion characteristics, the amount of advance required will be *reduced.*

Very often this ignition requirement is overlooked, but it can mean a lot of extra performance. For example, I remember of one instance when a well-tuned kit produced a boost of about 100 horsepower before the ignition was optimized (for the nitrous), but when the ignition timing was properly adjusted to compensate for the nitrous injection, the boost jumped to 135 horsepower. (The engine was running on high-octane pump gasoline.) And no matter how you look at it, 35 horsepower is a big performance gain.

Typically, each 50-horsepower increment in nitrous boost will require about 1 or 1.5 degrees *less* total advance. This seems to be true irrespective of the amount of nitrous injected to the engine. However, when only 25 to 50 horsepower of nitrous boost is used, the difference in the timing requirement is small and may be insignificant. Remember, though, that this is a rule of thumb, and not an absolute fact. Some testing will be required to determine the best timing curve for a specific engine, but in almost all cases, it is worth the effort to retard the advance (as compared to the total advance used without nitrous injection) to determine if there will be a significant improvement in output.

Also, when an engine needs relatively less total advance without nitrous, less "retarding" is necessary to compensate for the nitrous. For instance, many late-model production engines have relatively high intake-charge temperatures and, consequently, won't stand much total advance. In stock form some of these engines run as little as 25 degrees total advance. Under these circumstances, the ignition timing may not need to be retarded. Even if power is boosted by as much as 125 horsepower—this is about the maximum boost level that such an engine could reasonably tolerate—the optimum advance would probably not change, simply because 25 degrees is not a lot of total advance to begin with. In this case, the chance of "over-advancing" the engine during nitrous operation is small (assuming, of course, the engine shows no signs of detonation on the plugs when the nitrous is used).

The major ignition problems arise in racing engines that may have as much as 38 to 45 degrees of advance. Adding a 150-horsepower nitrous kit to a high-power engine will dramatically alter the optimum ignition timing. With nitrous, best power may result when the advance is reduced to as little as 23 to 25 degrees. If such an engine produces best power with a lot more advance than this, the fuel-to-

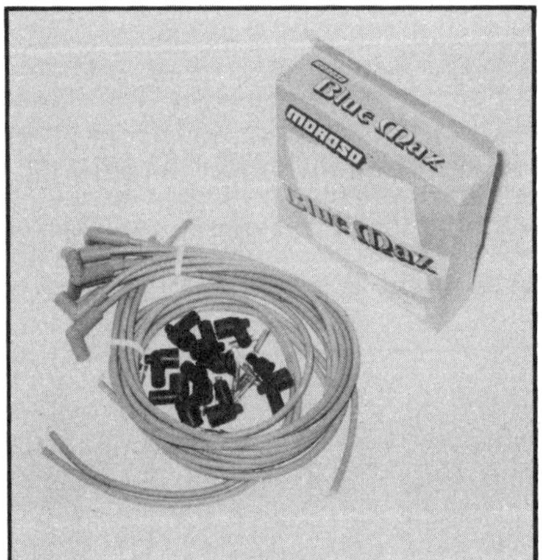

Ignition crossfire will quickly lead to disaster in a nitrous engine. Every performance engine should be equipped with heavily insulated (8mm), silicone-jacketed plug wires that are carefully loomed to prevent induction or short-circuit crossfire.

nitrous ratio should be checked. It could well be that the mixture is excessively rich—causing fuel saturation—which may inhibit combustion.

When the need for retard is determined, the next problem is to devise a simple and reliable method to appropriately reduce ignition advance whenever the nitrous system is in operation. Many late-model cars have computer-controlled ignitions and most specialty ignitions use electronic amplifiers of one sort or another, so the problem can be somewhat difficult. However, one of the easiest ways to solve the problem is to use an MSD Ping Control. This device works with the MSD ignition—it was originally designed to compensate for low-octane gasoline—and allows the driver to manually decrease or increase the advance by as much as 15 degrees (this is usually more than enough for a street or racing nitrous system). The Ping Control can easily be connected to a throttle switch that will activate the Ping Control—retarding the ignition—when the nitrous is in operation.

There may be even a simpler solution for certain all-out racing engines. Many racing engines currently use "crank-triggered" ignitions that have a fixed amount of advance. These systems are sometimes fitted with more than one trigger sensor—one is used for maximum advance and one is offset slightly to retard the ignition during startup. The engine is started on the "retarded" sensor and the driver simply switches to the "advanced" sensor once the engine is running. A similar arrangement—but in reverse—can be adapted to the nitrous injection. When the nitrous is activated, the ignition can be switched to a retarded sensor that will reduce the total advance to the required amount for best peak power.

There are, of course, several variations of this general theme. With some ingenuity the reader can devise a simple and reliable retard that will answer the specific needs of the engine and operational conditions.

HEADERS

Selecting headers for a nitrous engine is simple: The increased exhaust flow created by the nitrous injection dictates a large-diameter header. This applies especially to racing applications, but if the vehicle is used for daily transportation, consider the amount of time that the engine is operated without nitrous compared to the time with nitrous. Remember that large-diameter headers tend to reduce mileage, and typically, a street machine will give better day-to-day performance if the headers are selected to give maximum horsepower when the nitrous is not being used. When the engine is built for full-time racing the headers should be 1/8- to 1/4-inch larger than would normally be the case.

EXHAUST SYSTEMS

Back pressure in the exhaust system of an engine spells lost horsepower—whether the engine is nitrous-injected or not. Because nitrous-oxide produces such large quantities of exhaust gas, make certain that the exhaust system can handle the increased flow. Ignoring this area can result in 50 or more lost horsepower. If modifications are limited by emission requirements, the only option may be to build a custom large-tubing, dual-exhaust system using two high-flow catalytic converters (or two per side in parallel) and two efficient mufflers. Make sure the system includes a crossover pipe ahead of the mufflers, as this will substantially increase flow in any dual-exhaust system.

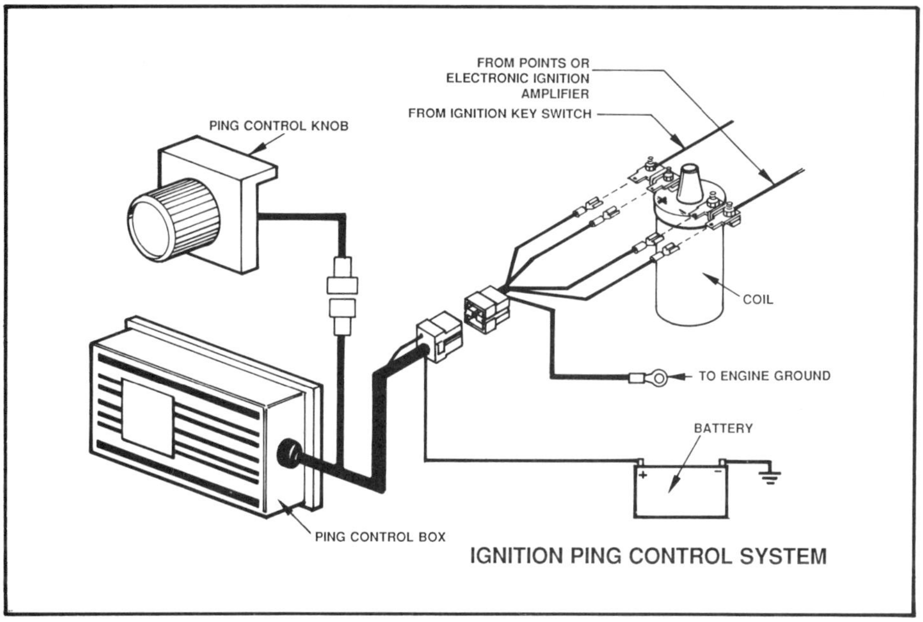

FIGURE 10-1: An MSD "ping control" system allows the timing to be varied by simply turning the dash-mounted control knob. This system is compatible with almost all vehicles (including many late-model systems) and can optimize the timing for operation with or without nitrous.

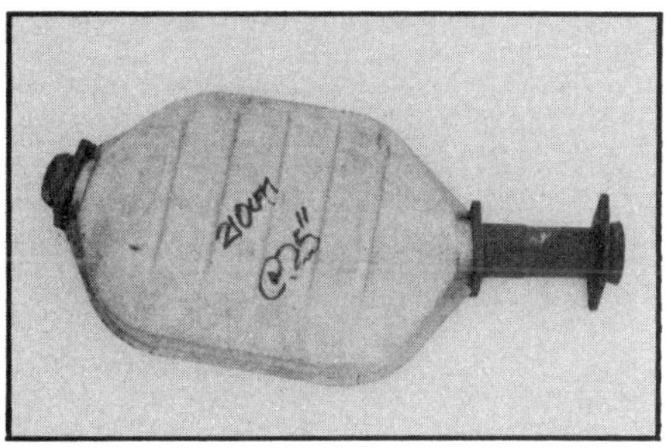

Restrictive catalytic converters inhibit the exhaust efficiency of an engine. During nitrous operation the volume of exhaust gas increases dramatically; a restrictive exhaust system will severely limit peak output.

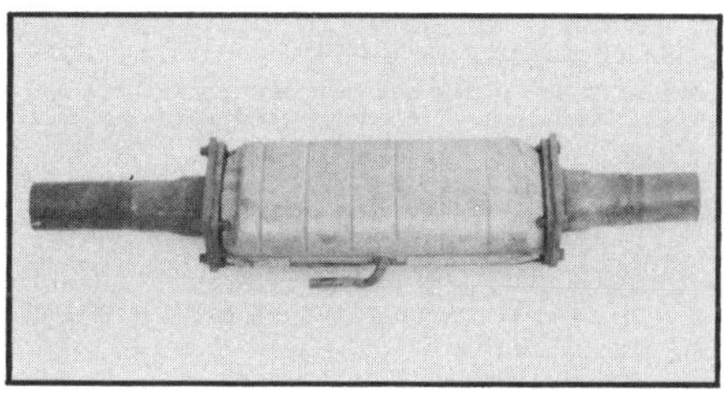

This General Motors high-flow catalytic converter is a good example of a cost-effective design that can legally improve engine output. Although it is expensive, this converter can add 30 horsepower to a non-boosted 305cid engine and as much as 50 horsepower when nitrous is used.

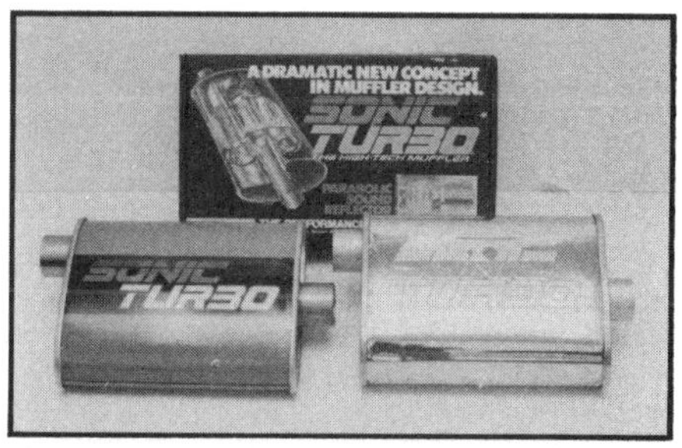

The final key to efficient exhaust flow is the design of the muffler. At the time of this writing, these high-flow "turbo mufflers" are among the most effective and efficient street-legal mufflers available.

BUYERS GUIDE

NITROUS-OXIDE INJECTION SYSTEMS

10,000 RPM SPEED EQUIPMENT
1922 Gladwick Street
West Compton, CA 90220
213-638-7780--Order & Tech
Retail Catalog: $3.00

MARVIN MILLER MFG./CHETAH SYSTEMS
7745 S. Greenleaf Avenue
Whittier, CA 90602
213-693-8235--Order & Tech
Retail Catalog: $2.00

NITROUS-OXIDE SYSTEMS
5930 Lakeshore Drive
Cypress, CA 90630
714-821-0580--Order & Tech
Retail Catalog: Free

RAM AUTOMOTIVE/ICE SYSTEMS
201 Business Park Blvd.
Columbia, SC 29203
800-845-2383--Order & Tech
Retail Catalog: $4.00

AIRCRAFT HOSE & FITTINGS

EARL'S PERFORMANCE PRODUCTS
825 E. Sepulveda
Carson CA 90745
213-830-1620
Retail Catalog: $4.00

RUSSELL PERFORMANCE PRODUCTS
6301 East Alondra Blvd.
Paramount, CA 90723
213-602-1202--Order & Tech
Retail Catalog: $5.00

AIR CLEANERS

K&N ENGINEERING
561 Iowa Avenue
PO Box 1329
Riverside CA 92502
800-858-3333--Outside CA
714-684-9762
Retail Catalog: $3.00

CAMS/VALVETRAIN

BILL MITCHELL RACING CAMS
800 Tanglewood Road
West Islip NY 11795
Retail Catalog: $3.00

CAM DYNAMICS
530 Fentress Blvd.
Daytona Beach, FL 32014
904-258-8845
Retail Catalog: $3.00

COMPETITION CAMS
3406 Democrat
Memphis TN 38118
901-795-2400
Retail Catalog: $5.00

CRANE CAMS
530 Fentress Blvd.
Daytona Beach FL 32014
904-252-1151
Retail Catalog: $4.00

CROWER CAMS & EQUIPMENT
3333 Main Street
Chula Vista CA 92011
619-422-1191
Retail Catalog: $3.00

ENGLE RACING CAMS
1621 12th Street
Santa Monica CA 90404
213-450-0806--Order & Tech
Retail Catalog: $2.00

ERSON RACING CAMS INC.
550 Mallory Way
Carson City NV 89701
702-882-1622
Retail Catalog: $4

ISKENDERIAN RACING CAMS
16020 S. Broadway
Gardena CA 90248
213-770-0930
Retail Catalog: $3.00

LUNATI RACING CAMS
4770 Lamar Avenue
P.O. Box 18021
Memphis TN 38118
901-365-0950--Order & Tech
Retail Catalog: $3.00

RACER BROWN
12111-1/2 Brandford St.
Bldg. C-4
Sun Valley CA 91352
818-897-4044
Newsletter: Free

SCHNEIDER RACING CAMS
1235 Cushman Ave.
San Diego CA 92110
619-297-0227--Order & Tech
Retail Catalog: $3.00

STAHL CAMS, INC.
1513 Mt. Rose Avenue
York, PA 17403
717-846-3123--Order & Tech
Retail Catalog: None

CARBURETION & FUEL INJECTION

BRASWELL CARBURETION
1650 E. 18 Street, Unit P
Tucson AZ 85719
602-884-7282
Retail Catalog: None

CARTER AUTOMOTIVE CO. INC.
(Carter Carburetors)
9666 Olive Street Blvd.
St. Louis MO 63132
314-997-7400
Retail Catalog: available at Federal-Mogal dealers; for location call above number.

FUEL INJECTION ENGINEERING
25891 Crown Valley Parkway
So. Laguna CA 92677
714-582-1170--Order & Tech
Retail Catalog: $2.50

HOLLEY REPLACEMENT PARTS DIV.
11955 E. Nine Mile Road
Warren MI 48089
For technical information, hard-to-get parts, and literature, call: 615-859-4924
Retail Catalog: $3.00

MIKE JONES CARBURETION
7602 Talbert Avenue, #6
Huntington Beach CA 92647
714-848-5505--Order
714-848-5500--Tech
Retail Catalog: $2.00

WALBRO CORPORATION
Automotive Products Group
630 Columbia Street
Caro, MI 48723
517-673-7727
Retail Catalog: Free

CYLINDER HEAD & VALVETRAIN

MONROE'S PORTING
2626 S. Bedford Street
Los Angeles, CA 90034
213-836-3214 &
213-837-2475--Order & Tech
Retail Catalog: None

MULLEN & CO.
348-C East Carson St.
Carson CA 90745
213-835-0686

HEADERS

CYCLONE EXHAUST
19007 S. Reyes Ave.
Compton CA 90221
213-639-6211
For Catalog: 216-398-8300, ext. 333
Catalog Price: $3.00

DOUG THORLEY HEADERS
1561 Commerce St.
Corona CA 91720
714-735-7280
Retail Catalog: Free

EAGLE HEADERS
19007 S. Reyes Ave.
Compton CA 90221
213-639-6211
For Catalog: 216-398-8300, ext. 333
Catalog Price: $3.00

HEADERS BY ED
2710-SA 16th Avenue S.
Minneapolis MN 55407
612-729-2802
Header Catalog: $3.95
Header Parts Catalog: $2.95

HEDMAN MFG.
9599 W. Jefferson Blvd.
Culver City CA 93021
213-839-7581
Retail Catalog: $3.00

HOOKER HEADERS
1024 W. Brooks St.
Ontario CA 91762
714-983-5871
Retail Catalog: $4.00

STAHL HEADERS
1515 Mt. Rose Ave.
York PA 17403
717-846-1632
Retail Catalog: Free

WALKER MANUFACTURING
1201 Michigan Blvd.
Racine WI 53402
414-632-8871
Retail Catalog: Free

IGNITION

ACCEL IGNITION
Echlin Road
US Route 1
Branford CT 06405
203-481-5771--Order & Tech
Retail Catalog: $4.00

ALLISON AUTOMOTIVE
720 E. Cypress Ave.
Monrovia CA 91016
818-303-3621--Order
800-325-2159--US Tech
800-325-5864--CA Tech
Retail Catalog: $2.00

AUTOTRONIC CONTROLS CORP.
MSD IGNITION
1490 Henry Brennan Dr.
El Paso TX 79936
915-857-5200
Retail Catalog: $2.00

GENERAL NUCLEONICS
SPEEDATRON
2807 Metropolitan Place
Pomona CA 91767
714-593-4985
Retail Catalog: None

MALLORY IGNITION
550 Mallory Way
Carson City NV 89701
702-882-6600
Retail Catalog: $4.00

MIDWAY INDUSTRIES
15116 Adams St.
P.O. Box 980
Midway City CA 92655
714-898-4477
Retail Catalog: $3.00

ROTO-FAZE IGNITIONS
23136 Mariposa
Torrance CA 90502
213-325-8844
Technical Info: Free
Offers nitrous-curved distributors

MANIFOLDS

CLIFFORD PERFORMANCE
500 West Harrington St., Unit H
Corona CA 91720
714-734-3310
Retail Catalog: $3.00

EDELBROCK CORPORATION
411 Coral Circle
El Segundo CA 90245
213-322-7310
Retail Catalog: $2.00

HOLLEY REPLACEMENT PARTS DIV.
11955 East 9-Mile Road
Warren MI 48090
For technical information, hard-to-get parts, and literature, call: 615-859-4924
Retail Catalog: $3.00

OFFENHAUSER SALES CORP.
5232 Alhambra Ave., PO Box 32218
Los Angeles CA 90032
213-225-1307
Retail Catalog: $3.00

PACER PERFORMANCE PRODUCTS
5345 San Fernando Road West
Los Angeles CA 90039
213-245-3654
Retail Catalog: None

WEIAND AUTOMOTIVE INDUSTRIES
2316 San Fernando Road
PO Box 65977
Los Angeles CA 90065
213-225-4138
Retail Catalog: $3.00

PISTONS/MAJOR ENGINE COMPONENTS

APT
(Automotive Performance Technology)
561 Iowa Avenue
Annex E
Riverside CA 92502
714-783-0344
Nitrous cams, pistons, rods, cylinder heads, and other related parts

ARIAS INDUSTRIES INC.
13420 S. Normandie Avenue
Gardena CA 90249
213-770-0055--Order & Tech
213-532-9737--Pistons
213-538-2505--Engines
Retail Catalog: $3.00

BATTEN HEADS, INC.
27554 Wick Road
Romulus MI 48174
800-233-1591--Order
313-946-9850--Tech
Retail Catalog: None

BROOKS RACING COMPONENTS
7091 Belgrade Avenue
Garden Grove CA 92641
800-824-4754--CA Order
800-854-6476--US Order
714-893-0595--Tech
Retail Catalog: $4.00

CHILDS & ALBERT
11030 Sherman Way
Sun Valley CA 91352
818-765-0988
Retail Catalog: $4.00

HANK THE CRANK INC.
7253 Lankershim Blvd.
N. Hollywood CA 90241
818-765-3444--Order
213-877-0347--Tech
Retail Catalog: $4.00

JAHNS QUALITY PISTONS
2662 Lacy Street
Los Angeles CA 90031
213-225-8177--Order
213-225-1568--Tech
Retail Catalog: $3.00

JE PISTONS
15681 Computer Lane
Huntington Beach CA 92649
714-898-9763--Order & Tech
Retail Catalog: $3.00

MANLEY PERFORMANCE PRODUCTS
13 Race Street
Bloomfield NJ 07003
201-743-6577--Tech
800-526-1362--Order (No direct sales)
Catalog: None

ROSS RACING PISTONS
11927 S. Prairie
Hawthorne CA 90250
213-644-9779--Order
213-644-9770--Tech
Retail Catalog: $2.00

SPEED-O-MOTIVE INC.
12061 E. slauson Avenue
Santa Fe Springs, CA 90670
213-945-2758
Retail Catalog: #4.00

SPEED-PRO/SEALED POWER CORP.
100 Terrace Plaza
PO Box 299
Muskegon MI 49443
616-724-5011--Tech
616-724-5266--Order
Retail Catalog: $3.00

TOTAL-SEAL PISTON RING CO.
2225 W. Mountain View, #17
Phoenix AZ 85021
602-242-9421
Retail Cagalog: Free

TRW PERFORMANCE PARTS
8001 East Pleasant Valley Rd
Cleveland OH 44131
Contact nearest TRW dealer to order.
800-352-2273--Tech, Ex Ohio
800-992-2273--Tech, Ohio
Retail Catalog: $5.00

VENOLIA PISTONS
2160 Cherry Industrial Circle
Long Beach CA 90805
213-636-9329
Retail Catalog: $4.00

TRANSMISSION/ TORQUE CONVERTERS

B&M PERFORMANCE PRODUCTS
9152 Independence
Chatsworth CA 91311
818-882-6422
Retail Catalog: $4.00

HURST (Mr. Gasket)
8700 Brook Park Road
Cleveland, OH 44129
216-398-8300
Retail Catalog: $4.00

TRANS-DAPT
16410 Manning Way
Cerritos CA 90701
213-404-2985--Order CA
800-420-6751--Order US
213-404-2988--Tech
Retail Catalog: $3.00

TRANS-GO
2621 Merced Ave.
El Monte CA 91733
818-443-7456
Retail Catalog: $1.00